D0130199

Risk, Health and

# Health Care

## A QUALITATIVE APPROACH

Edited by

**Bob Heyman** BA, PhD

*Professor of Health Social Research in the Faculty of Health, Social Work and Education at the University of Northumbria at Newcastle, UK*

MERTHYR TYDFIL COLLEGE
LIBRARY

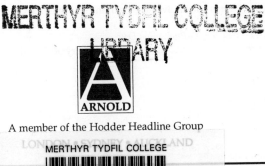

ARNOLD

A member of the Hodder Headline Group

LONDON SYDNEY AUCKLAND

MERTHYR TYDFIL COLLEGE

14198

£18.99
362
14198N

First published in Great Britain in 1998 by
Arnold, a member of the Hodder Headline Group
338 Euston Road, London NW1 3BH
http://www.arnoldpublishers.com

© 1998 Arnold

All rights reserved. No part of this publication may be reproduced or
transmitted in any form or by any means, electronically or mechanically,
including photocopying, recording or any information storage or retrieval
system, without either prior permission in writing from the publisher or a
licence permitting restricted copying. In the United Kingdom such licences
are issued by the Copyright Licensing Agency: 90 Tottenham Court Road,
London W1P 9HE.

Whilst the advice and information in this book is believed to be true and accurate
at the date of going to press, neither the author(s) nor the publisher can accept any legal
responsibility or liability for any errors or omissions that may be made.

*British Library Cataloguing in Publication Data*
A catalogue record for this book is available from the British Library

*Library of Congress Cataloging-in-Publication Data*
A catalog record for this book is available from the Library of Congress

ISBN 0 340 66201 8

Publisher: Clare Parker
Production Editor: Wendy Rooke
Production Controller: Rose James

Typeset in 10/12pt Palatino by Saxon Graphics Ltd, Derby
Printed and bound in Great Britain by J W Arrowsmith Ltd, Bristol

To Ruth, Michael, Anna, Daniel, Jess and the Soul of Bonzai

*These definitions [of quantitative risk assessment] begin with risk as the probability that **a particular adverse event** occurs during a stated period of time, or results from a particular challenge. As a probability in the sense of statistical theory risk obeys all the formal laws of combining probabilities.*

The Royal Society (1992) *Risk: Analysis, Perception and Management* p.2. (Bob Heyman's emphasis.)

*He preveth folk al day, it is no drede,*
*And suffreth us, as for oure exercyse*
***With sharpe scourges of adversitee***
*Ful ofte to be bete in sondry wise;*
*Nat for to knowe our wil, for certes he,*
*Er we were born knew al oure freletee;*
*And for our beste is al his governaunce;*
*Lat us than live in vertuous suffraunce.*

Chaucer, G. (1387–1400) 'The Clerk's Tale', *Canterbury Tales*, lines 1155–62. Edited by Skeat (1972). (Bob Heyman's emphasis.)

# Contents

# Contributors

**Joan Aarvold** is a principal lecturer, responsible for the BSc (Hons) European Health Sciences Programme at the University of Northumbria. She has been working with a range of users and providers of maternity services for more than twenty years. Through her involvement in Education for Parenthood programmes in schools, she developed and organised a support group for school-age girls.

**Richard W. Barker** qualified in social work in 1974, and was employed as a social worker and manager in social services departments. He is now a principal lecturer at the University of Northumbria. His current research interests include child-protection issues and child and family social work. His PhD thesis formed the basis for a book, *Lone Fathers and Masculinities* (Avebury, 1994).

**Charlotte L. Clarke** has worked with older people and in nurse education for nine years. She is currently employed as a research fellow in practice development at the University of Northumbria, with funding from the NHS Executive (Northern and Yorkshire). Her research interests include dementia care, family caregiving and the development of health-care practice.

**Glenda Cook** is a senior lecturer in nursing research at the University of Northumbria. She is currently seconded within the University on to a nursing research infrastructure support post financed by the NHS Executive (Northern and Yorkshire). Her research interests include risk-taking in the rehabilitative care of older persons, medical litigation and the moving and handling of patients/clients.

**Chris Corkish** qualified as a registered nurse for the mentally handicapped (RNHM) in 1983. He has worked in a long-stay hospital, in a small group home, and as a community nurse. He currently holds a half-time research fellowship with the University of Northumbria, funded by the NHS Executive (Northern and Yorkshire), and is evaluating the process of community relocation for adults with severe learning disabilities. His research interests include the needs of people who have severe or profound learning disabilities, and human and sexual relationships for people who have learning disabilities.

**Maria Davison** is Head of the Midwifery and Neonatal Care Subject Division at the University of Northumbria. She practised both as a nurse and a midwife before moving into education, and now teaches on both pre- and post-qualification midwifery programmes. Her teaching interests include curriculum design, assessment and multiprofessional learning. Her main research interests are adolescent pregnancy and consumer choice in health care.

**Chris Dracup** is a Chartered Psychologist and a principal lecturer in the Division of Psychology at the University of Northumbria. His main teaching and research interests are in the areas of individual decision-making, and psychological research methods and statistics.

**Elizabeth Handyside** worked as a senior health promotion officer, specialising in HIV/AIDS. She has undertaken research projects concerned with HIV services, the needs of people with mental health problems, and the sexual health of people with learning difficulties.

**Mette Henriksen** is a registered midwife, and works on the neonatal intensive care bank. She has a research studentship at the University of Northumbria, funded by the NHS Executive (Northern and Yorkshire). Her PhD research is concerned with the risk perceptions of pregnant women and the health professionals who care for them.

**Bob Heyman** is Professor of Health Social Research at the University of Northumbria. He played a major role in the development of the MSc Health Sciences, which is designed primarily for health professionals who wish to undertake practice-relevant research. His research interests include the needs of people with learning difficulties and perspectives on health risks. He has published one previous book: *Researching User Perspectives on Community Health Care*.

**Mick Hill** is a senior lecturer at the University of Northumbria, specialising in the sociology of health and illness. His academic interests include contemporary social theory, ageing and age structures.

**Sarah Huckle** worked for three years, at the Unversity of Northumbria, on the research project concerned with the needs of people with learning difficulties which is discussed in Chapter 9. She is currently writing up a PhD based on this study. She has worked on a project which evaluated the impact of market forces on the provision of support services for children with special needs, also at the University of Northumbria, and is presently teaching health and social policy in further education.

**Mike Kingham** is a principal lecturer, specialising in medical sociology, at the University of Northumbria, and Programme Director for the Diploma/MSc Health Sciences. He has edited the British Sociological Association's *Medical Sociology News*, published research on the culture of drug use, and contributed to AIDS initiatives. His main research interest is the portrayal of health issues in cinema drama.

**Tony Machin** is a senior lecturer at the University of Northumbria. He has a background in community mental health nursing, and academic interests in research methods, the sociology of health and illness and addiction.

**Susan J. Milner** is Subject Leader in Health Promotion at the University of Northumbria. She had previously worked as a nurse and health promotion specialist, becoming Regional Health Promotion Officer for the Northern Region.

**Margaret Moran** qualified in social work in 1979, and has worked for Barnardos and Newcastle Social Services. She has been employed at the

University of Northumbria since 1986, and is now a principal lecturer specialising in child protection and systemic practice.

**David O'Brien** is Head of the Acute and Critical Care Nursing Subject Division at the University of Northumbria, and teaches clinical nursing to undergraduate and postgraduate students. His research interest is the application of nursing theory to practice.

**Susan Procter** is Professor in Nursing Research at the University of Northumbria. She has been working in academic nursing and research for 15 years. Previously, she was employed as a ward sister on a medical ward in a busy London district general hospital. For a number of years she has been involved in the development of post-registration diploma, degree and masters courses for nurses. Her research interests include developing patient-focused nursing services, action research and practice development. She has published two books, both with Jan Reed: *Nurse Education: A Reflective Approach* and *Practitioner Research in Health Care*.

**Jan Reed** graduated in nursing in 1982, and worked with older people until she became a lecturer in nursing at what was to become the University of Northumbria. She held a Department of Health postdoctoral research fellowship from 1993–1995, when she undertook the study discussed in the present book. She is currently Reader in Nursing at the University of Northumbria, and founding editor of the journal *Health Care in Later Life*.

**Jacqui Russell** is Programme Director for the BSc (Hons) Nursing Science programme and the ENB Higher Award at the University of Northumbria. Her main teaching and research interests are related to reflective practice and practice development.

**Heather Scott** is Head of the Subject Division of Primary Health Care and Community Health at the University of Northumbria. A mental health social worker, she has been involved in the professional training of social workers for 15 years, most recently as manager of the North East Programme for Approved Social Work Training. Her interests include mental health in Europe, housing and community care, and women's mental health.

**Ann Smith** is Programme Director for the BSc (Hons) Nursing Studies/Registered Nurse Programme at the University of Northumbria. Her main teaching and research interests centre around the articulation and development of nursing knowledge through reflection.

**Bill Watson** is currently employed as a researcher at the University of Northumbria, funded by the NHS Executive (Northern and Yorkshire), and is undertaking a PhD which explores family involvement in the self-management of diabetes. He has worked previously in surgical, medical and high-dependency nursing, and has developed a special interest in diabetes care. He was involved in a random control trial of a structured education scheme for people with diabetes, and has undertaken a number of studies concerned with the self-management of this condition.

# Acknowledgements

I should particularly like to thank the following: Mick Carpenter, of the University of Warwick, for a superb critique of the opening chapters; Mr Bent Henriksen and Rabbi Francis Berry for allowing me to draw on their expert knowledge; my wife, Ruth, for her support and help with the draft; my son, Daniel, for his visual representation of risk; colleagues from the Division of Behavioural and Contextual Studies at the University of Northumbria for their advice and encouragement; health professional students on the MSc Health Sciences, for providing a continuing stream of ideas and enthusiasm; Mette Henriksen for a willingness to replace material lost by the editor which went beyond the obligations of a co-author; and the cartoonists who have allowed their work to be published in this book, mostly without charge, namely Steve Bell, Garland, Les Gibbard, Jak, Gerald Scarfe and Posy Simmonds. Responsibility for the content rests entirely with the named authors.

*Bob Heyman*
*August 1997*

# Introduction

## Bob Heyman

*We are all proselytes of science. And, in contrast to the followers of other religions, we can no longer bridge the gap between ourselves and the priests. Problems arise when we stumble on an outright lie.*

Høeg, P. (1993) *Miss Smilla's Feeling for Snow*, p. 375.

## From 'scourges of adversitee' to 'the probability' of 'an adverse event'

Chaucer's concern with adversity and that of the Royal Society (1992), quoted on the dedications' page, face each other across a 600-year period of modernisation. Chaucer, writing at its dawn, seems, at first sight, to accept a personalistic idea of the universe, since he suggests that human suffering should be cheerfully accepted as a divine test. However, irony can easily be detected underneath the surface of his words. If God knows all our frailties, why does He need to 'exercyse' (test) us, Chaucer asks. The Royal Society's treatment of adversity, in contrast, rigorously excludes intentionality, since adversity is explained by the impersonal workings of blind chance.

Chaucer appears uncertain about his world view, at a time when the authority of the Church over all forms of knowledge was beginning to weaken. The Royal Society (1992) exudes a confidence based on more than half a millennium of scientific and material progress. This book will explore some of the ground between these two positions in relation to lay and professional perspectives on health risks.

The human stock of knowledge has expanded immensely since the medieval period, thanks largely to the application of scientific methods. This development has been associated with a considerable improvement, however temporary, in life quality for people living in those societies which technology has transformed. But contemporary Western science suffers from systematic limitations. Traditionally, it has performed much better in reducing entities to simpler elements than in understanding their totality. It works more impressively in simplified laboratory conditions than in real life where, as a result of design faults, buildings sometimes collapse, aeroplanes crash, billion dollar stealth bombers lose their radar-avoidance coatings in the rain, and pharmaceuticals damage health. Science cannot accurately predict most biographical outcomes, answer questions about values, or provide convincing solutions to the mind–body problem (see Chapter 18).

Many of these issues come to a head in the management of health risks. It will be argued below that the notion of probability, which underpins the idea of risk, does not provide a rigorous scientific tool, but only a heuristic, rule-of-thumb device which has both utility and limitations; and that the assessment of 'adversity' entails weighing up values in ways which, sometimes, are contested. This book will explore the accounts which lay people and health professionals give of their sometimes overlapping and sometimes distinct approaches to the management of health risks.

The relationship between health professionals and lay people should not be represented as a battleground since the wider public have been heavily influenced by medical culture, and health professionals are affected by the same natural shocks as lay people. Nevertheless, as will be seen in the pages that follow, lay people apply considerably more scepticism to risk analysis than does the Royal Society in its definition of risk, (although, the last two chapters in the study group report, produced by social scientists, provide a more problematic treatment of risk).

## Scope and structure of the book

In the late 1990s, managing risk has become 'a priority in the health service' (Bowden, 1995, p. 1). The main thrust behind this new focus can be judged by the title of the first paper in Bowden's publication, namely 'Pathways to litigation' (Vincent, 1995, p. 1). Similarly, the first chapter in a recent guide to good practice in risk assessment and management (Kemshall and Pritchard, 1996) invites professional readers to worry about 'risking legal repercussions' (Carson, 1996, p. 3). At the same time, service-users have become increasingly willing to take legal action when they feel that they have suffered because the health-care system negligently placed them at risk.

The title of a following paper in Bowden (1995), 'Guidelines to reduce risk and improve the quality and cost-effectiveness of care' (Lloyd, 1995, p. 5), brings out the association between the current concern for risk management and intensifying pressure on health-care resources. The title claims that those who master the new technology of risk assessment and management can provide simultaneously, safer, cheaper and better care: a remarkable feat!

This book will focus not on legal or economic pragmatics, but on the lay and professional rationalities which underpin risk-accounting. The contributors examine these rationalities across a wide range of health and social care settings. We explore the ways in which they constitute, complement and contradict each other, giving rise to alliances, negotiations and power struggles between people with health needs, significant others and professionals.

Consideration of this topic can be practically justified, at minimum, on the grounds that individuals respond to the risks which concern them, not to those which trouble the experts. For this reason, health professionals need to inform themselves about clients' risk perspectives, even if they dismiss them as erroneous or unscientific. However, stronger claims about the status of popular risk knowledge *vis-à-vis* that of health professional experts can be made. A position on the delicate question of risk reality will be sketched out later in this Introduction, elaborated in Chapters 1 and 2, and worked through in the interpretation of research results in the chapters that follow. Assumptions about the ontological and epistemological status of risk provide a major element in the framework within which concrete transactions between health professionals and clients take place. For example, the view that risks exist objectively and can be discovered through science legitimates an 'undelimited' model of expertise (see Chapter 1) which assumes that professionals know best. Professionals, however immersed in the concrete detail of practice, cannot, ultimately, escape from philosophical questions.

The book is divided into three parts. Part One analyses risk conceptually, with particular reference to the implications of philosophical issues for the practice of health care. This Introduction discusses the origins of the book; analyses the concept of risk; provides a preliminary outline of forms of lay and professional risk rationality; offers a sketch-map of current risk research; and explores the wider cultural context for risk concerns. The Introduction provides a discursive overview, while the chapters that follow will be more tightly focused. Chapter 1 considers the problems of defining and assessing value in the management of health risks. Chapter 2 dissects probability. Both chapters are concerned with the ways in which health professionals and service-users approach, and account for, their relationships to the future. These chapters draw in some detail on those that follow, offering a framework for understanding risk concerns in a wide range of health and social care settings. The rest of Part One considers health risk from cultural (Chapter 3), sociological (Chapter 4) and psychological (Chapter 5) perspectives. This last chapter takes a quantitative, experimental approach to risk-reasoning. However, the ideas which it introduces, for example hindsight effects and probability heuristics, can be applied to the more situated analysis found in other chapters.

Part Two provides a series of research-based case studies of risk management in health care. The contexts covered include maternity (Chapters 6 and 7) and diabetes care (Chapter 8), services for adults with learning difficulties (Chapters 9 and 10), care for people with dementia (Chapter 11) and for older people (Chapter 12), and nursing (Chapters 13 and 14).

Apart from Chapter 14, which examines nurses' knowledge and practice of blood-pressure measurement, all the studies discussed in these chapters used qualitative self-report methods. The authors were asked not to dwell on methodological issues, but to use the limited space available to explore service-user and professional accounts of health-risk management. The studies suffer from the standard limitations of this type of design. Small, context-specific samples limit generalisation, and the data can only provide information on communicated, mostly retrospective, accounts of risk management. However, an exploratory, transverse view (Schrag, 1992), across a wide range of health and social care sectors, of the reasoning embedded in accounts of concrete incidents can provide a starting point for understanding the ways in which professionals and lay people approach health risks.

Part Three contains broader analyses of risk-management dilemmas in specific areas of professional activity. Chapter 15 considers the dilemma of autonomy versus safety in nursing. Chapters 16 and 17 discuss the management of risk in the political, culturally sensitive areas of child protection and mental health care, spheres in which professionals risk becoming victims of hindsight effects. Chapter 18 looks critically at health promotion from a perspective which refuses to ignore the intractable mind–body problem.

## Origins of the book

My own academic interest in risk was stimulated by research exposure to the perspectives of people with learning difficulties and their carers (Heyman and Huckle, 1993a, 1993b). This research aimed to explore the ways in which adults with learning difficulties saw their lives, and to compare their views with those of family and day centre carers. Our interest was quickly directed by the interview content to the ways in which people with learning difficulties and their carers understood the risks they saw facing them, as will be explained below.

Reading transcripts of our first interviews, we were immediately struck by the strong sense of danger which most conveyed. Although attitudes differed, a majority of adults with learning difficulties, and their family carers worried about the adult wandering around their local 'community', fearing, variously, that they might be verbally abused, run-over, kidnapped, mugged, raped or killed.

Turning to the learning difficulties research literature for guidance about a research topic which we had not, initially, intended to investigate, we found to our surprise that very little had been written about everyday risks for people with learning difficulties. Moreover, the limited available material seemed to assume that people with learning difficulties **ought** to take more risks. Perske (1972) wrote a widely quoted paper entitled 'The dignity of risk and the mentally retarded', while Richardson and Richie (1989), nearly two decades later, discussed the difficulties parents felt about 'letting go'. Such work suggested that family carers overprotect, and, by unexamined implication, that they decline to take acceptable risks, an opinion shared by day centre staff who participated in our research.

However, parents and other family carers vigorously rejected this view of the risks faced by their relative with learning difficulties. Most believed that this person could not lead a normal life without being exposed to unacceptable risks, and had reached the limits of their capacity to learn to manage hazards safely. We tried to suspend judgement about the rationality of the opinions held by the two sides to this dispute, and to explore the ways in which the various parties approached the dilemma of risk avoidance versus autonomy (see Chapter 9).

This book adopts a similar approach to risk management for other health matters. The contributors are all interested in the ways that those dealing with health issues, including service-users, patients, relatives, professionals, managers, policy-makers and politicians, conceptualise, assess and respond to health risks.

## The concept of risk

### DEFINITIONAL MATTERS

Risk will be defined, for the purposes of the present book, as '*the projection of a degree of uncertainty about the future on to the external world*'. This definition, justified and developed in Chapters 1 and 2, treats risk as a  simplifying heuristic which can provide a useful guide to action, but which can also systematically mislead. It may be contrasted with 'objectivist' formulations which, like the Royal Society definition, represent risk as a property of the world rather than of our knowledge.

As already noted, The Royal Society (1992, p. 2) has defined risk as '*the probability that a particular adverse event occurs during a stated period of time, or results from a particular challenge*'. It is often pointed out that the widespread use of the term risk dates back only to the eighteenth century, and was associated with the 'ventures' which merchants undertook when they entrusted a cargo of valuable goods to the sea (Bernstein, 1996, p. 93). The underpinning concept of probability emerged in the seventeenth century, and only became possible because the scientific revolution brought about a transformation in the way the world was understood (Hacking, 1975). This shift will be outlined in Chapter 2. Originating in the associated developments of modern science and capitalism, usage of the term 'risk' has spread into the wider culture. In doing so, it has, inevitably, been transformed. The risk concept is, at the same time, 'owned' by sciences such as epidemiology and economics, and a cultural resource employed in modern negotiations of everyday life, as when the editor tries to persuade his young son to wear his bicycle helmet, or cautions his older daughter about returning home alone, late at night, from the Newcastle club 'scene'.

Risk analysis provides a methodology for attempting to predict and control the future. Considered as a form of future management, it can be detected throughout recorded history. It reflects a fundamental yearning in humans, and perhaps all self-conscious beings, to know what will be. The Royal Society joins a mainly disreputable historical company which includes oracles, seers, practitioners of human sacrifice, prophets, astrologers, necromancers and witch-doctors. Defenders of scientific progress may feel insulted by such comparisons.

They can point out, correctly, that our knowledge, for example, about the risk of bacterial infection represents a straight gain over medieval beliefs that the plague was caused by Jews, witches or God's punishment. Nevertheless, attempts to describe risks objectively lead to fundamental difficulties, five of which are considered below, in relation to The Royal Society definition.

## Five difficulties with The Royal Society definition of risk

First, the notion of an 'event' requires an act of classification of heterogenous phenomena, and entails a decision, often implicit, both to discount differences within a class and to accentuate those between classes. Even a medical disaster like lung cancer takes various forms with different prognoses, and can develop earlier or later in life. The impact of Down's syndrome on the quality of life, discussed in Chapter 1, varies considerably from case to case. Medicine rests on largely unexamined taxonomic assumptions, even if these are enshrined in widely used systems of conventions such as the *International Classification of Impairments, Disabilities and Handicaps* (WHO, 1980).

Second, as will be argued in Chapter 1, the notion of an *'adverse event'* externalises adversity on to events, rather than locating them in the values which individuals or social groups place on event classes. Where those involved in risk assessment evaluate events in similar ways, they can communicate as if adversity appertained to events. However, when service-users and professionals differ in their value priorities, and professionals uncritically externalise their own values on to events, service-users will immediately reject professional expertise as oppressive. This process can be seen in a number of the chapters that follow: when a pregnant teenager refuses to have her pregnancy terminated (Chapter 6), or an older pregnant woman declines testing for Down's syndrome (Chapter 7); when carers of people with learning difficulties object to the professional line on normalisation, on the grounds that the benefits are not justified by the risks (Chapter 9); or when a carer of a relative with dementia rejects medical advice to have a loved relative institutionalised (Chapter 11).

Third, the idea, within The Royal Society definition, of *'a stated period of time'* begs the question of the temporal frame in which risks are considered. Most people worry less about future health adversities than about more imminent ones. However, decisions about personal risk-taking will depend very much on the time frame and discounting procedure which an individual adopts. They cannot be externally *'stated'*. This issue will be further considered in Chapter 1.

Fourth, The Royal Society definition treats probability as unproblematically given. Difficulties with the concept, and their implications for concrete transactions between health professionals and clients, will be explored in Chapter 2. In brief, probability can refer to fundamentally random, quantum events, to enigmas of human intentionality, to knowledge limitations about the complexities of physical and biological systems, or to any combination of these three sources of uncertainty. *'Probability'* involves an externalisation of uncertainty (Thompson, 1986) in the same way that *'adversity'* entails an externalisation of value. Chapter 2 argues that probability, as applied to the behaviour of complex systems, provides no more than a heuristic predictive tool. Rational observers can correctly attribute many probabilities to the same event. However, the strong tendency to externalise uncertainty in science-based cultures creates a cognitive illusion that multiple probabilities of the same event are logically impossible.

Fifth, and finally, The Royal Society definition focuses on single *'adverse event'* classes, the probability of which can be predicted in terms of a complex of interacting variables. Such a way of thinking fits comfortably with scientific specialisms, oriented towards the investigation and management of isolated problems. Academic papers are published, and medical consultancies granted, on the basis of such knowledge. However, individuals who manage personal risks are not usually concerned with predicting the probability of one form of adversity in terms of multiple indicators, but with its obverse. They seek to predict the multiple consequences, positive and negative, of a single type of action. For example, the young mothers, who are discussed in Chapter 6, understood the health risks for themselves and their babies associated with smoking, but continued to smoke because they wanted to avoid putting on weight, and because smoking helped them to cope emotionally.

The negativity of The Royal Society approach to risk can be explained, in part, by its focus on the multiple causes of a single adverse event class, rather than on the multiple consequences of a single cause class. However, focus on multiple consequences raises two issues which require *a priori* value judgements, namely the selection of consequences and the calibration of qualitatively different outcomes. Since choices have theoretically infinite consequences, prior selection of some for rational consideration cannot be avoided. For example, patients may be more concerned with the immediate consequences for their wider lives of health problems such as diabetes (see Chapter 8), while health professionals focus on the risk of long-term medical complications.

The results of risk appraisal will depend on which consequences are selected, over what time scale they are considered, how they are evaluated, and how qualitatively different positive and negative consequences are combined in an overall picture of the future. Assumptions about these matters provide the pre-rational foundations on which any risk analysis must be based. Where the parties to a possible health transaction begin such analysis from different but unarticulated starting points, then trouble, latent or overt, can be expected.

## Risk-reasoning

This section will briefly debate some analytical questions concerning risk-reasoning which will be taken up in the following chapters. The utilitarian calculus, the relationship between reasoning and acting, the 'reality' of risks and their temporal dimension will be introduced.

### THE UTILITARIAN CALCULUS

The implicit or explicit calculation of expected value through cost-benefit analysis lies at the heart of a utilitarian rationality which enables general principles to be applied to concrete decision-making in science-based cultures. Utilitarianism thus provides the pragmatic centrepiece of such cultures. It stands in contrast to fatalistic, personalistic and hedonistic approaches to future management, discussed in Chapter 2.

In order to evaluate alternative courses of action (or inaction), the utilitarian will try to calculate their expected value by identifying a set of practical choices, and in relation to each choice: first, identifying its possible consequences; second, assigning a more or less positive or negative value to each consequence; third, estimating the probability of each consequence occurring; and fourth, computing expected value by summing the products of values of consequences multiplied by their probabilities. The cost-benefit equation can then be applied to each choice identified, and the action line which maximises expected value selected. Such an approach allows the risks associated with the multiple consequences of a line of action to be reduced to a single numerical quantity (Fischoff, Watson and Hope, 1984). Utilitarian reasoning attempts to combine scientific knowledge, expressed as probabilities, with value judgements in order to provide a rational basis for decision-making.

Such reasoning predominates in the modern Western culture which arose out of the Enlightenment in the seventeenth century. Pascal, for example, attempted to prove the rationality of religious belief by using utilitarian arguments. He reasoned that even if the probability of God existing was very low, faith in Him might confer infinite benefits on the believer, while living a good life would cost little to those who were virtuously inclined regardless of divine incentives. Thus, faith would generate greater expected value (a low probability of an infinite benefit), in a cosmic lottery, than disbelief (Hacking, 1975, p. 69).

The utilitarian approach requires a neat separation between values and facts about the probabilities of effects (Rescher, 1983, p. 31). Facts, on this view, are to be described by science while values belong in the personal and political domain. However, making expected values calculable requires a raft of supporting presuppositions, outlined above: about the selection of consequences to be considered, and their spatial and temporal boundaries; about time-discounting; and about the terms of trade of qualitatively different values. This book will attempt to demonstrate that critical health-care incidents involving contention between service-providers and users can often be illuminated through comparisons of such presuppositions.

## REASONING AND ACTING

Our focus on cost-benefit analysis will encompass a wide range of degrees of formality and articulation of decision-making. A health authority might decide, after a lengthy formal assessment, to close a local accident and emergency unit. In contrast, a new couple might, in the heat of the moment, have sex without using a condom. The former decision might be based on extensive investigation, consultation, deliberation and documentation. The latter might simply happen, without an explicit phase of reflection, negotiation and deliberation. Nevertheless, those involved might, after the event, justify their conduct in terms of an informal, retrospective cost-benefit analysis. For instance, they might convince themselves that sexual intercourse without a condom was safe for them (Woodcock, Stenner and Ingham, 1992).

Research approaches which attempt to uncover *'situated rationality'* (Bloor, 1995, p. 23) by asking individuals about their reasons for taking or not taking risks may systematically underestimate their negotiated, socially structured character while, at the same time, overestimating their deliberateness. The male prostitutes studied by Bloor had sex without condoms simply because they lacked the social power to insist on their use. Conversely, the surface rationality of deliberative decision-making often conceals unexamined assumptions and hidden agendas. Although relationships between action choices and accounts of decision-making should always be questioned, the latter are worthy of study in their own right.

## ARE RISKS REAL?

The status of risk knowledge will be explored in some detail in Chapters 1 and 2. The present discussion aims only to briefly signpost the position to be developed. Risk appraisal can be decomposed analytically into considerations about values and about probabilities, although, in decision-making, the two types of judgement mutually affect each other (see Chapter 5). A weakly subjectivist position towards health values (considered in more detail in Chapter 1) will be offered, based on three considerations.

First, human nature is sufficiently fixed for certain common values to be widely shared. People, regardless of their culture, will mostly prefer longevity, absence of disease and impairment, self-esteem and contentment over their opposites. For this reason, diseases such as cancer and the plague can be characterised, only slightly facetiously, as 'fairly real dangers'.

But, second, health values, like all others, must be deemed ultimately subjective. Although generally valuing health, cultures, groups and individuals differ in the meanings they attach to the term, and in the priority they give to health as they understand it. Modern Western cultures value highly individual longevity and freedom from diseases, although they do not necessarily promote these ends in practice. But this premium value placed on health is historically specific, and not universally shared in other cultures. For example, medieval religious activists had other priorities when they chose to be bricked-up so that their suffering could contribute to the glory of God, as did pugilistic aristocrats who prized 'honour' earned on the battlefield above life and limb. Shakespeare's Falstaff anticipated a more modern view, not shared by his social betters, when he asked, rhetorically:

> Can honour set to a leg? no: or an arm? no: or take away the grief of a wound? no.
> Honour has no skill in surgery, then? no. (Henry IV, Part I, Act IV, Scene ii)

Third, and most importantly for the kinds of risk analysis which follow, difficult decisions about risks entail weighing-up and trading-off qualitatively different values, for example autonomy versus safety, or quality of life against longevity. Such trade-offs of finely balanced but incompatible ends require value judgements which individuals and social groups make differently, and which cannot be meaningfully aggregated or anticipated. The persons most directly concerned in a health decision may have difficulty in deciding or even predicting what they would do. Health professionals who wish to help clients to manage risk need to grasp the complexities involved in such reasoning: an important theme of this book.

It might be supposed that scientific objectivity rests on safer foundations with respect to probability (discussed in Chapter 2), but its solidity can be questioned. In brief, the most common form of health-risk reasoning involves reducing uncertainty by attributing observed aggregate properties of a category to individuals within that category (Rose, 1985a), and therefore entails acceptance of the ecological fallacy. For example, the probability of a particular woman of a certain age having a baby with Down's syndrome might be defined in terms of the observed frequency of that condition among women of a similar age. This form of prediction can provide useful glimpses of the future, but only at the cost of simplification which will sometimes systematically mislead. Probability statements do not provide descriptions of 'real' events, only of our limited knowledge about them. To put the matter bluntly, you will either die horribly in a road accident, or, hopefully, you will not. After your eventual death, we can see retrospectively that the odds on this particular adverse event were 'really' either 1 or 0.

Individuals can be categorised in an indefinite number of different ways, many of which make at least some predictive sense. Their probability of experiencing a particular event will depend on how they are classified, and classification involves choice. Therefore, the same person can be subject to many probabilities of the same event. This apparent impossibility is justified in Chapter 2 through the redefinition of probability as the projection of uncertainty on to the world.

It is not being argued, relativistically, that all risk-groupings are equally useful. Some will work better than others in the sense of differentiating low- and high-risk groups as much as possible. For example, the risk of lung cancer can be better predicted by subdividing populations into smokers and non-smokers than by separating-out those whose names begin with a consonant and a vowel. Nevertheless, in complex cases of partially unknown multiple causation, many classification schemes will work well enough, and will generate different risks for individuals. In such unclear conditions, classificatory choices will, inevitably, be influenced by social attitudes, for example towards stigmatised groups, as will be shown in Chapter 2. Moreover, the evolution of classification schema, and the location of particular individuals, both depend on what is known. For example, as will be shown in Chapter 2, a woman's risk of carrying a baby with Down's syndrome will change after she has taken a genetic test. Readers who find this notion perverse are invited to reframe 'probability' as 'uncertainty'.

It can be concluded, therefore, that a particular event may have many different plausible probabilities, and that, in this sense, probabilities, like values, can only be regarded as fairly real! Demoting probability, in risk analysis, to the status of a heuristic allows its analysis to occupy the much sought after, but little realised, middle ground between positivism and social constructionism (Stevenson and Cooper, 1997). Probability statistics cannot be regarded as '*signs from God*' (Prior Roger Schulz of Taize, cited by Hood and Jones, 1996, p. 84). Neither do they '*only exist in the* **mind** *of the beholder*' (Toft, 1996, p. 101, Toft's emphasis). What they do is to provide glimpses, which go beyond present detailed knowledge, of complex futures. The price which must be paid for such leaps of prognostication is acceptance of the simplifying assumption that the properties of a class which the observer has defined can be validly attributed to the individuals within that class. Probabilities occupy a messy, but useful, epistemological position between *'brute'* and *'institutional'* facts (Searle, 1995, p. 34).

However, once socially established, risks take on a life of their own, despite their indirect relationship to underlying causal processes, leaving behind their tenuous, debatable origins. They become subject to processes of reflexive recursion, whereby thinking about and responding to a risk changes it. Reflexive recursion can drive service-users up or down risk escalators, systems of care of increasing or declining intensity. An extended consideration of the concepts of reflexive recursion and risk escalators will be offered as the climax to Chapter 2.

## THE TEMPORAL DIMENSION OF RISK MANAGEMENT

Since probabilistic reasoning involves predicting the future on the basis of experience of the past, temporal elements are crucial. Table 0.1, below, subdivides lay and professional risk appraisal in relation to the time position of adversity. Although important differences between professional and lay risk assessment can be identified, both confront a similar set of issues. The considerations which come into play when the risk of future adversity is being contemplated differ from those which would be thought about after an adverse event has happened.

**Table 0.1** Lay and professional risk appraisal

| | Lay perspectives | Professional perspectives | Critical issues |
|---|---|---|---|
| **Future oriented** | Lay decision-making | Professional decision-making | *Hazard selection* |
| | | | *Cost-benefit analysis* Choice identification Selection of consequences Utility calculations Social action |
| **Past oriented** | Lay accounting | Professional accounting | *Inquiry* Outcome assessment Explanation Counterfactual appraisal Moral attribution Hindsight effects |
| | | | *Responding to adversity* Damage assessment Over the edge experiences Coping, normalisation and medicalisation Selection of new hazards |

## Risk and managing the future

Risk assessment provides one means of attempting 'colonization of the future' (Giddens, 1991, p. 111) both for individuals managing their own lives, and for professionals who supply risk expertise.

Risk analysis generally is, and should be, an element in a decision-driven activity. Individuals will only engage in future oriented risk appraisal if they identify both hazards and choices about how to respond to them. They may then undertake a more or less systematic cost-benefit analysis for available choices, for example about contraception (Chapter 6), genetic testing (Chapter 7), accepting services for a relative with dementia (Chapter 11) or moving into an old people's home (Chapter 12). Much of the material which follows in the book will be concerned with this form of risk appraisal.

## Risk and managing the past

Past oriented risk appraisal involves consideration of accountability for outcomes which have come to pass, and of lessons for the future. Theoretically, this form of appraisal may be triggered by positive as well as negative occurrences. For instance, a midwife, quoted in Chapter 13, described her good feelings, in the retrospective light of a positive outcome, about supporting a family who wanted a home birth for a post-mature baby. More usually, given the role of risk as a forensic device (Douglas, 1990) in modern societies, retrospective appraisal is used to negotiate and attribute responsibility for adversity, as with the inquiries into killings carried out by persons with serious mental health problems which are discussed in Chapter 17. The pregnant teenagers whose views are considered in Chapter 6, felt, looking back, that they had not really reflected on the risks associated with the non-use of contraceptives, or had drawn incorrect inductive conclusions from a period of infertility. They wanted, with the benefit of hindsight, to advise other girls to avoid making similar mistakes. Such retrospective accounting requires counterfactual consideration of alternative histories, of what might have happened if different choices had been made, and is influenced by hindsight effects (see Chapter 5).

If adversity has occurred, then those involved have to assess the damage and decide how to deal with it. 'Over the edge' experiences arise from a sense that a disaster, for example cancer, has occurred, perhaps despite all the preventive efforts which were taken. The world acquires new, alien, emergent qualities. A fissure opens up both with the personal past, and with others who, however sympathetic, cannot understand experiences they have not shared. One parent described the experience of discovering that their child was seriously ill as 'like walking through the gates of hell' (Cohen, 1993, p. 83). Such experiences are accentuated, if not constituted, by a preventive culture which treats adversity as avoidable, and neglects the needs of those for whom prevention, anomalously, has failed.

Alternatively, or subsequently, the adversity may be minimised and normalised. For example, some family carers of people with dementia (Chapter 11) emphasised signs, however slight, of their relative's retained capacity to relate to others. Newly diagnosed diabetics (Chapter 8) and women needing adjuvant therapy for breast cancer (Cowley, 1996) may reassure themselves that others are worse off than themselves. Some diabetic patients (Chapter 8) and carers of relatives with dementia (Chapter 11) attempted normalising strategies which conflicted with medical advice, and led to non-compliance. Instead, those afflicted by health adversity may, like another of the diabetic patients considered in Chapter 8, cope by enthusiastically embracing the medical regime, perhaps with overoptimistic expectations.

Health adversity gives rise, Janus-like, to new hazards requiring future oriented risk appraisal. For example, family carers may drastically restrict the autonomy of adults with learning difficulties in order to protect them from danger, or give them freedom at the cost of considerable anxiety (Chapter 9). Some family carers of people with dementia (Chapter 11) took risks which horrified professionals, such as allowing an elderly man to wander around his local community, on the grounds that restrictions might make his condition worse.

## Introduction to risk research

### RISK AS A TOPIC

The reader can now explore an extensive research and analytical literature on risk, and on the underpinning concept of probability. This work draws on a range of academic disciplines, including philosophy, mathematics, statistics, systems theory, epidemiology, economics, psychology, sociology, anthropology, social policy history, and communication, legal and management studies. Much of this material focuses on health issues. Hayes (1992) found over 100 000 references to risk in the Medline database in the seven years between 1985 and 1991. He estimated that about 5 per cent of all references in the database contained the term 'risk'.

Despite this voluminous literature, chapters on risk and related topics did not appear in social science health texts produced during the 1980s and early 1990s, either in health sociology (Stacey, 1988; Gerhardt, 1989; Rogers, 1991) or health psychology (Gochman, 1988; Niven, 1989; Sarafino, 1990). Risk appears only briefly even in the indexes of these texts. Since the mid-1990s, chapters on risk have been included in at least one health sociology (Nettleton, 1995) and one health psychology (Stroebe and Stroebe, 1995) textbook. The latter frames risk as '*self-protection*', thus prejudging the argument about risk dilemmas in favour of officially sanctioned safety.

A time lag in the emergence of risk as a core focus results, in part, from a catching-up process, as the social sciences latch on to a health service qualitative shift towards a risk orientation. This shift has itself resulted from heightened concern with litigation (Bowden, 1995), as already noted, and from a refocusing of health and social services on preventive screening of populations, rather than on the needs of individuals (Castel, 1991).

Moreover, social scientists have had some difficulty in packaging risk as a standard topic on a par with subjects like social class or attitude change, for two related reasons. First, they have, traditionally, been mainly concerned with trying to explain, and so reduce, uncertainty about social behaviour. But the study of risk involves analysis of uncertainty management, not its abolition. An orientation towards prediction and control, perhaps, makes risk an uncomfortable topic for social scientists to digest. However, the recent development of the science of complexity (Reed and Harvey, 1994) has legitimated the new social scientific focus on uncertainty. Second, serious analysis of risk requires the social scientist to straddle uncomfortably the academic cultural divide between art and science, and between qualitative and quantitative paradigms. Risk analysis involves both engagement with the numerical complexities of probability, and consideration of philosophical questions, such as what makes a probability probable or an adversity adverse.

Even articulate critics of the tyranny of numbers in risk analysis can go astray. Hansson (1993, p. 20) asserts that *the reliability of risk analysis depends on the absence of systematic differences between objective probabilities and experts' estimates of those probabilities*. However, probabilities depend on the observer's knowledge, and so can never be objective, as will be argued in Chapter 2. The concept of probability is considered further in Chapter 5, and its implications for health-care practice will be explored throughout this book.

## A TAXONOMY OF HEALTH-RELATED RISK RESEARCH

A taxonomy which may help the reader to locate health-related risk studies is provided in Table 0.2 below. Like all taxonomies, it inevitably oversimplifies.

### Studies of health risks

Studies of health risks focus on specific hazards, which are viewed as natural phenomena, the probability of which can be assessed through epidemiological research, as shown in the first cell of Table 0.2. Studies of health risk, in contrast, raise critical questions about the concept of risk, and its use within specific historical and cultural contexts.

As already noted, the volume of epidemiological work has expanded rapidly since the 1960s, and has been ironically characterised by Skolbekken (1995) as *a risk epidemic*, of particular virulence in the areas of obstetrics

Table 0.2    A taxonomy of health-related risk studies

| Study focus | Studies of health risks | Studies of health risk |
| --- | --- | --- |
| Risk phenomena | Epidemiological studies | The social construction of risk |
| Risk perceptions | Lay misperceptions of 'objective' risks | Comparisons of lay and official risk perceptions |
| Risk-management concern | How to maximise compliance with official risk assessments based on utilitarian quantification | How to negotiate social power in order to encompass pluralistic values |

and gynaecology. Two features which Skolbekken notes in the risk epidemic give away its character. First, terms with related meanings, namely 'hazard', 'danger' and 'uncertainty' did not show an increase in usage to match that identified in the risk epidemic. Second, the risk epidemic has been largely confined to research on non-iatrogenic risks. Terms such as 'uncertainty', 'probability', 'risk', 'hazard' and 'danger' carry significantly different shades of meaning, and the preference for 'risk' reflects a much wider world view, based on uncritical acceptance of the authority of 'scientific' medicine. The same world view leads to relative research neglect of iatrogenic illness.

The second cell in the 'Studies of health risks' column focuses on lay risk perceptions. This approach compares 'perceived' with 'objective' risks, in order to assess and explain lay 'errors'. For example, Avis et al. (1989) found a systematic tendency for lay people to underestimate their risk of a heart attack, as estimated by a formula derived from epidemiological research. Those at highest risk, according to the formula, were most likely to underestimate their risk. Such research implicitly takes for granted the superiority of expert over lay knowledge, and treats communication as a one-way process in which risk experts educate lay people (Bradbury, 1989).

Risk management, within this approach, is therefore equated with increasing conformity with expert advice, despite the generally low rates of public compliance with health-education initiatives. Avis et al. (1989) concluded that the impact of feeding back the 'objective' appraisal of an individual's risk of coronary heart disease varied considerably. Some research participants judged their levels of risk to be **less** after they had been informed that they were at high risk. Without a methodology for investigating the qualitative detail of lay people's own rationalities, such apparently perverse findings can only be explained pathologically.

## Studies of health risk

While those who investigate health risks are keen to use the concept as a tool to analyse problems of interest, students of health risk wonder about the tool itself. Despite the 'epidemic' of studies of health **risks**, far less research has been done on health **risk**. Studies concerned with this issue investigate the ways in which risks are identified and assessed by experts and lay people, and used pragmatically to negotiate and manage events. For example, Roberts, Smith and Bryce (1993) concluded that parents living in a socially deprived environment were primarily worried about environmental risks to their children, such as road traffic, while caring professionals focused on individual parental behaviour. Professionals may home-in on individuals because they lack control over the wider environment (Crawford, 1977).

By implication, researchers who study risk adopt a more critical stance towards the use of the concept than do those who study risks (Skolbekken, 1995). Although acknowledging the pragmatic need to assess risks as systematically as possible, the contributors to this book fall into the former camp.

# The wider cultural context of risk

Although this book is concretely concerned with the management of health risk, the issues that arise can only be understood in their cultural context, for example in relation to wider value systems, ways of relating to the future and attitudes towards expertise. The following section outlines the cultural backdrop to health-risk concerns, and provides a frame for the more focused material which follows. It begins with an anecdote intended to illustrate the interconnection between technical health-risk analysis and broader sociopolitical concerns. Social attitudes towards risk are then explored through a sketch of the so-scalled 'risk society' (Beck, 1992).

## RISK AND ANOMALY: IS MELATONIN A DANGEROUS DRUG?

In August 1996, a representative of the Inspection and Enforcement group of the Medicines Control Agency (MCA), accompanied by police, visited the offices of Pharma Nord (UK) Ltd. They were investigating the sale of a banned substance, melatonin, which they regarded as potentially dangerous, and proceeded to confiscate the company's entire stock. Melatonin, a natural substance found in all living organisms, had been sold freely in the UK for a number of years, and can be purchased as a dietary supplement, without restriction, in the USA.

As a result of the press publicity describing its potential as a sleeping aid, the MCA decided to classify melatonin as an unlicensed medicinal substance, and to ban its free sale as a food supplement. This decision was based on their interpretation of a European Union directive stating that full pharmaceutical licensing was required for any substance used *'with a view to making a diagnosis or to restoring, correcting or modifying physiological function in human beings or animals'* (Medicines Control Agency, 1995, p. 6). The MCA had become concerned about the long-term side effects of taking doses considerably higher than would be ingested from natural sources such as oats and bananas (Lazarides, 1996, p. 2).

This example appears to illustrate the rigour with which the authorities protect the public from health risks. However, it can be used to raise some critical issues. Uncertainty about the long-term side effects of increased doses of melatonin, and about the costs and benefits of using this and other expensive vitamin supplements, cannot be discounted. But animal toxicity trials suggest that melatonin lacks toxicity even in gigantic doses (Barchas, DaCosta and Spector, 1967). Up to 10 million Americans have taken melatonin daily for some years, with no reported side effects. Concerns about possible health damage apply equally to all dietary supplements, genetically engineered foods, widely used mood-altering drugs such as tobacco, alcohol and coffee, herbal remedies, and many medical procedures. For example, the long-term consequences of hysterectomy have not been systematically assessed despite evidence of possible serious side effects (Hill *et al.*, 1994; Hartmann *et al.*, 1995; Luoto *et al.*, 1995; Namnoum *et al.*, 1995).

In the case of melatonin, an uncontrolled, implicitly safe, dietary supplement became a risky drug simply because lay people started to employ it for a new 'medical' purpose, as an aid to sleeping. The expense of the licensing procedure permanently precludes its use for naturally occurring, unpatentable medicines, which, therefore, can never be deemed safe. Senior scientific staff from the MCA, a commercial agency, are mostly associated with the pharmaceutical industry, the main source of the necessary expertise. But the discovery of a safe, effective, unpatentable sleeping aid would threaten one of this industry's main markets. Hence, the source of risk expertise is tainted by the possibility of self-interest.

Cultures provide ways of classifying the world. Properties are attributed to categories, rather than to single items, and define the ways in which members of a class should be approached. Difficulties arise with anomalous or ambiguous entities which do not neatly fit into a given classification system. Western, science-based cultures draw a distinction between foods and medicines. Foods, under lay control, are presumed, *a priori*, to be safe and 'natural', and to provide vitamins and trace elements necessary for general health maintenance. Medicines, under expert control, are considered to be 'artificial', to be potentially dangerous, and to have specific therapeutic functions.

Douglas (1966, Chapter 3) undertook a detailed feat of detection concerning the abominations of Leviticus. She asked why Old Testament law prohibited Jews from eating certain apparently harmless foods, and concluded (p. 54) that *'holiness is exemplified by completeness. Holiness requires that individuals shall conform to the class to which they belong. And holiness requires that different classes of things shall not be confused.'* Pastoralists, used to keeping cloven-hoofed, cud-chewing, ungulate, domestic animals, such as goats and cows, rejected pigs, for example, not for hygienic reasons, but because they were not ruminants.

Cultural anomalies, for example foods with pharmaceutical properties, seem dangerous. Similarly, Aarvold (Chapter 6) discusses the views of pregnant teenagers about being treated as medical risks, and so irresponsible. Many parents treat the sexuality of adults with learning difficulties as dangerous because they regard their relatives as physically mature but mentally childlike (Heyman and Huckle, 1995c). Kingham, in Chapter 4, discusses jokes and imagery associated with the idea of AIDS as a gay plague. Moran and Barker (Chapter 16) analyse the risk-management problems arising from heightened public and media sensitivity to cases of parental harm to children. Disproportionate social concern with sexually active children, men who have sex with men, or parents who harm their children, relative to cool acceptance, for example, of road accidents and poverty-related deaths, suggests that the anomalies in the former cases touch raw cultural nerves.

## THE RISK SOCIETY

### Risk alarm

As the Western world counts out a second millennium, the news is alarming. The public is asked to worry about an ever-expanding list of present and future hazards: collisions with asteroids; destruction of the ozone layer, the greenhouse effect, the exhaustion of natural resources, the elimination of species, and poisoning of the air, water, land and food supply; genetic engineering, repetitive strain injury, and information-fatigue syndrome; war, crime, traffic gridlock, the collapse of the moral order, unemployment, poverty and illicit drug-taking; declining sperm counts, antibiotic resistant microorganisms, uncontrollable infections, cancer, heart disease, asthma, AIDS, BSE, Alzheimer's disease, arthritis, depression and suicide.

This heightened concern with diverse hazards seems to reflect both changes in life conditions and in cultural preoccupations (Lash, Szerszynski and Wynne, 1996, p. 6). A form of modernisation in which the polluting consequences of industrial activity, dismissed by economists as 'externalities', are not paid for by those who profit from them has gathered pace over the last two centuries, with ever-more destructive effects. Beck (1992, p. 11) anticipates that '*in its mere continuity industrial society exits the stage of world history on the tip-toes of normality, via the back stairs of side effects*' (Beck's emphasis). In the UK, the value of further modernisation has been widely questioned in the fields of genetic engineering, road building, nuclear-power generation, open-cast mining and digital television.

Beck (1992) aims to discern the shape of a new modernity which possesses two main features: reflexivity and individualisation. As industrial societies modernise, the benefits of economic growth become ever-more marginal, while side effects, and their attendant risks, continually accumulate. At some point, a cultural phase shift occurs. The benefits of modernisation are no longer taken for granted, and become contested at every point, leading to heightened risk consciousness. The same modernisation process weakens wider social bonds such as those associated with family, class, occupation and religion. Individuals have to face the demands and perils of the risk society without their support.

Giddens (1991) has characterised Western advanced industrial societies, in similar terms, as 'late modern'. This concept, again, implies a phase shift from earlier stages of modernisation, when the value of technological progress was largely taken for granted. Late modern societies, according to Giddens, are affected by rapid continuous changes in social structures such as the family, work organisations and welfare systems, with an attendant rise in personal insecurity; a switch in emphasis from production to consumption resulting from the automation of routine manufacture; heightened but selective anxiety about the risks arising from modernisation; and a reduction in the social distance between experts and non-experts, as trust in the former weakens, and sources of knowledge become more accessible to the latter. This book will work through the implications for health professional/client relationships of these last two changes, namely heightened risk consciousness and the dethronement of expertise.

Risk has become a central consideration in a more critical stance towards modernising activities which have uncertain collective and individual consequences. Nobody knows how many people will die in the UK as a result of the BSE fiasco, or who those individuals will be; what long-term impact oestrogen-imitating industrial chemicals will have on male fertility, or who will become infertile; what effects increased air pollution from motor traffic will have on the population, or who will succumb. At the same time, the accelerating pace of economic change has given rise to a more diffuse social anxiety, as indicated, for example, by increased parental reluctance to allow young children to make solo journeys (Hillman, Adams and Whitelegg, 1990), and heightened fear of crime (Forde, 1993). Such concerns impact on the health and social care system, as when older people seek institutional care because they do not feel safe in their own homes (see Chapter 12); or when child protection (Chapter 16) and mental health professionals (Chapter 17) must respond to intense media attention to rare but catastrophic outcomes.

The same rapid development of scientific knowledge which made modernisation possible also created a powerful challenge to a prevailing cosmology based on the argument from design. The Darwinian, evolutionary explanation of human existence has replaced divine planning with blind chance. Those who accept the Darwinian view can hope, like The Royal Society (1992), to influence their future only by trying to use their knowledge to weight the dice in favour of the individual, group or species. Hence, the ecological alarm associated with later stages of modernisation, which Beck (1992) has so vividly analysed, dovetails with Darwinian ideas. In combination, they lead to heightened risk consciousness.

Paradoxically, however, heightened risk consciousness coexists with the highest ever levels of life expectancy for most groups currently residing in advanced industrial societies, although mortality has increased for some of the poorest groups unlucky enough to live in the more unequal United Kingdom of the 1990s (Phillimore, Beattie and Townsend, 1994). Three possible, non-competing explanations of this paradox can be offered. First, current safety may have been achieved at the expense of mortgaging the middle-distance future, as economic growth challenges natural life-support systems. Second, accelerating socioeconomic change, associated with modernisation and globalisation, may provoke a widespread but diffuse sense of insecurity which is culturally channelled into concerns about individual health. Third, as human life becomes more secure and prosperous, its value increases, placing health systems on a treadmill of rising expectations. Our modern Pharaohs await medical advances, mummified in cryogenic suspended animation.

## Variations in risk attitude

Attitudes towards risks differ more than Beck's concept of the risk society might suggest. Risk enjoyment, risk acceptance, and individual, subcultural and cultural variations in risk sensitivity can be identified in advanced industrial societies. Responses to the risks which concern professionals must be understood in the context of the socially mediated accounts people give of their own lives and the choices open to them. The alarm continually expressed in the mass media about ecological and individual risk is not universally shared. Signs of increased risk-taking, and risk enjoyment, can be identified. Risky sports such as mountaineering have exploded in popularity, and sedentary spectators are untroubled by the high risk of injury accepted by their sporting heroes. The popularity of gambling has reached new heights in the UK since the advent of the National Lottery in 1995, although, for the majority of punters, the hoped-for individual financial gain will never materialise, while the social benefits will pass them by, directed mainly towards the concerns of the cultural élite. Children are experimenting with smoking, sex and alcohol at younger ages (Woodroffe et al., 1991) in defiance of official health-promotion messages. More young people may be committing crimes and taking illicit drugs (Rutter and Smith, 1995), although historical comparisons are always problematic.

People accept risks either because they enjoy them, or because they believe, intuitively or calculatively, that, on balance, the expected benefits outweigh the possible costs. Lay and professional uses of cost-benefit analysis as a guide to individual decision-making will be considered in Chapter 1, and throughout this book. In general, cost-benefit analysis can be used to justify any number of decisions about risk-taking, opening up the potential for individual and cultural variation. Those who dismiss defiance of official preventive advice about smoking, the use of illicit substances or sexual contact as non-compliance risk overlooking or misunderstanding decision-makers' own rationality.

A story titled 'Ukraine hit by outbreaks of cholera and bravado' (*Guardian*, 16/08/95) noted that young people continued to swim in a heavily polluted river despite cholera outbreaks, and major preventive efforts by the authorities, including notices, the deployment of soldiers and fines. At first sight, this example appears to illustrate the poor understanding and irresponsibility which health professionals sometimes attribute to the public. However, the article points out that local people know that cholera can be easily cured by a readily available, cheap powdered drink. To those who, like the editor, value beyond price the experience of swimming in clear water, the bathers' behaviour, although in no way recommended, makes sense in terms of an informal cost-benefit analysis.

Pluralistic attitudes to matters of health and illness can be expected in complex, multicultural societies (Unschuld, 1986). Cultural filters influence the selection of what risks to worry about (Adams, 1995, p. 42). For example, German parents are much more likely to allow young children to travel to school on their own than are parents in England (Hillman, Adams and Whitelegg, 1990). In contrast, UK beef consumption recovered rapidly after news about the BSE fiasco broke in 1996, while Germans were, two months later, still eating 50 per cent less beef (*Guardian*, 15/05/96). Despite the relative similarity of the two societies, their cultural filters select different types of risk. Scott, in Chapter 17, argues that UK media anxiety about rare incidents of violent crime committed by the severely mentally ill is not found in other European countries, or even in the USA.

Attitudes towards specific risks, and towards risk in general, can be expected to vary with age, gender, social class, religious affiliation and ethnicity. Misunderstanding and intolerance may be anticipated where professionals and service-users employ different cultural filters, particularly in multicultural contexts (see Chapter 3). In Chapter 2, the historical and cultural specificity of the idea of risk is discussed, and risk analysis is compared with alternative orientations towards the future which cultures or individuals may adopt, including personalism (belief in a just, divinely created universe), fatalism (regarding the future as unalterable) and hedonism (discounting the future).

## LAY AND PROFESSIONAL RISK MANAGERS

The term 'lay' will be used to refer to people who attempt to manage risks in their own lives, or in those of significant others, and the term 'professional' to reference those who are paid to employ their expertise in order to help lay people to manage such risks. The distinction between lay and professional risk-managers reflects a division of labour in modern Western societies.

As with any simple classification of complex phenomena, it crumbles at the edges. Lay people develop their own understanding of the health-care culture, through direct experience and exposure to the mass media, and will variably identify with or reject aspects of the medical model. Professionals belong to a wider culture, and have to confront much the same hazards for themselves and their loved ones as do lay people. They also face personal risks arising out of their work, such as litigation, infection, or attack by violent service-users (MacKay, 1994). Instructive accounts given by professionals who have 'crossed over' to become users of the services they provide are considered in Chapter 1. Different professional groups, and individuals within groups, will hold discrepant views, as can be seen throughout the book. Nevertheless, their socialisation, organisational and occupational position, and experience of human suffering as work (Strauss and Corbin, 1988) partially blind professionals to client views.

The term 'professional', in the context of health-risk management, will be used broadly, to include people who, because of the expertise in predicting and controlling health futures ascribed to them, are paid to help others to manage health risks. Examples considered in this book include health promotion specialists, child-protection workers, day centre staff working with people with learning difficulties, and nurses working with elderly or diabetic clients. All active professionals are practitioners, even if their practice primarily involves giving advice, but practitioners, for example care assistants and home helps, are not necessarily professionals. The definition deliberately leaves open questions about the credibility of the implicit and articulated knowledge base on which professional claims to expertise are based.

This formulation does not entirely correspond with the classical sociological definition of professional status in terms of occupational attributes such as high social standing, decision-making autonomy, self-defined and enforced ethical standards, monopoly over particular forms of expertise and the power to control entry into the profession (Bond and Bond, 1986, p. 283). Such a clear-cut status depends on a social consensus which has eroded in the late modern era, as all forms of specialist knowledge, and professionals' claims to ethical disinterest, have lost credibility. While 'semi-professions', such as nursing (Hammond, 1990) and social work (Aldridge, 1996), still aspire to full professional status, the standing of professions like medicine, which they seek to emulate, has itself become uncertain (Lupton, 1994a, p. 54).

In a less cynical age, professionalism could be defined in terms of the disinterested ethical standards which the professional was presumed to adopt. Today, most people outside a particular professional group take it for granted that its members will venally promote their own interests unless systematically prevented from doing so. For example, the NHS and Community Care Act of 1990 aimed to curb medical power by removing decisions about the allocation of resources from the control of providers. A highly critical report about maternity care (DOH, 1993) has argued that an over-hospitalised system meets the career needs of obstetricians, in the name of risk avoidance, but not those of most pregnant women. Despite such concerns, the Caesarean section rate continues to rise inexorably (Francome *et al.*, 1993, p. 5). Doubting service-users may judge professionals' credentials as much by their position in the labour market, and the interests which these give rise to, as by their claims to knowledge and probity. Since all claimants to expertise, including those who write academic books, have careers to promote, their credibility will depend on the extent to which they are seen as tied to selling particular products.

The question of how health professionals and lay people have responded to this more critical atmosphere will be considered in the latter part of Chapter 1. Health-risk expertise, which will be analysed in some detail, is based on the claimed ability to predict the probability of various future health trajectories becoming a reality for a given individual. Since health professionals will see many of these probabilities as conditional on choices taken by clients, those around them, or the wider society, prediction becomes bound up with control. The health professionals' crystal ball, although providing only cloudy, probabilistic glimpses of possible futures, through the methodology of epidemiology, leads them into attempting to manage risks on behalf of their clients.

## Conclusion

This Introduction has sketched out an overview of the role and significance of lay and professional health-risk reasoning. Inevitably, the discussion has been somewhat wideranging, discursive and impressionistic. The reader is promised a more structured approach to value judgement and probability assessment in Chapters 1 and 2 respectively.

Three key arguments can be carried forward. First, risk management in the health and social care sectors is affected by the wider cultural context of late modern personal insecurity, heightened risk consciousness and selective alarm.

Second, health transactions depend on mutual trust and co-operation between professionals and clients. Professionals cannot hope to gain such trust unless they can understand the ways in which clients reason and feel about risks. Research into lay accounts of health-risk reasoning can generate information which helps professionals to better appreciate the complexities of client perspectives, although it cannot provide the last word on risk behaviour.

Third, the status of professional, science-based risk knowledge can be questioned. The aims of health care depend on the values which underlie them. Commonly, health decisions require a balance to be struck between conflicting values, for example between safety and autonomy, or the prevention of disability and care for the unborn child. Professionals need to understand clients' aspirations because such dilemmas cannot be solved by scientific evidence. They can only be managed through personal choice which clients must, ultimately, make for themselves. At the same time, probabilistic predictions, although derived from evidence, do not have a simple one-to-one relationship with 'reality'. Professionals need to appreciate the limitations of the risk heuristic, and to understand the ways in which their clients reflect on and attempt to manage their future health. To these issues we now turn.

# PART ONE

# Risk rationality

# Values and health risks

## Bob Heyman and Mette Henriksen

> *Your child has been born ... and, mercifully, has died.*
>
> *Children are life renewing itself, Captain Butler. And when life does that, danger seems very unimportant.*
>
> Gone with the Wind (MGM Studios, 1939)

## Introduction

The current Western, medical orthodox position (Lupton, 1994a, p. 91), by no means universally accepted even by doctors, maintains that individuals should draw on medical expertise in order to postpone mortality, and avoid morbidity as far as possible; that the locus of control for health outcomes rests primarily with individuals through their lifestyle choices; and that the impact of mental on physical processes can be discounted (see Chapters 2 and 18).

This chapter will consider the ways in which the complexities of lay value systems subvert official medical orthodoxy. It will be argued first, that discrepancies in health choices often arise from differences in the initial selection of consequences to be included in the cost-benefit equation, so that like is not compared with like; second, that the constitution of diseases as entities entails decisions, not always universally accepted, to discount differences within disease categories; third, that qualitatively different values cannot be meaningfully summed at the nomothetic, group level; fourth, that values vary multidimensionally, so that the 'same' effect may be judged differently, depending on the assessment of its severity, distribution, imminence, direction, voluntariness, moral acceptability and other attributes; and, fifth, that judgements of value and probability interact in non-linear ways.

The complexity of health-value judgements provides foundations for many different cost-benefit analyses. The starting point for lay and professional calculations tend to differ systematically because professionals operate in an organisational context which is not shared by service-users. Discussion of this fundamental divide will lead into the last section of the chapter, which considers the problematic and contested status of health-risk expertise.

Probability is dissected in Chapter 2. Values have been separated from probability, in different chapters, purely for analytical convenience. It is argued, in Chapter 2, that the same health phenomenon can be validly assigned many different probabilities, which can be used to support numerous *a priori* value positions.

## Selecting consequences for risk analysis

The following section will focus on variability in selective attention to health risks. To become a source of concern, a possible source of future adversity must first, be identified; second be seen as controllable; and, third, be judged to have significant consequences. In general, people will not worry about health risks unless they believe that some causal connection exists between a given present state and a future outcome, that they can exert some control over their present state, and that the future outcome matters.

### PREDICTION, CHOICE AND VALUE

Individuals must first recognise possible hazardous consequences before they can consider them further (Weinstein, 1988). For example, debate about the costs and benefits of sweetening wine with lead could not take place until its poisonous properties were recognised in the seventeenth century, after millennia of use (Eisinger, 1991). Conversely, most doctors in Victorian England regarded male masturbation as both a serious health hazard and a moral abomination (L.A. Hall, 1992). Few doctors today would think of starting a risk appraisal of this practice.

Second, individuals who have identified a hazard source must decide whether they can avoid it. Bolivian tin-miners (Nash, 1979, p. 200), homeless people (Health Advisory Service, 1995, p. 25) and young male sex-workers (Bloor, 1995) may understand that they are drastically shortening their life expectancy. But, in conditions of social powerlessness, they may judge that they have no alternative. The absence of perceived choice makes weighing-up the options futile.

Third, cost-benefit analysis can be undertaken for actions which are believed to entail preventable risk. Theoretically, actions generate an infinite number of consequences, and all events in the history of the universe interconnect. Since the world is replete with consequences, cultures, groups and individuals have to choose which ones to worry about, specifying an event '*horizon*' (Hansson, 1993, p. 18) before calculating expected utility. The boundaries we place around consequences depend on what we know, choose to investigate, and value.

The appreciation of differences in the selection of health consequences for cost-benefit analysis requires some imagination. For example, Reed (Chapter 12) found that one of the main considerations motivating elderly people to give up their independence and move into residential care was fear of dying alone. Patients with serious diseases may worry more about the social than the medical consequences. One diabetic patient's principal concern was that he would be unable to continue to work as a taxi-driver (see Chapter 8). Another was most worried that he might be unable to pursue flying as a leisure activity. The pregnant teenagers interviewed by Aarvold (see Chapter 6) feared side effects from using the contraceptive pill, and experienced difficulty in negotiating the use of male condoms. One girl rejected the femidom, female condom because '*they look funny*'. Members of a focus group of 14–16-year-olds who were asked about sexual risks (Tim Gristwood, personal communication), were most worried that their parents might return home unexpectedly, and catch them *in flagrante*. Some young people living in Western societies, particularly women, starve themselves voluntarily, placing their health at risk, so that their bodies may conform to cultural icons of thinness. Not smoking at age 15 was best predicted, in one study (McGee and Stanton, 1993), by the dislike of immediate negative effects such as taste and smell, at age 13.

This finding suggests that health promotion might more effectively focus on such medically trivial factors, rather than on the long-term risk of deadly diseases. Even the editor of this book has been observed to risk not wearing the riding hat which he uses to protect his brain when cycling, because he cannot face comments from passing children about its unfortunate resemblance to a First World War German military helmet.

The prioritisation of non-medical considerations is not confined to lay people. Burgess (1996, p. 47) criticised student nurses for risking injury to themselves and their patients in their efforts to prevent patients from soiling their clothes when being lifted on and off the commode. However, these concerns can be understood in the context of strong associations between personal cleanliness and the dignity of the individual in Western cultures. Similarly, one man, looking after his mother, who had dementia, particularly welcomed professional help in maintaining her personal hygiene (see Chapter 11). Such caring, although physically unproblematic, would have violated strong cultural taboos about proper transactions between adult children and opposite-sex parents. Adversity can only be understood in its cultural context.

## CONSEQUENCE SELECTION AND RISK DECISIONS

Contrasting decisions may result from differential selection of consequences for appraisal, rather than from discrepancies in the assessment of the same consequences. Moran and Barker note, in Chapter 16, that social service departments, established in the UK in 1971, were, at first, more concerned with juvenile delinquency than with child protection, later to become their main priority. Henriksen and Heyman (Chapter 7) found that 'older' pregnant women who had rejected amniocentesis focused on their aversion to termination, and the risk that the procedure could cause a spontaneous abortion of a healthy fetus. In contrast, women who had opted to have the test, and who intended to terminate in the event of a positive result, considered the impact on their other children of having to look after a child with Down's syndrome. Rapp (1993), similarly, outlines the case of an American Catholic supporter of the right-to-life movement who decided to abort following a diagnosis of Down's syndrome for her baby, because she wished to protect her daughter from having to look after a disabled sibling after her own death. Hence, women who take different decisions about genetic testing may not be considering the same effects or time frame. The implicitly consensual 'social values' which Fischoff, Watson and Hope (1984, p. 128) require in order to calculate expected utility are likely to be contested. These authors invite critics to begin cost-benefit analysis by selecting consequences, but do not explain how this can be done rationally.

Social amplification theory (Renn *et al.*, 1992) suggests that public concern about risks is closely related to exposure via the mass media. However, the mass media themselves belong to the wider culture, and reflect its concerns. According to the cultural theory of risk (Douglas, 1966), the dangers which a culture chooses to emphasise reflect its values and sense of the anomalous, as noted in the Introduction. For example, in Western Europe, the murder of children provokes shock and news headlines (see Chapter 16), while the regular killing of many times that number of children in road accidents is treated as a routine event. Road accidents have been normalised as a relatively acceptable consequence of an individually mobile way of life. Deliberate harm to children seems, in contrast, to threaten our contemporary notion of childhood as a protected time of innocent happiness.

## Value externalisation in the management of health risks

The Royal Society (1992) definition of risk as the probability of an adverse event externalises adversity on to events, just as it externalises uncertainty into probability, as will be argued in Chapter 2. However, one person's meat may be another's poison. We '*ascribe values to negativities*' (Rescher, 1983, p. 27). Because many of these values arise from our common human inheritance, they will be widely shared even across cultures. Nevertheless, when they come into conflict, groups and individuals may prioritise them differently. Contention, overt or covert, can only be avoided because, in a particular social group, we share similar values. Hamlet may have been exaggerating when he asserted that '*There is nothing either good or bad, but thinking makes it so*' (*Hamlet*, Act II, Scene ii). However, 'thinking' strongly affects the way an adversity is experienced and rated relative to other considerations. Even a serious illness such as cancer can have some positive aspects, leading to enhanced appreciation of time, life and interpersonal relationships (Kennedy *et al.*, 1976; Novakovic *et al.*, 1996).

Adversity is, ultimately, not a property of events, but of our ways of thinking about them. Providing that the parties to a health transaction share similar values, externalisation of adversity on to events provides a firm pragmatic basis for action, and should not lead to conflict, although it may reduce awareness of alternative perspectives. However, where the parties to health transactions hold fundamentally different values, or prioritise values differently, their externalisation on to events will lead, variously, to power struggles, miscommunication and covert conflict.

The embedding of contentious values in apparently naturalistic descriptions of the world impedes understanding of the other's point of view, which appears to defy 'common sense'. Thus, one person's 'substance use' is another's 'drug abuse'. What one person considers 'pornography', another regards as 'adult material'. A pregnancy may be 'terminated', resulting in the loss of a fetus, or 'aborted', leading to the death of a child. Family carers of people with learning difficulties who see themselves as 'responsible' may find their actions denigrated as 'overprotective' (see Chapter 9). The snake-handling preacher in Tennessee, when told that the author of *Salvation on Sand Mountain* (Covington, 1995, p. 1) did not have any snakes in his car, asked *'What's the matter with you boys? ... Are you crazy?'*.

The prepackaging of values with description only becomes explicit when values are disputed, as illustrated by the following quotation from one of the interviews with pregnant women discussed in Chapter 7.

> And I said, 'Well, if they find out that there's anything wrong with the baby, I can have the pregnancy stopped, you know.' And she [woman's mother] says, 'That's an abortion.' And I says, 'But they don't use it like that, you know,' I says, 'It's not the same.'

## THE PRICE OF A HUMAN LIFE

Economists' attempts to price human life in dollars illustrate the absurdity of treating value as an intrinsic, measurable property. At worst, this approach can smuggle technically driven values into numerical descriptions which the producers would almost certainly disown if they were not cloaked in the respectability of science. For example, environmental economists working for the UN's Intergovernmental Panel on Climatic Change (IPCC) calculated the value of human life by estimating how much communities were currently paying to prevent a death, a standard procedure in economic analysis. Their conclusion, pricing a life at $1 500 000 in the richest countries, but at only $100 000 a snip, in poorer countries, provoked intense controversy (*New Scientist*, 19/08/95). The authors have refused to modify their report, on the grounds of upholding 'scientific' over 'political' correctness. However, this type of formal cost-benefit analysis suffers from major problems.

Members of Western, science-based cultures tend to defer uncritically to numerical representations, regardless of their epistemological and empirical basis. But estimates of the monetary value of life differ widely, even in studies using a similar methodology. For example, occupationally based estimates of its value in developed countries have varied from just over $500 000 to more than $15 000 000 (Viscusi, 1992, p. 52). Wider consideration suggests that the average amount spent on saving a life depends massively on the social context. The reader is invited to guesstimate the 'value' of a life, in terms of the investment spent to save one, of Cabinet ministers, fighter pilots, inhabitants of Death Row in the USA, and very young or elderly people in the UK vulnerable to hypothermia because of poverty and poor home insulation.

This whole shaky edifice only works if we agree to determine values through extrapolation from existing safety expenditure. However, cost-benefit analysis could equally well be based on different *a priori* values, for example that market economies systematically undervalue collective long-term health. The 'scientific' correctness of cost-benefit analysis based on current expenditure rests on an unexamined political leap from 'is' to 'ought'.

Additional assumptions are required to spatially and temporally delimit consequences such as global warming in order to make them calculable. For example, the deaths caused by extra storm damage will be suffered globally, and will not be confined to the industrial societies which produced most of the carbon dioxide. Classical economics dismisses the wider negative and positive effects of industrial activity, such as pollution and the multiplier effect, on employment, as 'externalities' which can be excluded from calculations of expected value because they would make quantification too complex. Those who live downwind of emissions, or lose their jobs in secondary industries, tend to disagree with such simplification.

Problems arise in moving between the individual and aggregate level. We need to ask whose life is worth how much to whom? A suicidal person may value their life negatively, while Richard III, according to Shakespeare, was willing to trade his whole kingdom for a horse in order to save his skin. Jaymee Bowen, an 11-year-old schoolgirl who, in March 1995, was refused NHS treatment for leukaemia on the grounds of low survival chances and unnecessary suffering, commented that '*If you give up, you will end up with nothing left. I'd rather have gone through more suffering to live than not go through anything and die*' (*Guardian*, 26/10/95).

The calculation of generalised value, like estimation of probability (see Chapter 2), requires heuristic acceptance of the ecological fallacy that aggregated measures can be attributed to individuals. Averages involve much more than summary descriptions of numerical data, and we need to consider the relationship between the mean and the individual values they represent. The IPCC Report, discussed above, chose to average life-preserving expenditure separately for developing and developed countries. But we could also calculate the value of human life for groups or individuals within those societies. If costed in terms of the amount spent on their preservation, the lives of richer individuals (who, for example, invest in private health-care insurance) must be valued more highly than those of poorer people. It would follow that health services could improve their cost effectiveness by being targeted at prolonging the lives of the wealthy. We end up with a pseudo-scientific justification for the inverse care law. By choosing to aggregate the value of life calculation separately for developed and developing countries, but not within such countries, the authors of the IPCC report unreflectingly reproduce the prevailing world order.

The **general** 'risk-dollar' trade-off advocated by Viscusi (1992, p. 51) means nothing in cultures which do not have a market in lives. Readers who doubt this are invited to name the price at which they would be willing to sell their own life. Failure to find absurd the value inversion involved in estimating the dollar cost of human life reflects the hopefully temporary historical hegemony of market ideology in Western cultures, a hegemony accentuated by the collapse of the Soviet bloc and the current lack of credible alternatives. A marked historical shift from collective to individual values has occurred over the last 30 years, at least in the USA (Rokeach and Ball-Rokeach, 1989) and other Anglo-Saxon societies, but may be now unravelling.

## The constitution of consequences as risk entities

The categorisation of a type of event involves an act of classification of the dissimilar. Delineated events take on a life of their own, and are soon experienced as part of the natural world, while the pragmatic considerations which gave rise to their invention become lost. Values become embedded in the categories themselves. Hence, a consequence can only get into the cost-benefit equation through a double prior judgement, usually implicit, that it constitutes an homogenous entity, and that it falls within the event horizon for consideration, as discussed above.

Although the discussion which follows will focus on Down's syndrome, a similar point could be made about many other medical or social 'conditions'. Providing clear-cut criteria for the categorisation of schizophrenia is notoriously difficult (Kringlen, 1994). Jackson, Sanders and Thomas (1995) note that the term 'child abuse' covers a variety of behaviours, such as neglect, physical and sexual abuse, differing in subtype and dangerousness. Hence, the epidemiologies of schizophrenia and child abuse are, themselves, predicated on the amalgamation of heterogenous events into a single category (see Chapters 16 and 17). Patients with angina may be treated with drugs which have mainly palliative benefits, or with surgical intervention such as angioplasty or bypass surgery, depending on the severity of the condition. However, MacDermott (personal communication) has been assessing the quality of life of angina patients, as part of the RITA clinical trials comparing drug treatments, angioplasty and bypass surgery (Greenhalgh, 1993). He has found that the symptoms of patients treated with drugs vary considerably, and show less stability over time than their categorisation in a group not needing surgery might suggest.

All forms of analysis entail classification of the dissimilar. But constant critical challenges to the apparently natural status of disease entities and risk factors serve the function of preventing them from becoming undebated transmitters of social attitudes. This point is illustrated below through a more detailed consideration of Down's syndrome as an adverse event.

## IS DOWN'S SYNDROME AN ADVERSE EVENT?

This section considers differing perspectives on the wider meaning of Down's syndrome. It is argued that researchers, doctors who deal with medical complications, parents and people with Down's syndrome themselves may evaluate 'allowing' a person with the condition to be born quite differently. The nature and severity of the adversity, if any, associated with the condition cannot be divorced from wider societal responses, for example stigmatisation, segregation, provision or lack of provision of supportive resources.

### Medical perspectives

The impact of Down's syndrome varies considerably, leading to different degrees of intellectual, medical and functional impairments. Pregnant women who receive genetic counselling are presented with 'facts' about the risk of their baby being affected by the syndrome at a given maternal age. This analysis requires a numerator and denominator, and, therefore, entails some form of classification which homogenises those included in the numerator of the risk ratio, while differentiating them from the total population, in the denominator. The category then becomes not just a convenient shorthand label for a variable phenomenon, but a cultural product with socially shared meanings, associations and imagery attached (see Chapter 4). The tag 'Down's syndrome' thus becomes an *'iconic description'* (Rapp, 1988b, p. 150).

Once constituted as a natural event, Down's syndrome becomes a potential target for nomothetic research comparisons of averages in groups of people who do and do not have the syndrome. Such comparisons have generated a litany of adversity over and above intellectual disability, illustrated in Table 1.1, with examples of supporting research.

### Parental perspectives

The medical research illustrated in Table 1.1 can be used to paint a catastrophic composite picture of Down's syndrome, built up from a series of disparate group comparisons. More holistic approaches generate a sharply different assessment. Bailey (1996) argues that Down's syndrome children rarely experience pain or distress, and that professional concern has been directed primarily at the impact on parents of caring for such children. However, parental accounts suggest that they cope well. Black (1979) found that 45 out of 47 parents who had had a mentally handicapped child (Down's syndrome and unknown) reported that they had coped at least fairly well, despite common initial feelings of shock, anger, denial, sense of loss and guilt. Looking after a child with Down's syndrome appears to impact little on parental quality of life (Branholm and Degerman, 1992). Many mothers of Down's syndrome children feel that they benefit from a loving relationship with the child (Black, 1979).

A composite picture of parental evaluations of having a child with Down's syndrome can be built up from studies such as those discussed above, and from the views of pregnant women considering genetic testing, analysed in

**Table 1.1** A view of Down's syndrome based on medical research

| Developmental deficits | Physical problems | Functional disabilities |
|---|---|---|
| Child mortality (Bell, Pearn and Firman, 1989) | Smaller brain size (Raz et al., 1995) | Hearing difficulties (Davies, 1988) |
| Disturbed lung growth (Schloo, Vawter and Reid, 1991 | Disfunction of the central nervous system (Vieregge et al., 1992) | Visual problems (Hestnes, Sand and Fostad, 1991) |
| Reduced physical growth (Anneren et al., 1993) | Congenital heart disease (Marino, 1993) | Speech disfluencies (Devenny and Silverman, 1990) |
| Age-related decline in cortical functioning (Soininen et al., 1993) | Atherosclerosis (Ylaherttuala et al., 1989) | Attention deficits (Green, Dennis and Bennets, 1989) |
| Age-related deterioration in receptive language skills (Cooper and Collacott, 1995) | Breathing difficulties (Aboussouan et al., 1993) | Child hyperactivity, sleep disturbance and disobedience (Pueshel, Bernier and Pezzullo, 1991) |
| Premature ageing (Roeden and Zitman, 1995 | Obesity (Prasher, 1995) | Depression (Cooper and Collacott, 1994) |
| | Liver diseases (Ruchelli) et al., 1990) | |
| | Thyroid disorders (Dinani and Carpenter, 1990) | |
| | Leukemia (Mili et al., 1993) | |
| | Immune system deficiencies (Nespoli et al., 1993) | |
| | Susceptibility to infections (Anneren et al., 1992) | |
| | Periodontal diseases (Modeer, Barr and Dahllof, 1990) | |
| | Spinal problems (MacLachlan et al., 1993) | |
| | Skin problems (Brugge et al., 1993) | |
| | Hip defects (Shaw and Beals, 1992) | |
| | Dementias and Alzheimer's Disease (Collacott, Cooper and Ismail, 1994) | |
| | Epilepsy (McVicker, Shanks and McClelland, 1994) | |

Chapter 7. This picture is summarised in Table 1.2. Individual perspectives vary, and the table presents a range of considerations which influence parental decision-making, rather than a typical perspective. This catalogue of perspectives excludes the opinions of people with Down's syndrome about the value of their own existence.

## Comparison of medical and parental appraisals of Down's syndrome

A gap can be seen between the medical composite view of Down's syndrome as a severely adverse 'event', and family perceptions (Diachuk, 1994, p. 257). Several reasons for this gap can be suggested.

First, most epidemiological studies have considered single conditions, and inform us only about how an aggregate group of people with Down's syndrome compares with some other 'control' group. Such nomothetic research tells us little about the variable quality of life for individuals because problems may be concentrated within a subset of the population under investigation. McGrother and Marshall (1990) identified 71 serious or fatal medical conditions suffered by 56 children with Down's syndrome during a 10-year period from their birth. However, an undiscussed footnote to their paper shows that a further 51 children, 48 per cent of the sample, did not have any recorded condition whatsoever. Perhaps as a result of the specialised organisational structure of medicine, a large volume of research has investigated associations between Down's syndrome and specific diseases, but the overall health of real individuals has been largely ignored.

Second, many of the consequences of Down's syndrome can be mitigated. Medical advances have led to a dramatic improvement in life expectancy for people who have the syndrome. For example, the survival rate up to five years of age has been estimated as 42 per cent for children born in 1940 and 79 per cent for those born in 1976 (McGrother and Marshall, 1990). But such advances have to be paid for. Similarly, the adverse effects of Down's syndrome on learning ability cannot be separated from the learning environments to which individuals are exposed, and may be mitigated through appropriate but expensive educational interventions (Wishart, 1993). Thus, some of the adverse 'consequences' of Down's syndrome fall on the wider

Table 1.2    A view of Down's syndrome based on research into parental perspectives

| Reasons for not aborting fetus with Down's syndrome | Reasons for aborting fetus with Down's syndrome |
| --- | --- |
| Children tend to be loving | Effects on other children |
| Normal baby | Quality of life of child with Down's syndrome |
| Intellectual impairment not seen as problem | |
| Variation in levels of disability | Want first child to be perfect |
| Emotional trauma of termination | Inexperienced as parent |
| Rights of the unborn child | Unable to cope |
| Religious beliefs | Too old to cope |
| Social disapproval of abortion | Social disapproval of creating societal 'burden' |

society which acquires an obligation to compensate for its effects. Parents may exclude such concerns from their cost-benefit analysis more readily than do health professionals who have to provide services, and who may sometimes view people with long-term disabilities as a burden.

Third, health problems can appear quite different from a medical perspective than from the point of view of those personally involved. One woman in Black's study (1979) felt that consideration of termination for fetuses with genetic abnormalities made her own child 'abortable', violating its rights. Rothman (1988) discusses a paraplegic woman, reluctant to have amniocentesis, who mentioned several paraplegic friends who might have been detected by the test, and so never born. This respondent emphasised the variable nature of the impairment associated with paraplegia, thus showing awareness that diagnostic categories provide only simplifying iconic devices.

Medically, death may be an enemy to be fought. But in an uneven struggle, which medicine, for the forseeable future, is doomed to endlessly lose, 'normal life expectancy' must be accepted as the best which can be achieved. Shorter, more disease-prone lives, relative to current historical standards, should not be dismissed as intrinsically not worth living. Stainton (1992) gives the example of a woman suffering from a very serious heart disease whose baby died six days after being born. She regarded these six days as '*a gift*', but medicine, in its narrowest terms, had failed.

## Comparing qualitatively different values

Real-life choices affect the probability of occurrence of multiple consequences, and therefore require the decision-maker to weigh up the importance of qualitatively different values. Practice can only be straightforwardly 'evidence based' when all but one outcome parameter can be held constant, for example, if two therapeutic options produce very similar results, but one costs less than the other. Even in this simplest case, only aggregated outcomes can be assessed, and the best treatment for patients on average may not be optimal for some individuals. Real-life therapeutic options, particularly for complex, chronic and disabling conditions, vary multidimensionally, in terms of their cost, impact on the life quality of those with health problems and their families, their effect on life expectancy, and their consequences for the safety of service-users, relatives and the wider public.

Many health decisions will not involve dilemmas for most people belonging to a particular culture. For instance, in Western societies, few people, other than those who object on religious grounds, would find it difficult to decide whether to allow their GP to remove a small melanoma under local anaesthetic, or whether to accept an operation to prevent glaucoma causing blindness. However, such 'simple' problems generally involve secondary, curative prevention without side effects. Both primary prevention, avoiding health problems, and tertiary prevention, managing difficulties associated with long-term impairment, usually entail societal, family and lifestyle changes. Such 'wicked' problems (Rittel and Weber, 1974; Kingsley and

Douglas, 1991; Heyman, (1995a, p. 2) require the management of dilemmas, do not have optimum consensual solutions, and cannot be resolved solely through the use of 'evidence'. Because dilemmas cannot be solved, service-users must be allowed to make their own decisions, as already argued.

Since the multiple consequences of health-related decisions will be mostly uncertain, decision-making requires judgements about different probabilities of qualitatively distinct outcomes. For example, a smaller chance that a condition will kill prematurely after medical intervention might have to be balanced against a higher probability that such action will adversely affect life quality. Older men with prostate cancer face this dilemma because an operation intended to prolong life carries a risk of sexual disfunction (Ofman, 1995). Those who seek to 'sell' medical interventions may unconsciously underplay their downside. Russell and Smith, in Chapter 13, discuss a critical incident in which a nurse expresses her concern that an elderly man, advised to accept long-term dialysis, was not told how tired and ill he would feel. The nurse did not feel able to communicate this concern to the patient or medical staff, a reflection of the influence of health-service power structures on clinical decision-making.

Much of the difficulty involved in decision-making about risk, explored in Parts Two and Three of this book, arises from the requirement to weigh up varying probabilities of qualitatively different outcomes. Contraceptive choices can involve many considerations, including protection against pregnancy and against infection, cost, availability, ease of use, negotiation, preparation and maintenance requirements, pleasure, side effects, reversibility, consistency with religious principles and ecological consequences (see Chapter 6). In deciding whether to have amniocentesis, pregnant women have to choose between the risk of having a baby with Down's syndrome and the increased risk of miscarriage associated with the procedure (see Chapter 7). Diabetics must balance the immediate impact on their lives of dietary and alcohol restrictions against the increased risk of future health problems if they do not strictly control their insulin levels (see Chapter 8). People with learning difficulties, and their carers trade-off risks against autonomy in different ways (see Chapter 9). Professionals who look after institutionalised people with severe learning difficulties face a similar dilemma, and must balance safety for the majority against restrictions for the most able minority (see Chapter 10). Family carers have to set the safety of a relative with dementia against further damage to that person's already deteriorating mental state if their normal life patterns are disrupted to protect them (see Chapter 11). Older people balance the risks they associate with choosing to live independently, for example becoming a crime victim, against the effect on their life quality of moving into an institution (see Chapters 12 and 15). Social work and other professionals must weigh the risk of child abuse against the likelihood of damage to families placed under protection orders (see Chapter 16). The risk that people with serious mental health problems might harm themselves or others must be set against the damaging effects of institutionalisation (see Chapter 17). The public have to balance the potentially health-damaging effects of worry caused by taking public health scares seriously against possible risk to their physical health if they do not (see Chapter 18).

Professionals sometimes face the difficult task of making such decisions without time for reflection. One of the critical incidents described in Chapter 13 required a nurse, confronting a suicidal patient holding a razor blade, to choose between the risk of being attacked if she approached the patient and the risk that the patient would harm herself if she did not.

## QUALITY ADJUSTED LIFE YEARS (QALYs)

The problems associated with QALYs (Quality Adjusted Life Years) illustrate the difficulties involved in comparing different kinds of value. QALYs (Cubbon, 1991; Petrou and Renton, 1993; Mason, 1994) represent an attempt to establish the equivalence between costs and benefits arising from mortality and morbidity. A QALY is a ratio of 1 (a year of perfect health) adjusted for reduced life quality. Thus, a QALY of 0.9 would indicate that, because of pain or disability, a year of life for a given individual is 'worth' 90 per cent of its value to a person in perfect health. The benefits of a health-care intervention can be quantified by estimating the average number of QALYs which it will save, and this benefit can be related to its economic cost, to give a cost-benefit ratio. If valid, QALYs would provide policy-makers and managers with an empirical, value free, means of allocating resources between different treatments, such as heart transplants and hip replacements. If they are invalid, as will be argued below, QALYs simply provide scientistic legitimation for the administrative retention of power.

The calculation of QALYs requires a procedure for establishing the terms of trade between different conditions. These are worked out in a variety of ways, based on the opinions of 'prospective' patients (Carr-Hill, 1989, p. 472). For example, the 'time trade off' method involves asking respondents how much shorter a life in good health they would accept to be free of a given health problem. The 'equivalence of numbers' method requires respondents to judge how many more people would have to be cured of a milder condition for the outcome to be comparable to treating a smaller number of people with a more severe condition.

Two complicating factors must be taken into account before QALYs can be calculated. First, a way must be found to discount time, to give a reduced value to outcomes, positive or negative, which will occur further into the future. This is usually done through using the 'real' (inflation adjusted) rate of return in financial markets to reduce the estimated value of future benefits (Viscusi, 1992, p. 55). Second, since health outcomes are usually uncertain, attitudes towards risk need to be incorporated into the calculation. For example, 'prospective' patients might not judge a low probability of a highly negative outcome equivalent to a higher probability of a less negative outcome (see Chapter 5). In order to make the calculation of QALYs manageable, it must be assumed that individuals have a constant attitude towards risk, the assumption of risk neutrality (Fischoff, Watson and Hope, 1984, p. 131).

Psychological research suggests that this assumption may be unjustified. It must also be assumed that individual attitudes towards risk are not affected by health status (since 'potential' patients are used as informants).

Carr-Hill (1989) identifies many methodological and epistemological problems with QALYs. The survey method can, at best, determine nomothetic averages for the terms of trade between different conditions. Individual and subgroup differences in values are not taken into account. The meaningfulness to hypothetical patients of the comparisons they are asked to make can be seriously questioned. For example, how realistically can a healthy person make an imaginary choice between a shorter healthy life and a longer disabled one? Time cannot be validly discounted at real market rates. Its value to individuals depends on their personal projected futures. Future years might have a completely different value to young parents, scientists working on a lengthy project, those imprisoned for life, and single, socially isolated and permanently unemployed persons. Carr-Hill (1989) emphasises that he accepts the need to carefully weigh up the costs and benefits of different kinds of health-care intervention, using as much empirical evidence as possible, in order to make choices about the use of scarce resources. But empirical data can only be translated into action plans through the injection of value judgements, whether implicit and buried in complex calculations, or explicit and publicly debated. Different kinds of valued outcome can be compared only through the judgements of individuals and groups.

## Weighing positive and negative consequences

This section elaborates the argument made previously, that risk decisions will, almost invariably, entail balancing qualitatively different values. No generalised rubric can be provided for taking such decisions. Health professionals need to understand the complexity of the considerations which clients take into account when they attempt to manage health in a wider life context.

### COMPENSATIONS AND SIDE EFFECTS

Risk analysis needs to take account of the probabilities of positive as well as negative consequences of individual, group and collective human actions. At the collective level, exponential economic growth in a small number of industrialised societies has created appalling long-term risks for the future of human life, and vehicles choke cities. Yet economic growth and private transport confer obvious benefits.

At the individual level, many people enjoy, variously, smoking, drinking alcohol and coffee, consuming illicit substances which affect their mental state, eating fatty foods and having unprotected sex with multiple partners (although not usually at the same time). Research, in so far as it can detect causal effects within complex tangles of covariation, suggests that such activities produce more complex mixtures of health effects than the health-education propaganda war sometimes allows. We do not seek to promote activities such as smoking or unprotected sex with multiple partners, only to argue that actions with multiple consequences, almost invariably, confer a mixture of advantages and disadvantages.

Moderate alcohol consumption may prevent heart disease (Criqui, 1996). Cholesterol serves vital physiological functions, and reduced levels have been linked with the increased risk of health problems, including depression and suicide (Zureik, Courbon and Ducimetiere, 1996), lung cancer (Chang, Barrett-Connor and Edelstein, 1995) and colon cancer in men (Kreger et al., 1992). Even the generally lethal habit of smoking confers some emotional benefits (Graham, 1987), can be used for weight control (see Chapter 6), and has been linked to the reduced risk of Alzheimer's disease (Lee, 1994, but see below) and of endometrial carcinoma in postmenopausal women (Weiss, 1985).

On the other hand, officially health-promoting activities have possible downsides. Long-term intense sporting participation may cause osteoarthrosis of the hip in men (Vingard et al., 1993) and increase the risk of sudden cardiac death, as well as preventing longer-term heart problems (Burke and Virmani, 1994). Even breathing has its detractors, because it creates destructive free radicals which can only be partly mopped-up by anti-oxidants such as vitamins C and E (Anzueto et al., 1992).

The direction of causality in the above relationships can be seriously questioned (see below). The benefits of disapproved activities may be swamped by costs, as with smoking, or the costs of approved activities outweighed by benefits. Nevertheless, the above examples do suggest that all human activities confer mixed blessings.

## DEFENCE OF THE HEALTH-PROMOTION LINE

Challenges to the standard health-promotion line, that individuals can control their health risks through correct lifestyle choices, invariably provoke heated controversy. For example, low serum cholesterol levels may be caused by cancer (Delahaye et al., 1992) rather than vice versa, and possibly have a protective function against incipient disease (Buchwald, 1992). The apparent preventive benefit of smoking with respect to Alzheimer's disease could, in theory, result from differential survival, i.e. smokers destined to develop the disease excluding themselves from research samples by dying younger (Riggs, 1996). Dutch researchers (New Scientist, 19/04/97, p. 13) have recently concluded that smokers and ex-smokers are at increased risk of Alzheimer's disease and other dementias. They argue that previous research systematically excluded people suffering from heart disease and strokes. When such individuals are included in the research sample, the apparent benefits of smoking are reversed. These hypotheses, if accepted, would, in each case, rescue the health-promotion position.

However, because the power of epidemiology to establish any causal connections is notoriously limited (Skolbekken, 1995), largely confined to nomothetic, multivariate correlations of weak accuracy, and subject to constant revision, the general public may suspect that investigative efforts are biased towards sustaining the official line. For example, the American National Academy of Science, eager to dispute a postulated iatrogenic causal association between maternal abdominal X-rays and Down's syndrome, has argued that sick women might be both more prone to receive X-rays and to produce children with Down's syndrome (Rose, 1994). In contrast, the causal status of the relationship between maternal age and the risk of Down's syndrome has been taken for granted even by critics of the view that having a baby after the age of 35 entails the acceptance of high risk (Mansfield, 1988).

Individuals and groups would not accept avoidable risks unless they anticipated some benefits. It may be even more difficult to weigh-up qualitatively different positives and negatives than to just compare negatives. How do people balance autonomy against safety, or the pleasures of unprotected casual sex against the risk of HIV? Comparison of incommensurables depends on concrete value judgements involving real, context-specific decisions. Weighing-up expected values in particular cases does not always generate a clear preference, as anyone who has agonised over a finely balanced major life decision can testify.

Attempting to change behaviour involves enough problems without having to admit that everything we do carries a mix of costs and benefits. Professionals, therefore, will tend to present their advice in terms which avoid shades of grey, while lay people, who have to live with good and bad consequences, may be less willing to oversimplify when asked to abstain from enjoyable activities. As Stone (1986, p. 672) wryly noted, the initial 'missionary' zeal of preventive specialists has provoked a 'colonial revolt'.

## Value complexity

### THE MULTI-DIMENSIONALITY OF VALUES

To complicate expected utility calculations still further, judgements of the positivity and negativity of individual consequences themselves involve multidimensional considerations. Rescher (1983, p. 24) proposes that negativities can be compared in terms of severity (the badness of the consequence), distribution (how many people are affected) and imminence (how quickly they will occur). These dimensions can be used equally well to categorise judgements about the benefits of risk-taking.

Comparisons of values which vary on more than one dimension are complex and unwieldy. How do we compare, for example, a severe consequence for a smaller number of people with a milder effect on a larger population, for instance the cancer-inducing potential of a polluting industrial plant against the health-damaging effects of unemployment if the plant is not built? Moreover, aggregate statistics differ in variability as well as central tendency, further complicating comparisons. For example, lung cancer usually kills, but strokes can have many outcomes including complete recovery, more or less severe impairment, and death.

Unfortunately for those with a powerful urge to quantify values, further dimensions can easily be identified (Hansson, 1989). Three important additional dimensions, namely cost-benefit direction, voluntariness and moral acceptability, will be briefly considered below.

Moral and political issues concerning risk are often bound up with questions about who suffers and who gains, and so about what risks are acceptable to whom. Cost-benefit direction assesses the extent to which those seen to benefit from risk acceptance match those perceived to bear its costs. In the case of vested interest, the main beneficiaries of a risky activity, such as those who work in the tobacco industry and governments which obtain tax revenues, differ from those who suffer its adverse consequences, such as children who smoke. On the smaller scale of health and social care transactions, service-users will make judgements about the extent to which proposed therapeutic options involving risks serve the interests of providers. For example, some of the parents of adults with learning difficulties interviewed by Heyman and Huckle (1993a) believed that formal carers at adult training centres encouraged attenders with learning difficulties to take outside jobs because they wanted to clear places at the centre. The parents opposed this move, which they felt benefited the centre rather than the adult, because they feared that they, not service-providers, would be left to pick up the pieces if anything went wrong.

Differences in perceived control of an outcome require a fifth dimension of values. Individuals tend to evaluate the same negative consequence less unfavourably if it has arisen from their own choices (Slovik, 1987). Conversely, patients may receive less sympathy if they are judged responsible for their own condition, for example through smoking, alcohol or illicit substance use, or attempting suicide (Stockwell, 1972; Lorber, 1975; Jeffrey, 1979).

A sixth dimension involves the moral acceptability of a risky activity. Adversities, such as the death while climbing of a top mountaineer, or sports injury to a professional footballer, seem less severe because they are culturally legitimated. Historically established hazards become accepted as 'natural' (Hansson, 1989). AIDS-related deaths, popularly associated with activities such as homosexuality, intravenous drug-taking and prostitution which the wider culture questions, may be judged more adverse than more 'innocent' fatalities. Professionals sometimes see both younger (Chapter 6) and older (Chapter 7) pregnant women as facing more severe risks than those who have children at the 'proper' age, relative to prevailing cultural notions about motherhood: an attitude which both younger and older women may strongly resent. The difference they saw between themselves and the professionals can be understood in terms of different background assumptions about the 'natural' age span for having babies.

Since each of the multiple positive and adverse consequence included in a cost-benefit calculation may vary in perceived severity, distribution, timing, direction, voluntariness, moral probity and other attributes, apparently similar contingencies may be judged entirely different because they differ on one dimension. For example, a devoted mother might judge asthma resulting from smoking to be less bad than lung cancer for herself, but view asthma for her child as worse than lung cancer for herself. In this example, the perceived direction of adverse consequences affects their judged severity. Such combinative effects cannot be understood except in relation to individuals' self-identities and wider values, such as the predominant importance to many women of motherhood. A simplistic quantitative approach to value is hopeless because it reduces complex patterns of individual judgement to single numerical values.

## CALIBRATION PROBLEMS

Those involved in managing a health risk need to make decisions, finding a way through the complexities of weighing up qualitatively different values. Thus, a patient might decide to accept a prostate operation to reduce the risk of cancer, or to decline such an operation to avoid the risk of sexual disfunction it would entail. Such decisions require implicit or explicit calibration of different values. Outcome A is deemed better than outcome B, or a balance is struck which allows some combination of A and B which reflects their relative worth. For instance, family carers of people with learning difficulties (Chapter 9) developed differing compromises between autonomy and safety for their relative which reflected the relative weight they gave to these two, often conflicting, considerations.

These decisions will be more or less weighted for probability, to allow for the possibly greater acceptability of a less likely adverse outcome or a more likely positive one. Again, no uniquely correct method of adjusting calibration to allow for probability can be established. Individuals have to decide such matters for themselves.

The expected utility model implies that calibration involves a bottom-up reasoning process. However, everyday observation suggests that top-down processes are at least as important. We calibrate consequences to support judgements we have already made. For example, the case of severely brain-damaged Thomas Creedon, whose parents wanted him to be allowed to die, provoked intense media debate in the UK (Kay, 1996). The parents maintained that the child was suffering severe pain, and could not look forward to any quality of life. Pro-lifers argued not only that failing to sustain life (through intravenous feeding) was wrong, but that a good life quality for such children could be achieved. Hence, each side calibrated life quality in a way which supported their wider judgement.

Expected utility cannot be validly derived from the product of value and probability. We need to know how individuals meaningfully combine probability and value for a set of identified consequence into an overall judgement in particular cases.

## The organisational context of health professional values

This section discusses the effects of the organisational context on the appraisal of risk values. Our consideration of the organisational context of health care is designed to show that, in appraising risks, professionals and service-users do not evaluate the same set of contingencies. Lay people approach services because of personal concerns, for example to preserve life or to enhance its quality for a loved relative with disabilities. Professionals seek to help clients to manage their futures and to promote their wellbeing. But they do so from within an organisational context that exerts pressures which their clients do not encounter. Three such influences, namely accountability considerations, resource constraints and professional identity are considered below. Because of their impact, professionals and clients employ different 'event horizons' (Hansson, 1993, p. 18). Professionals may be concerned about censure if adversity results from risk-taking, consumption of limited caring resources which could have benefited others, or threats to the power and influence of a profession with which they identify personally.

## PROFESSIONAL ACCOUNTABILITY, LITIGATION AND RISK MANAGEMENT

Late modern health-care systems are characterised by increased individual accountability for adverse events which possibly could have been prevented, and heightened concern about litigation.

Annandale (1995) observed, in the context of consumerism in the health service, and developments such as the Patients' Charter, that nurses felt individually vulnerable to complaints and litigation, even though they had little personal control over what happened to patients. Their fear was reinforced by apocryphal 'horror stories', for example of a confused patient who had groundlessly accused his nurses of abusing him. As a result, nurses were strongly motivated to maintain written records, and to avoid situations in which they might be deemed to have acted beyond their certified competence.

Heightened concern with litigation may yield mixed benefits for service-users. The chance of serious medical errors may be reduced, but the balance of risk assessment is shifted towards caution. For example, women may be given Caesarean sections in low-risk cases simply to avoid the risk that a hospital would be sued if anything went wrong with a more natural birth. In the UK, some hospitals now insist, for legal reasons, on the presence of a doctor during birth. Strategies for avoiding litigation thus defeat the policy aim of making maternity services more midwifery-led and woman-friendly.

## RESOURCE CONSTRAINTS AND PROFESSIONAL RISK MANAGEMENT

The management of accountability in health-service organisations has to be balanced against the need to make decisions about the allocation of scarce resources such as time, money and transplant materials. Professionals cannot meet all the demands made on them. However, service-users, immersed in their own lives, may have difficulty accepting that options for their personal futures have been excluded because, in relation to the general picture, they have been given low priority. The father of one adult with learning difficulties, interviewed for the study discussed in Chapter 9, knew that he was dying of heart disease, and that he would not be offered a transplant because the limited number of hearts available would go to younger people. Although he accepted this situation, it caused him visible distress. A divide could be seen between the personal value of an individual's life, on the one hand, and the problems of resource allocation to populations, on the other.

The connection between resource constraints and the representation of risks is explored below in relation to the management of genetic testing for unborn children. It will be argued that the dividing line between 'low' and 'high' risk maternal ages is resource-driven, but becomes redefined in health-care practice as a natural risk boundary. However, doctors may not, in their practice, respect such arbitrary borders consistently. Service-users find out about these discrepancies, making fragile the whole edifice of categorising and prioritising a high-risk group.

## The organisational derivation of prenatal genetic risks

The potential for clashes between the professional requirement to allocate resources and clients' personal involvement in their own futures creates a tactical problem for professionals in terms of how they represent their decisions and policies. This issue will be illustrated through a discussion of decision-making about the offer of fetal genetic testing in the hospital used for the research discussed in Chapter 7. Since the risk of having a baby with a genetic abnormality increases with age, the cut-off point, if any, at which genetic counselling is offered must be arbitrary. Because counselling and testing have economic, emotional and medical costs, its analysis illustrates the processes through which organisations allocate scarce resources to prevention, and draw lines below which the probability of an adverse event will be accepted.

The commonly used cut-off point, at 35 years, was originally justified on the grounds that the risk of having a baby with Down's syndrome matches the risk of amniocentesis causing a miscarriage at this age. But the use of this criterion requires a value judgement that a miscarriage and having a child with Down's syndrome carry similar degrees of adversity. The 35-year cut-off has also been linked to the capacity of laboratories in the USA to carry out screening at the time that genetic screening was introduced (Donnenfeld, 1995). Despite its arbitrary, resource-driven, origin, the age of about 35 has now acquired the status of a natural boundary for the maternal risk of Down's syndrome. A colleague of Mansfield (1988, p. 446), aged 34, was advised to choose between pregnancy and sterilisation 'to avoid crossing the biological boundary and becoming a high-risk patient'. The editor's wife was told by her GP that she did not need to worry about the risk of Down's syndrome because she was only 35. Thus, organisational policies and constraints are projected on to the natural world.

However, given the arbitrary nature of this dividing line, its operation in clinical practice varies considerably. The dividing line for genetic counselling used by doctors in the hospital site for our research ranged between 32 and 37 years. Individuals tended to project their own idiographic norms on to organisational policy. One doctor said, during genetic counselling, that 'we offer to [screen] mothers who are over 30 or 32'. A pregnant woman quoted the doctor who counselled her as saying 'I just thought it [screening] might have been on your mind, but we don't normally offer it until you are 37.' A similar projection of idiosyncratic norms on to imagined hospital policies may be seen in the case of routine hospital blood-pressure reading, discussed by O'Brien and Davison in Chapter 14. Burroughs and Hoffbrand (1990) found that about 80 per cent of nurses wrongly believed that their blood-pressure reading practice followed hospital policy. Hence, in both cases, professionals legitimated idiosyncratic customs as expressions of a wider social order.

Consultants and registrars did not apply even these personal rules consistently. One consultant said he would sometimes underestimate a woman's age if she looked young, and forget to check her notes, or might be distracted if the phone rang during the counselling session. The study found examples of women, sometimes puzzled or angry, who had not been offered testing even though they met the registrar or consultant's own criteria. This combination of screening according to risk factors with an idiosyncratic, case-by-case, approach may result from health services being currently in a historical transition phase from patient-centred to population-based systems of care (Castel, 1991).

Two consultants told pregnant women, during counselling, that they wished to offer this service to all women, but were unable to do so because the health-purchasers would not provide funding. A follow-up interview with one woman and her husband shows that this information concerned them, and that they had wondered why they had not been offered counselling for a previous birth, when the woman was younger. Professionals may avoid such bluntness, and represent decisions about whom to screen as based on clinical need, rather than on the requirement to allocate resources so as to minimise risk for populations.

## Fences and stable doors

Some aspects of organisational procedures for allocating resources to hazard management can be understood in terms of the contrasting metaphors of 'putting a fence round the law' and 'closing the stable door after the horse has bolted'. Given their natural inertia, complex organisations may possess an in-built tendency to gravitate towards one of these two extremes, or even to alternate between them (see Chapter 15).

Forbidden by biblical injunction from eating kid cooked in its mother's milk, on the grounds that it entailed gratuitous cruelty, Jews were then prohibited from consuming goat cooked in any milk in case they accidentally used the mother's milk. To make sure that the latter did not happen, eating any combination of meat and milk was banned. To guarantee that milk and meat were not accidentally consumed together, Orthodox Jews were then forbidden from ever using the same utensils, plates and cutlery for milk and meat. This system has remained essentially intact for more than 2000 years, although it has had to be constantly updated to cope with new situations, for example the creation of new foodstuffs through genetic engineering.

The process described by Jewish theologians as 'putting a fence round the law' can be compared to the gradual building of a series of walls around an area in order to defend it. Each wall is designed to protect the one within, but, over the course of time, the initial defensive objective may be lost sight of. Martin (1994, p. 25) reproduces just such an image from a hygiene text of around 1920 to illustrate attitudes towards health maintenance in a pre-immunological age. Keeping the kitchen clean reduces the risk of germs getting on to people's hands, while hand-washing removes any organisms that pass through the first line of defence.

Those operating the modern health-care system, still mainly oriented towards secondary prevention, may continue to see themselves as fighting a war. One of the nurses whose accounts of critical incidents are discussed in Chapter 13 felt distressed that an elderly lady with leukaemia 'would give up without a fight'.

As a descriptive device depicting one approach to risk management, the military defence metaphor oversimplifies in two respects. First, individual practice of any institutionalised custom usually varies far more than outsiders realise (Douglas, 1966, p. 90). Second, the defensive system may acquire functions other than those initially intended. Sustaining military defences provides jobs, and dietary restrictions helped Orthodox Jews to defend their cultural distinctiveness in the hostile Diaspora. Similarly, O'Brien and Davison argue, in Chapter 14, that routine but inaccurate blood-pressure measurements for hospital inpatients give little medical protection, but provide a reassuring ritual display of the nurse's commitment to patient safety.

Putting a fence round the law stands in contrast, at the other extreme on a continuum of protectiveness, to 'closing the stable door after the horse has bolted'. The latter involves holding an inquiry after a disaster has happened in order to apportion blame, and attempting to prevent the disaster from recurring. Such a strategy minimises the requirement for protective resources, but has two drawbacks. First, adverse consequences have to be suffered before a preventive strategy is contemplated. Second, individual disasters provide a poor guide to underlying probabilities. In contrast, a fencing strategy requires a heavy investment of preventive resources, and acceptance of a high frequency of missed opportunities to make choices which would not have led to adverse consequences had they been selected (Adams, 1995, p. 55). For example elderly people may miss opportunities for social contacts if they do not go out because they fear being mugged (see Chapter 12).

Comparisons of the hazards which societies or social groups deal with maximally, through a system of defensive barriers, and those which they manage in a minimal reactive mode, can tell us much about their underlying but implicit cultural values.

Most Western cultures, including the UK, have selected HIV infection and 'drug abuse' as dangers meriting maximal defensive responses. Thus, a blanket prohibition against illicit 'drugs', i.e. all those which happen to be currently illegal, has been justified on the grounds that partial legalisation would send the wrong 'message'. Putting a fence around the law worked for Orthodox Jews because the process arose out of a sense of the fragility of human intentions, was linked to the sacred, and fitted into a wider system of cultural values. The lack of success of 'safe' sex campaigns with young heterosexuals (MacDonald and Smith, 1990) and defeat in the drug 'war' result from them being none of the above.

Conversely, government responses, during the 1990s, to risks associated with the practices of the meat industry appear to illustrate the drawbacks of a stable-door policy. In early 1997, at the time these words were written, the Conservative government was struggling to cope with the electoral consequences of multiple deaths from BSE and E-Coli infection which many voters blamed on its deregulation policy. The government's health-risk management strategy had, for the first time, become a significant general election issue in the UK.

## PROFESSIONAL IDENTIFICATION AND RISK MANAGEMENT

Another set of pressures on practitioners arises from their identification with the values and historical traditions of a particular profession such as nursing, midwifery, physiotherapy or medicine. Faith in the efficacy of the service offered by their own professional group becomes a matter both of personal self-esteem and occupational self-interest.

Professional values influence judgements about the probabilistic aspect of risk. Schuman and Marteau (1993) found that obstetricians rated birth as significantly more risky than did pregnant women, who judged it more risky than did midwives. Greater differences were observed in both professional groups among those who had served longer in their profession. Each group appears to have assessed risk in a way which enhanced its own sphere of activity: the obstetricians by maximising medical complications, and the midwives by minimising them. Individual practitioners had become increasingly immersed in their professions over time. In consequence, the longer they had worked, the more their risk assessment diverged from that of their clients.

Similarly, Grande, Todd and Barclay (1995) found that GPs and district nurses differed significantly in their ratings of the difficulty of controlling symptoms in terminally ill patients. GPs rated symptoms for which they could give pharmaceutical treatment, such as sleeplessness and pain, as easier to manage than did district nurses. In contrast, district nurses rated symptoms which would receive mainly nursing interventions, for example incontinence, as less difficult to deal with than did GPs. In comparison to patients, GPs significantly underestimated the presence of symptoms, and a strong correlation was found between GP ratings of the difficulty of controlling a symptom and their tendency to underestimate its prevalence. The authors offer two related explanations of the findings of this important study. They suggest that doctors may be less willing to ask about symptoms which they believe they cannot control, while patients may avoid mentioning such symptoms if they think the doctor will be unable to help them. However, as stated above, doctors' judgements of treatment difficulty were influenced by their medical orientation.

A faith in the efficacy of their own nostrums which is not shared by others prevails in most professional groups, a side effect of specialisation. For example, health-promoters continue to believe in the efficacy of education, since they cannot change structural factors such as poverty through their professional activities. They maintain this faith despite a lack of evidence both that individual behaviour strongly affects public health, and that behaviour can be significantly changed by health education (Roberts, Smith and Bryce, 1993).

Public health physicians in Northern Ireland (Kee, Gaffney and McDonald, 1995) report they have been unable to shift consultants' confidence in andiograms, despite evidence of their unreliability, and note that both the rate of angioplasty and the proportion of cardiologists in the population of the province are twice those for England and Wales. These researchers found that patients with heart problems significantly overestimated the benefits, in terms of additional life expectancy, of angioplasty, suggesting that health professions may have successfully oversold their remedies, or, at least, have not dampened overoptimistic expectations which help them to market their wares.

Differences in orientation between professional groups can generate conflict, as illustrated by the following quotation, obtained for the research discussed in Chapter 9, from a worker in a day centre catering for people with learning difficulties:

> The doctors always need to have a label for them [people with learning difficulties]. I have had some hideous experiences in hospitals. Sheer ignorance. There was one lad who has a very severe physical disability, and the doctor actually asked us if he was worth saving. We come across that kind of thing all the time ... Most service-users have had years of abuse.

## Risk expertise

The section which follows analyses the ways in which service-users and risk professionals understand and negotiate risk expertise. Health-care transactions concerned with risk cannot be understood unless professional and lay views of the status of the professional's expertise, and the interrelationships between their views, are taken into account. Conversely, the difficult epistemological status of risk knowledge makes risk transactions particularly fertile ground for observation of late modern attitudes towards expertise.

### THE PROBLEMATIC STATUS OF EXPERTISE

Most of the issues discussed in this book revolve around the troubled and contested status of expertise in late modern cultures. Individual attitudes towards particular bodies of expertise will differ. However, these cultures have a collective ambivalence towards expertise, based on three ingredients. First, members of highly specialised, information-based societies cannot escape from **dependency** on experts whose knowledge they need to use in order to achieve their personal objectives, including the management of risks. Second, in order to belong to the mainstream economy, individuals have to **sell** one of the many extant bodies of specialist knowledge. Third, individuals need to maintain a substratum of **suspicion** about types of expertise they have to draw on, but which experts are required to sell in order to earn their daily bread.

Older readers may reflect back on their own *'substratum of trust'* (Giddens, 1991, p. 129) and consider whether it has changed over the last 20–30 years. The editor smoked in the 1960s, and, in the early 1970s, regularly took his young child to a beach near the Sellafield nuclear plant at which potentially lethal radioactive particles were subsequently discovered. At that time, he took it for granted that the authorities would not knowingly allow citizens to endanger their health. Looking back, such faith seems risible.

O'Riordan (*Times Higher Education Supplement*, 14/03/97) has reported the results of a recent survey which illustrates the extent of the general public's mistrust of risk experts. The survey found that a quarter of the sample or less would trust government, business or the media to tell the truth about risks such as sunbathing and genetic manipulation. Scientists were trusted by 60 per cent of the sample, while doctors, friends and family members were trusted by around 80 per cent or more. These findings provide a quantitative frame for the qualitative data to be discussed below.

Our research provides a more fine-grained, qualitative picture of attitudes towards doctors and other health professionals. This research suggests that the public feel ambivalent towards even the most trusted sources of professional expertise. The ideal expert, from a lay perspective, combines risk knowledge with both disinterest and personal qualities such as lived experience, wisdom and commitment. Health professionals may be seen as promoting occupational or organisational interests. On the other hand, their expert credentials may sometimes be established, ironically, through their personal qualities.

All professionals do not depend upon commission, but, nevertheless, their career prospects rely on societal valuation of their expertise. It becomes increasingly difficult for those who are immersed in a particular profession to criticise, or even be aware of, the bedrock assumptions on which their knowledge base depends. The exclusion of 'externalities' as too difficult to quantify in mainstream economics, and the treatment of states of being as mental 'diseases' in conventional psychiatry, provide examples of the blinding power of expertise. The trap of assumptions cannot be escaped in any structure of knowledge, including those encoded in academic, critical writing. But individuals who only live once cannot afford to rely too much on simplifying assumptions.

Herbivores will uneasily tolerate the presence of lions at the waterhole, but will startle at the slightest sign that the hunt is about to begin, because they know that a crafty carnivore will attempt to conceal its intentions from its prey as long as possible. After the immediate danger has passed, they will return calmly to the waterhole, as they need to drink. So, non-experts will treat the most minimal and qualified admission of the tiniest possibility of a small problem as an indication of oncoming, concealed disaster. For example, in the UK, the rapid but temporary abandonment of certain forms of contraceptive pills, associated with a higher risk of thrombosis, in 1995, and of British beef in 1996, both illustrate the value of the predator/prey metaphor of attitudes towards risk expertise.

The credibility of the knowledge base underpinning occupations such as social work (Aldridge, 1996) and nursing (Paley, 1996) has become a critical issue in discussions about their professional status. Paley (1996) used the debate around Benner's (1984) notion of intuitive nursing expertise to make some sharp points about the problematic status of professional knowledge. The often-quoted model for intuitive expertise involves an analogy with chess mastery. The chess expert can remember the position of a random set of non-chess pieces on a board little better than a novice, but can recall a real chess position much more accurately (Schneider *et al.*, 1993), suggesting that expertise generates qualitative perceptual shifts. Paley points out that clear criteria exist for defining a good chess-player, but not for defining a good nurse. The notion of expert judgement presupposes that optimal solutions exist and can be discovered. However, this view takes for granted the reliability, let alone the validity, of expert judgements. For example, experimental studies in which mental health specialists have been exposed to the same detailed evidence about a possible child-abuse case (Horner, Guyer and Kalter, 1993), have shown that individual experts can have high confidence about conflicting conclusions. Physicians appear similarly overconfident about the correctness of their own clinical judgements (Christensen-Szalanski and Bushyhead, 1981).

The self-validated decision-making alleged to underlie nursing and other forms of professional expertise cannot be pronounced free of contamination with self-interest (Sapolsky, 1990). Indeed, bodies of artists and scientists tend, notoriously, to honour received wisdom which protects their own paradigms. The public, wisely, feel sceptical towards such self-validating forms of expertise, apart from those they sell themselves.

## EXPERT/LAY RELATIONSHIPS

Experts are swayed by loyalty to their own careers; become desensitised to the harmful side effects of the application of their expertise; avoid looking in awkward directions in order to sustain the mantra of 'no scientific evidence'; use oversimplified models in order to sustain claims to be able to control the future; tenaciously resist being proved wrong; and ignore organisational complexities which generate systematic gaps between policies and practice.

However, representation of expert/lay relationships as a battleground arising from unbridgeable gaps in perspective gives an oversimple, partial picture. Expertise cannot be escaped in late modern cultures. The credibility even of damning exposés is itself based on trust in another kind of expert: journalists, who, in turn, have to rely on their own expert whistle-blowers. Paradoxically, the Green movement depends on information supplied by modern science, which it distrusts as the source of environmental problems (Yearley, 1992). Tension between views of the expert as callous exploiter and bearer of gifts leads to considerable intracultural variation. Although the aggregate societal attitude towards expertise can be characterised as ambivalent, individuals vary greatly in their general degree of suspicion of experts in general, of particular types of expert and of individuals.

Subcultural gaps between lay people and professionals must be balanced against commonalities (Heyman, 1995a, pp. 36–7). Health professionals and lay people belong to a wider culture, itself pluralistic and diverse. Research into priority-setting (Bowling, Jacobson and Southgate, 1993) suggests, ironically, that the public, fed on television dramas about medical emergencies, prioritise high-technology secondary prevention, while consultants and GPs give more emphasis, in surveys at least, to directing resources into community care. Thus, the public favour the medical model more than doctors.

Lay people think that they have some understanding of the world of health professionals. Conversely, their exposure to human suffering as paid work separates health professionals only partially from the wider social world. As well as sharing wider cultural values, health professionals have children, get depressed, become sick and eventually die. The slightly surprising quality of this truism is associated with the tendency, in a specialised culture, to separate out the professionals who are paid to manage health futures from the public who call on their assistance.

## How do health professionals manage risks to their own health?

The experiences of professionals who cross the floor to become users of the service they provide can offer important insights into the relationship between lay and professional perspectives on risk management. Interview data, obtained from the studies presented in Part Two of this book, suggests that professional training makes little difference to those personally involved with a health problem. One learning difficulties professional (Chapter 9) said that his expertise 'went out of the window' when he was trying not to overprotect his own son, who had learning difficulties. A student nurse (Chapter 13) described her fear of becoming infected from drinking tea while visiting the home of an AIDS patient, even though she knew 'that AIDS cannot be caught on the contact that I would be having with him'. A pregnant midwife (Chapter 7), was determined not to 'hear' about risks with which she dealt professionally. The quotation below suggests a partition between her expert and personal selves.

> Some people tell me about awful things when they hear you are pregnant ... And I say, well you try and tell me anything that I haven't seen as a midwife. But, nevertheless, I don't want to hear about it.

Another midwife had, prior to her pregnancy, wanted to do everything 'by the book', but became a 'non-complier'. She did not consider it necessary to attend the clinic because she felt so well, and believed that her body 'told' her what to do. In contrast, a third midwife, having her first child at the age of 31, said:

> Whether you are a midwife or not, you do feel vulnerable, so I put my boots back on [when instructed] like a good girl.

Some differences between the pregnant midwives and other expectant mothers were found. The midwives were more likely to worry about the risk of a stillbirth, while this possibility was rarely mentioned by the other women. Professionals did not, in general, discuss this risk with pregnant women because they believed they could not prevent it, and did not wish to cause unnecessary alarm. (One doctor did inform women who smoked during pregnancy that their habit increased the risk of a stillbirth.) But the rate of stillbirths, around 5 per 1000 (Silverton, 1993, p. 43) compares very closely with the overall rate of genetic abnormalities (Davidson and Rakusen, 1982, p. 75).

Midwives, unlike other pregnant women, could use informal contacts with colleagues in order to gain information and reassurance, and may have been treated differently because of their profession. In consequence, their pregnancies involved less of a journey to the other side than might otherwise have been expected. The midwife quoted below felt that she had learnt most about what it meant to be a patient during a brief incognito period. She may be considered as a modern version of such Shakespearean figures as, Henry V and Duke Vincentio in *Measure for Measure*, who wandered about disguised as ordinary people in order to investigate their subjects' real feelings about their reign.

> And that was the second occasion where I'd felt as if I was being treated like a paranoid midwife. But what worried me was the first 10 minutes, when I asked about the blood pressure and everything. They didn't know I was a midwife. I was an ordinary client asking what my blood pressure was, and I expected a straight answer, and I was really disappointed.

Nevertheless, some midwives found being on the receiving end illuminating.

> I feel that I have got more information [to give pregnant women as a midwife] from going through it myself ... I would stress more the dilemma of, like, the decision [about genetic testing] ... And, also, if you are against terminating the baby, then there is no point in having the bloods [serum-screening] done in the first place ... Not putting them through the trauma of having things done like that ... and the decisions you need to make.

The above quotation picks up the shortcomings of a purely nomothetic, 'evidence-based' approach to clinical decision-making involving dilemmas, the main theme of this chapter. This midwife had grasped through personal experience a point which her socialisation had, perhaps, obscured: that tests may serve little purpose if the client has clearly ruled out acting on their results.

One midwife, who felt, unlike the above, that the experience of giving birth had not changed her professional approach, expressed unusually critical opinions about women in labour:

> I would say I am absolutely no different because I have always been sympathetic with pain [in labour]. Looking after pregnant women, I get quite irritated when they start fighting or saying, 'I want it out' ... What really annoys me are scan defaulters. Yes, because I think, 'What a waste,' and, 'How can they not want to see the baby?'

This untypical example suggests the hypothesis that not experiencing a journey to the other side may be associated with a less questioning approach towards a form of expertise, and a more negative attitude towards service-users who do not comply with its demands.

Data presented in Chapter 7 will point up a possible discrepancy between health professionals' personal attitudes towards genetic testing and their advice to patients. Among 19 consultants, registrars and midwives whose views were assessed for our research, only three would accept, or would have accepted, serum-screening for their own baby. Hence, they almost universally rejected, for themselves, one of the main options which they gave to pregnant women. According to our questionnaire survey of 1000 women using the hospital-maternity service, serum-screening was taken up by about half of those to whom genetic testing was offered. Medical staff may see serum-screening as cost-effectively reducing the population prevalence of Down's syndrome, but resist using it personally because they know about the inaccuracy of positive results (see Chapter 7).

Professionals who became users of their own services frequently encountered complications in family negotiations which involved both their expertise and close personal relationships. One midwife felt that her husband had left the decision about genetic testing to her because of her presumed expertise.

> [Husband] left everything to me because, as he said, I'm a midwife, I probably know more about the statistics than him.

However, she put down her decision-making about testing to 'just instinct' and said that she had not wanted to look at the statistics on the age-related risk of Down's syndrome at the time of her pregnancy. This example illustrates the way in which individuals may avoid the probability heuristic. By relying on intuition, the respondent avoided placing herself in a risk category (e.g. that of older women) or needing to simplify the complexities of probabilistic reasoning. The price which she paid was loss of the fingerhold on the future which such categorisation could have provided. Another midwife explained her husband's deference to her expertise in terms of gender politics.

> He probably thinks that I knew what I was talking about [with respect to genetic testing], and leave it up to me, sort of thing, which I think that men do a little bit, don't they? They don't want to make hard decisions.

In contrast to the midwives, whose husbands respected their expertise, perhaps as an excuse for decision-defaulting, a man who worked with people with learning difficulties felt that his wife did not share his ideas about providing a stimulating environment and accepting risk. This conflict of perspectives had led to considerable family tension, limiting his ability to apply a professional, risk-tolerant approach to bringing up his own child.

> I said, 'People who aren't disabled get knocked down,' but that means you're deliberately putting him in a situation where he is at risk. I said, 'Well, you know, even people who are not deliberately put into a situation get knocked down,' but that leads to an argument [with wife].

## FORMS OF EXPERT STATUS

In order to work together, professionals and service-users have to negotiate the status and extent of each other's expertise. Their relationship may take a number of different transactional states, including reciprocity of perspectives, open conflict, or public compliance combined with private disagreement (Heyman, 1995a, pp. 16–17).

Three ideal types of claim to expert status, 'undelimited', 'liberal' and 'reflecting team', can be differentiated. A particular claim may be more or less shared by professionals and clients. For example, as will be illustrated below, clients may reject the expert's undelimited claim to be able to make decisions on their behalf, or may try to guess the real views of a liberal expert who is striving to empower them.

## The undelimited claim to expertise

The health professional who makes an undelimited claim to expertise feels able to give clients concrete behavioural advice, for example about genetic testing, sexual behaviour, or managing risks faced by vulnerable people. Such claims will 'work', in the sense of being accepted by both professionals and service-users as the taken-for-granted basis of their transactions, in so far as both parties see themselves as sharing the same therapeutic aims, and place confidence in the skills and knowledge which the professionals apply to achieving those aims. For example, Silverman (1987, pp. 24–8) found that many parents of very sick children were eager to follow the consultant's advice. The notion of medical dominance (Foucault, 1973) gives a misleading picture of professional–client relationships where both parties see knowledge as asymmetrical, and view each other as strongly motivated to achieve the same objective.

Any communication problems within professional–client relationships based on acceptance of the professional's undelimited claim to expertise will arise from their consensual foundations, and will involve the expert keeping clients thoroughly informed, discussing their anxieties, and being receptive to potentially relevant clinical information which they can provide. Although this latter form of communication might be seen as opening the door to client expertise, it can be compared to that which typically took place between Sherlock Holmes and a falsely accused client. The suspected client is enjoined to give as much precise, detailed information as possible, and to avoid interpretation. But only Holmes can see its significance. Dr Watson's bungling leaps to wrong conclusions serve only to reinforce the master detective's undelimited claim to expertise.

This model of expertise will tend to break down when professionals and clients contest therapeutic aims. There have been bitter legal disputes concerning the right to treatment of very sick children, as in the case of Jaymee Bowen, and equally intense disputes concerning the right of severely disabled children to die, as with Thomas Creedon, both previously discussed. Many people dismiss health-educators as 'health fascists' for their diatribes on smoking, fatty foods, exercise and the like. In such contests, questions of 'fact', involving the shaky ground of future prediction, inevitably become confounded with issues of value.

When clients do challenge an undelimited claim to professional expertise, overt or covert conflict can be expected since this form of expertise illegitimises lay challenges to its authority. A junior doctor told one older pregnant woman who participated in our research that she had to see the consultant before leaving the hospital because she refused genetic testing. After a lengthy wait, and developing a migraine, the consultant responded '*very sen-* *sible*' to her expressed wish not to have the test, thus illustrating the liberal position, outlined below.

The undelimited claim to expertise is undermined by evidence of expert inconsistency. Woody Allen's fantasy, in the film *Sleeper*, of waking up in a future time period and being instructed to smoke on medical grounds, may reflect wishful thinking, but illustrates the subversive effect of being exposed to conflicting but undelimited expertise. The editor's own faith in dentistry has never recovered from the shock of being informed, by a new dentist, that he was wearing his gums out, and that he could not grow new ones. For 25 years he had enthusiastically obeyed a previous dentist's instructions to brush his gums vigorously.

In a consumerist age, professionals who make undelimited claims to expertise risk facing empty waiting-rooms. One of the critical incidents discussed in Chapter 13 involved a woman who dismissed health concerns about smoking in pregnancy as '*a fad*' which would '*blow over*'. The nurse had felt unable to '*push*' the issues for fear of jeopardising her relationship with the patient.

Those who feel railroaded will simply reject professionals' orders. For example, as already noted, some family carers of adults with learning difficulties (see Chapter 9) resented pressure, as they saw it, for their relative to take additional risks. They also questioned the professional agendas underlying such advice-giving. One respondent, quoted in Chapter 9, feared that her child risked becoming caught up in the machinery of experimentation. The following extracts bring out another respondent's sense of an erosion of trust in expertise, through the contrast which he makes between a 'vocation' and a 'job'. Ironically, modern emphasis on 'evidence-based' practice in nursing and other professions may have contributed to this erosion by minimising the emotional and ethical aspects of care, traditionally encapsulated in the notion, however mythical, of vocation.

> I see them [professionals providing day services for adults with learning difficulties] to a large extent doing a job where I would like to see there is a vocation. If it was a vocational thing on their part, which is a strange word these days, then you could collaborate in a much more co-operative fashion ... Then [when staff change], you really are exposed to risk because you don't know what is happening. That is what worries me. You have got them [relative with learning difficulties] for life. For the person who is doing the job, it is only a stepping-stone in a career.

A number of the teenage girls, whose views are discussed in Chapter 6, had experienced negative attitudes towards their pregnancies. One girl's GP had told her that her youth meant that she was at high risk of losing the baby. However, when she refused to have an abortion, his attitude changed, and he told her that the risks were usually similar for everyone. The perception that professionals' use of risk propositions was biased by their moral disapproval of teenage pregnancy corroded these young women's faith in medical expertise.

Even when clients do feel that a professional's values conflict with their own, they may attempt to manipulate the professional in order to achieve their own ends, rather than resort to confrontation, an example of a process which Clarke (1995b) has described as 'interfacing'. One woman caring for a husband with dementia (see Chapter 11) minimised the severity of his symptoms in order to ensure that he was not taken into care. Presumably, she either felt powerless to prevent the professionals from taking the decision for her, or preferred to avoid a confrontation.

## The liberal claim to expertise

Many health professionals have responded to late modern scepticism about expertise by adopting a liberal stance. Patients, according to this model of expertise, are offered therapeutic choices, and the onus is placed on them to select from the options offered. Each choice should be presented objectively in terms of scientific knowledge about the balance of advantages and disadvantages. As one of the pregnant girls whose views are discussed in Chapter 6 said, *'they should tell and let you know everything, but I don't think they should advise you'*. A registrar, whose genetic-counselling session was recorded for the research discussed in Chapter 7, perhaps reacting to the tape-recorder, informed a pregnant woman nine times, during a 15-minute genetic-counselling session, that decisions about genetic testing were up to her, and mentioned the disadvantages associated with the various options on six separate occasions.

The liberal version of expertise gives rise to several problems. Health professionals must, inevitably, have their own private opinions both on clinical and wider social issues, for example with respect to abortion, sexual morality, disability and the optimum ages at which to have a baby. Presenting an unbiased view is notoriously difficult. Professionals who try to give both sides of the case risk being accused of covertly influencing client decisions.

A registrar, interviewed for our maternity research, who personally opposed abortion on religious grounds, responded to the implicit accusation of bias as follows:

> I do think that I am fair, non-judgemental, in giving my information, my facts. And, if I am asked direct questions, I state where I stand. And I don't think that I give biased information.

Meanwhile, the processes underlying the selection of the set of choices which health professionals offer to clients themselves lie unexamined in the background. Bailey (1996) argues that the very offer of genetic testing, and of termination as a 'treatment' for Down's syndrome legitimates abortion. Doctors do not offer infanticide, normal in many cultures, including Classical Greece and Rome, as a therapeutic option for babies with serious genetic abnormalities.

A liberal approach to expertise requires the professional to adopt a neutral stance towards available options for dealing with the future. But clients may suspect that the professional does have an opinion which they attempt to guess from more subtle clues. As one of the older pregnant women whose views are discussed in Chapter 7 put it:

> They didn't try to push me into having the test [amniocentesis] or vice versa. But just by the way they were speaking, I think they were more or less telling me not to have it.

Shiloh and Saxe (1989) found a positive correlation, with medically assessed risk controlled for, between parental assessments of the risk of their baby having a genetic abnormality and their ratings of genetic counsellor neutrality. Conversely, a woman receiving adjuvant therapy for breast cancer (Cowley, 1996, p. 131) interpreted her doctor's laconic approach to information-giving as a reassuring sign:

> *He was so matter of fact about it you know ... I was prepared for him sort of giving some nasty details, and the fact that he didn't, I thought, 'Oh well, I must be alright.'*

The liberal approach to expertise can thus lead to a guessing game in which neutrality is, variously, interpreted as either good news or the withholding of bad news.

## The reflecting team claim to expertise

The above analysis suggests that contemporary experts can sometimes find themselves in a 'no win' situation. Undelimited claims to expertise may provoke accusations of health fascism, while liberal claims are deconstructed to uncover implicit professional oppression, or lead to guessing games about the professional's 'real' opinion. Faced with this trap, professionals often display contradictory or shifting attitudes towards their own claims to expertise.

Silverman (1987, pp. 146-8) observed that consultants acted prescriptively with the parents of most children who were candidates for open-heart surgery, but adopted a liberal stance if a child had Down's syndrome, stressing parental choice, and the relevance of wider quality-of-life issues to medical decisions. This comparison suggests that medical staff implicitly gave less value to the life of a child with Down's syndrome. Ironically, 'demedicalisation' and parental empowerment were founded on a discriminatory attitude.

The reflecting team approach to expertise, as developed in family therapy, provides a possible way out of the impasse of expertise (Andersen, 1987; Stevenson, 1995). This approach is based on the idea that both professionals and clients bring different forms of expertise and values into therapeutic encounters. Therapy involves exchanges of information in which both professionals and clients can learn from each other. Open acknowledgement of the importance of the learning pathway from clients to experts is excluded from both the undelimited claim to expertise ('I know how to manage your future') and the liberal alternative ('I will spell out the options'). As applied to family therapy, the reflecting team approach (Andersen, 1987, p. 415) involves some members of the team watching family therapy from behind a one-way screen, discussing what has happened within the team, and then discussing this discussion with the family. The underlying epistemology is elegantly summarised by Andersen (1987, p. 416):

> *Because persons experiencing the same world 'out there' make different pictures of it, problems will emerge when they debate which picture is right: **either** mine **or** yours.*

Our acknowledgement of the recognition of learning pathways from clients to professionals in the reflecting team approach to family therapy should not be taken as an endorsement of its therapeutic value, about which the authors of this chapter lack expert knowledge.

Because the undelimited and liberal claims to expertise do not legitimate a learning pathway from clients to health professionals, the impact of client inputs on expert judgements tends to be unacknowledged, as illustrated by the following examples. Fielding and Evered (1980) found, using a vignette describing a patient with ambiguous symptoms, that medical students were more likely to judge the patient to be suffering from heart disease if told that he had a working-class background, and to diagnose his problem as psychological if his purported origin was middle class. The researchers argued that doctors make implicit assumptions about the acceptability of the diagnosis to the patient, and anticipate greater reluctance on the part of working-class patients to accept a psychological diagnosis. This assumption may reflect overall social class differences in attitude to psychological explanations of health problems (Blair, 1993). Similarly, the greater willingness of less-educated women to accept hysterectomies may explain their greater 'risk' of being told that they need the operation, and of receiving it (Santow, 1995).

Handyside's (1995) evaluation of new services for HIV-positive people in a rural area of the north of England illustrates the potential for professional experts to openly acknowledge learning pathways from clients to themselves. At the time of the study, in 1992, the area had a low HIV prevalence, and special services were only beginning to be developed. One consultant, from an unrelated speciality, came to be known as the local 'expert', but, in the interview, reported his own feelings of inadequacy. He felt that he acquired much of his information from patients:

> *HIV people are very well informed, and I can learn from them.*

He believed in expressing his own opinion overtly, and saw the issue of professional power as involving more than giving patients options, as in the liberal approach to expertise.

> *All treatment is discussed and negotiated with patients. I give them options, and tell them what I believe, but many will defer and say that you know best.*

He adopted an active strategy of trying to overcome the power difference between himself and patients.

> *When patients are ill, they are less objective about what you are saying. They just want you to get them better ... I consciously try not to let the power image get in the way. I don't pretend to the patient that I'm an expert.*

The consultant's openness to lay knowledge, and to the stickiness of professional power, were perhaps associated with his lack of formal training, the newness of HIV/AIDS as a health problem, and the gap he saw between his knowledge and the expert status which the outside world ascribed to him. This example suggests the hypothesis that the more socially entrenched is a form of expert status, as indicated, for example, by well-established training and a long tradition of practice, the less awareness experts will show of the implicit assumptions and value judgements on which their stock of knowledge is based. Strong forms of accreditation of expertise, as in the case of medicine, have tended to turn learning pathways from clients to experts into forbidden, unacknowledged territory. Epstein (1995) has argued that, in the

USA, the traditional boundary between lay and professional knowledge has been breached in the case of AIDS, although primarily through the colonisation of lay activists into medical culture. Forms of management of new diseases, unencumbered by history, reflect most accurately the ambivalence towards expertise which characterises the late modern age.

## THE ACCREDITATION OF EXPERTISE

### Expert status and individual competence

In deciding how much trust to place in the professionals on whom they depend, service-users have to make two different types of decision. One concerns the credibility of particular forms of expertise. The second involves questions about the competence of specific individuals or organisations. Well-publicised horror stories about negligent, unskilled or even murderous professionals, and about organisations which conceal poor practice, have heightened general concern about expert variability.

The television programme *Dispatches* (Channel 4, 27/03/96) discussed the case of a hospital in which 9 out of 13 babies given an arterial switch operation died, despite a national death rate of only 10 per cent. Reluctant to admit to problems, the Trust involved had continued with the operations despite warnings, including one from the Department of Health. When a new surgeon was appointed, the mortality rate dropped below the national average. One mother stated that the previous consultant had predicted a survival chance of 50 per cent for her baby at one session, and 67 per cent at the next. When asked why the odds had changed, he had replied '*I'm feeling optimistic today.*' Numbers, however spurious, carry great power in science-oriented cultures, but their aura of precision can undo those who shield behind them.

In an era in which professional status is no longer taken as an automatic indicator of competence and probity, professionals have to work to establish their credibility. As one registrar, interviewed for our research, said, in a pre-natal genetic counselling session:

> I know that I have never lost a baby with amniocentesis ... the people here doing them are well past the early learning curve.

This message was regularly echoed back by women in research interviews, suggesting that they sought indicators of professional competence:

> That [using a small number of surgeons] must help to lower the risk because they really are experts.

### Personal experience as a form of expert credential

Transactions such as those discussed above symbolically define an expert's individual credentials. However, risk management involves more than purely technical expertise, which does not indicate wisdom. Some of the women discussed in Chapter 7 drew on the doctor's personal characteristics for quality assurance:

*Well, I took the reassurance from the female doctor. I mean, she's a mother herself, and I have got faith in her.*

Professionals sometimes used themselves as exemplars in order to inspire confidence. A nurse whose child had suffered brain damage after a vaccination had moved into work with people with learning difficulties. She had found the period after this disaster traumatic, but felt that, because she and her husband had eventually coped, she could reassure others in the same situation:

*But I mean, the families [who have a child with learning difficulties] now, you just see so much of what you went through over and over again. And it's just a lovely feeling to let them know that I'm not just saying, 'I know what you mean.' I actually went through it and felt it.*

In contrast, a nurse supporting women with gynaecological cancers who had, herself, recently had a gynaecological tumour removed, reported (personal communication) that she did not feel able to share her experiences with patients, even though the tumour had turned out to be non-malignant. Professionals may feel more or less comfortable in drawing on their own experience in their work. These feelings will depend, in part, on the location of cultural and personal boundaries between private and public lives.

Examples of professionals utilising direct experience of health problems represent special cases of a more general process of synthesising expert knowledge and personal experience. For example, a staff nurse, quoted in Chapter 11, felt that knowing persons with dementia *'like your own mother or father'* helped her to understand them better. Whether or not professionals can realistically develop such personal knowledge on the basis of brief visits, the quotation does illustrate the way in which they attempt to draw on a wider cultural knowledge base. Similarly, personally trusted non-professionals who have experienced a health problem may be given the status of honorary expert. One diabetic woman, quoted in Chapter 8, went to a neighbour whom she regarded as a *'mother figure'* for practical advice because the latter's son had diabetes.

Service-users themselves may strive to obtain advice which combines personal wisdom with professional expertise. A pregnant woman, whose genetic-counselling session was taped for the research discussed in Chapter 7, asked the doctor, perhaps with a hint of desperation:

*In your personal or your professional opinion, what would you do [about genetic testing] if you were in my shoes?*

Professionals would not call on personal sources of quality assurance if they did not implicitly recognise both the limits of, and the need to sell, their expertise. Conversely, people with health problems and their family carers lack professional expertise, but can offer personal commitment and detailed idiographic knowledge. Signs that the professional does not support family carers' commitment can lead to instant rejection. For example, a wife caring for her husband, who had dementia, quoted in Chapter 11, had immediately decided that she *'didn't like'* her GP for suggesting that she *'have him put away'*. Her use of this phrase conveys anger at the professional's dehumanising disrespect for a person she loved.

Lay people managing personal health needs attempt to fine tune 'treatment' by drawing on detailed individual knowledge. For example, some of the diabetic patients, discussed in Chapter 8, tried to regulate their insulin levels by drawing on the personal experience of their own responses. One patient adjusted his insulin level to accommodate his expected eating patterns when going out socially. Another felt that she had learnt, through observing her own reactions, how much of a dangerous food, such as chocolate, she could eat. The daughter of a woman with dementia, quoted in Chapter 11, varied her mother's meals on the basis of detailed circumstantial knowledge *'according to how her bowels are, etc.'*. The emphasis which lay people put on the individual case may be contrasted with the current official emphasis on evidenced-based medical practice which can only deal in averages.

## Conclusion

This chapter has analysed the role of values in health-risk management, with reference both to studies presented later in the book, and to published research. Individuals, depending on their underlying values, the consequences which they choose to consider, and the ways in which they combine analytical elements, can value the same class of actions quite differently. Value differences come to the foreground particularly strongly when health decisions entail dilemmas, and valued ends have to be traded against each other. Such dilemmas, numerous examples of which will be considered in Parts Two and Three, can be expected whenever a health problem cannot be prevented or cured without significant cost. In situations of value conflict, service-users need to make their own, difficult decisions.

However, organisationally driven agendas may lead professionals to attempt to constrain client choices, through overt or more subtle means. The outcomes of health transactions will depend on the kind of expert authority which professionals claim, and the ways in which these are received by service-users. We have argued that the prevailing 'undelimited' and 'liberal' professional approaches to expertise are fraught with difficulty. Undelimited claims are rejected in a late modern, sceptical culture as soon as they challenge clients' values. Liberal claims lay professionals open to accusations of bias, and may generate guessing-games in which the client tries to infer the professional's 'real' attitude. Many clients, when faced with difficult human dilemmas, appear to crave expertise which combines technical risk knowledge with wisdom. If professionals are to begin to offer such a synthesis, they will need to reconsider the exclusivity of their expertise, and to openly acknowledge learning pathways from clients to professionals. The prevailing idea of evidence-based practice may need to be synthesised with the traditional notion of vocation if professional credibility is to be sustained in the late modern era.

This chapter has focused on the problems of defining and negotiating health values. As will be shown in Chapter 2, lay people may also understand probabilities in different ways, and may draw on non-probabilistic forms of rationality based on fatalism, divine justice or hedonism. The scene is set for misunderstandings between health professionals and lay people, particularly if the professionals, struggling to process masses of service-users within complex organisational contexts, believe their scientific expertise gives them privileged access to uniquely correct answers to problems of health cost-benefit analysis.

# Probability and health risks

Bob Heyman and Mette Henriksen

*Life is a gamble at terrible odds – if it was a bet you wouldn't take it.*
Stoppard, T. *(1968) Rosencrantz and Guildenstern are Dead,* Act III.

## Introduction

Having explored values in Chapter 1, we examine probability, the second analytical element in risk, in this chapter. In order to understand how professionals and lay people approach and manage health risks, we need to investigate and compare the ways in which they conceptualise and communicate about probabilities.

The availability of complex mathematical and statistical resources for the description of probabilities obscures confusion about the phenomena which the numbers refer to (Gigerenzer *et al.*, 1990), for example about whether probability statements refer to subjective uncertainty, or to the expected frequency of events. This chapter will probe this confusion, and explore its influence on the practical detail of health care.

Although we think of probabilities, and so risks, as natural, taken-for-granted phenomena, historians tell us that our modern machinery for thinking about probability was invented relatively recently. We consider briefly the modern history of the construct of probability. The difficulties associated with the externalisation of uncertainty on to probability will next be discussed. Probabilistic reasoning, reduced in status to one of many modes of relating to the future, will then be contrasted with personalistic, fatalistic and hedonistic alternatives. The chapter next explores the impact of the complexities of probabilistic reasoning on health-risk management. We consider the representation of probability in professional/lay communication; the ways in which conditional probabilities can be used tactically to manipulate risk acceptability through the differentiation and generalisation of aggregate statistics; and, finally, the management of reflexive recursion, processes in which the probabilities of health outcomes are affected by thinking about them.

## The history of probability

### ORIGINS OF THE TERM 'PROBABLE'

An historical perspective provides a valuable corrective to the view that probability refers to a natural property of the world, rather than to one way of understanding it.

The meaning of the term 'probable' has shifted qualitatively between medieval and modern times (Hacking, 1975, p. 1). In the Middle Ages, probable meant 'likely to be true' and this, in turn, meant 'supported by authorities'. The following quotation from Gibbon's eighteenth-century *Decline and Fall of the Roman Empire*, which seems nonsensical from our modern standpoint, illustrates the shift in meaning which has taken place:

> *Such a fact is probable but undoubtedly false.* (Gibbon, cited in Hacking, 1975, p. 19)

Hacking argues that medieval scholars relied on the opinion of authorities because they did not distinguish, in the way that modern scientists would, between signs and what they signified. For example, Paracelsus (1493–1591) knew that mercury in the right dose would cure syphilis, even though his colleagues were killing patients with incorrect doses, because syphilis was associated with the marketplace where it was caught, the planet Mercury was associated with the marketplace, and the chemical mercury bore the same name. A modern critic would feel that Paracelsus was confusing properties of the names of things with properties of the things themselves, and that his thinking was affected by the nominalist fallacy. In the above example, Paracelsus attributes medicinal properties to mercury because of its verbal association with syphilis.

Paracelsus believed that nature indicated the age of a stag by the ends of its antlers, and the influence of the stars by their names. Medieval thinkers did not distinguish signifiers and signified because they saw nature as a book written by God (Hacking, 1975, p. 42). The attempt to separate subject and object, observer and observed, became a defining characteristic of the science-based, modern Western, mode of thought which began to emerge at the end of the seventeenth century.

## THE MODERN CONCEPT OF PROBABILITY

According to Hacking (1975), the development of the modern concept of probability depended on a number of related shifts in the ways in which the world was understood. Its behaviour came to be seen as determined by natural laws, rather than as a story written by God. Internal evidence, from things themselves, was differentiated from external evidence, from authorities such as the Church. Induction (deriving conclusions from observation) became an important source of knowledge, not least in medicine. Although seventeenth-century thinkers such as Descartes wanted to connect religious and scientific knowledge, they initiated a process which, in most Western cultures, led to the former's long-term decline.

Historians agree that formal theorising about probability emerged quite suddenly in the Western world in the second half of the seventeenth century (Covello and Mumpower, 1985; Hacking, 1990), even though evidence of interest in odds and gambling, such as dice games, has been frequently found in the Ancient world. There is less agreement about why formal theorising did not occur earlier and about why it suddenly appeared at this time.

Hacking (1975) argues that the weakening of the power of the Church allowed its authority as the source of truth to be challenged. At the same time, as internal (empirical) evidence accumulated alongside external evidence (from authorities), the former gradually accumulated strength, and was differentiated from the latter. This process was mainly associated with developments in 'low' sciences, particularly medicine, which had to rely on induction (e.g. trying out remedies) rather than 'high' sciences such as astronomy which were able to develop mathematical laws. Bernstein (1996) suggests that the clumsy numbering systems used in the Classical world, and the lack of a zero, impeded numerical calculation: an interesting example of the dependence of thought on its symbolic representation. Arab texts, from the ninth century AD, discussed mathematical operations involving the modern number system. But, Bernstein argues (1996, p. xxxv), they did not explore probability because they believed, fatalistically, that the future was determined. Whatever the reasons, a concern with the nature of probability and risk emerged as a defining feature of the modern Western world, bound up with the associated developments of science, trade and capitalism.

Some historical imagination is needed to visualise a world view which did not take for granted our modern axioms about probability. For example, odds and pay-offs even in a simple game of dice could not be calculated before about 1650. The 'law of averages' was unknown because the mathematical average had not been invented.

Annuities were an important source of government revenue in the seventeenth and eighteenth centuries. But no British government before the end of this period thought to take account of the age of the person seeking an annuity in calculating a fair cost. Practitioners of risk, for example those selling insurance or annuities, resisted using newly developed statistical methods because they believed that each case had to be considered holistically and individually. For instance, a younger person in poor health might die before an older but fitter one (Gigerenzer *et al.*, 1990, p. 26).

The law of averages permeates our modern decision-making so much that we have difficulty imagining a world without it. Knowledge of average accident rates may persuade us to travel by aeroplane, and not to drive after drinking large amounts of alcohol, against the evidence of our senses in both cases. We can understand the relationship between unprotected penetrative sex and the risk of HIV, even though, in the majority of cases, infection does not result. Scientists in the USA are trying to persuade men not to have dangerous and expensive penis-enlarging operations by demonstrating that the average size of the erect penis is popularly exaggerated (Mestel, 1995). The law of averages even provides a counterweight against the well-known case of Auntie Nellie who lived to a ripe old age despite smoking, drinking, being overweight and never exercising, since averages apply to groups, not to individuals.

Although the law of averages is frequently misunderstood, such errors could not occur before the average was invented. A health policy academic colleague from North Karelia, Finland, predicted high summer temperatures for his chilly region, on the fallacious predictive grounds that they would bring the yearly temperature up to its normal average, following a cold spring. While in a 'brown café' in Amsterdam, the editor overheard some American (male) doctors discussing the risk of HIV infection from unprotected sex. One doctor stated that the risk of a man contracting HIV from unprotected sex with an infected woman was about 1 in 200. He interpreted this statistic as meaning that a man would have to have sex 200 times with infected women in order to catch HIV, and, by implication, that the first 199 episodes would not lead to infection. A midwife married to a university researcher (see Chapter 7) cited an exact, unrounded probability of older women like herself conceiving a fetus with Down's syndrome. She reasoned that her personal risk had to be less because relatively few older women became pregnant.

Rapp (1993, p. 188) notes that educated, middle-class pregnant women frequently *'fight with numbers'*, supporting a personal position on genetic testing with idiosyncratic statistical interpretations. However, fighting with numbers, without a statistical veneer, can also be observed among the less educated. A teenage girl who had conceived unintentionally (see Chapter 6) defended the safety of withdrawal as a contraceptive method on the grounds that *'not much goes inside you'*, overlooking the redundancy built into the reproductive system. These examples show how easily mistakes in reasoning about probability can be made. The HIV example illustrates the way in which social values influence the delineation of risk, a theme taken up below, since the probability of women being infected by men did not enter the discussion. However, such mistakes and value influences could not have arisen before the average became a taken-for-granted foundation of Western explanatory thinking.

## THE TESTIMONY OF PEOPLE IN MODERN PROBABILISTIC THINKING

It is tempting to regard the modern development of probabilistic thinking as simply a form of progress. Hacking (1975) expresses some disdain for the medieval, non-probabilistic thinking which he reconstructs so vividly. From a modern perspective, thinkers in medieval times seem overly reliant on evidence from authorities, and unable to distinguish between the external testimony of people and internal evidence from things. However, the technical–rational view of risk as something to be discovered and measured through the rigorous application of scientific methods has been widely questioned (Douglas, 1990).

The testimony of people is often embedded covertly in the assumptions on which probability statements are predicated, but sometimes becomes blatant. In the 1980s, British television viewers were treated to the sight of a Conservative government minister demonstrating the safety of sea water containing untreated sewage by paddling in it. Another minister, notoriously, tried to counteract the BSE scare by feeding his child a beefburger on television in order to 'prove' the safety of British beef. In the summer of 1995, a French general swam in a lagoon above the site of underground nuclear tests to demonstrate its safety. Although farcically counterproductive as public relations exercises, such displays tell us much about the medieval thinking of those in authority: namely that if a powerful person testifies to the safety of a suspected hazard, ordinary mortals will be reassured.

Knowledge about the natural world, and power to change it for better or worse, have progressed enormously since the medieval period. Underpinning this progress has been a mode of thought which attempts to split the observer from the observed in order to minimise the influence of the former. Although the attempted removal of the observer has proved impossible at the quantum level, modern, science-based cultures have valued objective over subjective knowledge of the larger-scale world. External evidence 'from things' is considered to be superior to internal evidence from the testimony of people. However, as Fischoff, Watson and Hope (1984, p. 124) argue:

> Along with these elements of objectivity in public opinion, there are inevitably elements of subjectivity in expert estimates of risk. Within the philosophy of science, 'objective' … typically means something akin to 'independent of observer' … However meritorious as a goal, this sort of objectivity can never be achieved.

The section that follows will attempt to demonstrate that the observer can never be removed from probability judgements.

## Probability, chance and uncertainty

### THE DUALISTIC CONCEPT OF PROBABILITY

Probability texts frequently claim, often in passing, that probability can arise from two sources: the randomness of events in the world, and ignorance. On this view, someone who chooses heads or tails has a 0.5 probability of being correct because of the inherent randomness of tossed coins. On the other hand, a person who loses their way and chooses to turn left or right has a 0.5 probability of going in the right direction because of their lack of knowledge.

Hacking (1975, p. 1) argues that the modern idea of probability which emerged around 1660 had two forms. It referred to the degree of belief warranted by evidence ('epistemic' probability) and the tendency of some chance devices to produce stable but irregularly sequenced relative frequencies ('aleatory' probability). Although Hacking mainly uses dice throws to illustrate the latter, he also refers to the probability of a person dying in a particular year (p. 123) as an example of aleatory probability. Field *et al.* (1994, p. 3) convey a similar dualistic notion with respect to uncertainty about illness when they assert that '*Uncertainty itself may be influenced by both the ambiguity and the complexity of the situation.*' Hood *et al.* (1992, p. 96), in their contribution to the Royal Society *Risk* report also promote the dualistic notion of probability. They cite Vesley and Rasmuson's (1984) distinction between 'physical' and 'knowledge' uncertainty and that of Blockley (1980) between 'parametric' (stochastic and measurement) and 'systemic' (risk model) uncertainties. Similarly, Casti (1992, p. 23) states that '*Roughly speaking, we can identify two main sources of the uncertainty we want to banish from our everyday lives: randomness and imprecision.*' As well as reproducing the dualistic version of probability, the last quotation also illustrates the prevailing view, in a science-dominated culture, that people 'naturally' want to reduce uncertainty.

The dualistic view of probability recurs frequently in the literature, but usually without critical examination. It faithfully reproduces that separation between subjective and objective on which so much of Western scientific thought has been based. Uncertainty about the future, from this perspective, may arise out of either the randomness of the world or our lack of knowledge. Gigerenzer *et al.* (1990, p. 8), who do criticise the binary notion of probability, note that classical probability theorists did not distinguish between subjective (cognitive) and objective (frequency) probabilities because the realms of the subjective and the objective were not at that time so sharply differentiated. These authors thus see the distinction between epistemic and aleatory probability as depending upon historically and culturally limited taken-for-granted epistemological assumptions.

To complicate matters still further, first-order uncertainty arising from observed frequencies must be distinguished from second-order uncertainty about these frequencies themselves. For example, the proportions of women of given ages who will carry a fetus with Down's syndrome are empirically well established. But this inductive knowledge leaves expectant mothers uncertain as to the genetic status of their own child. In contrast, the rates for contracting Creutzfeldt-Jacob Diesease (CJD) associated with different patterns of eating British beef during the 1980s cannot yet be inductively estimated because of the lengthy incubation period for the disease. Beef-eaters, thus, face an alarming double uncertainty, both about the risks they were exposed to and about their own individual fates, as did the general population in the early years of the HIV epidemic. Inductive frequencies can usually be estimated more easily for recurring health problems than for rare large-scale events, such as earthquakes and nuclear accidents, on which risk analysis has traditionally focused. However, as noted, second-order uncertainty provides a potent source of heightened alarm with respect to some health risks. Even where inductive frequencies have been clearly established, as in the case of the maternal age-related risk of Down's syndrome, second-order uncertainty, for example about a woman's precise age at conception, cannot be totally eliminated (see the section on *'Communication of probabilities in genetic counselling'* in Chapter 2).

It will be argued below that the apparent duality of probability breaks down on closer analysis. Probability statements entail the projection of uncertainty on to the world. This point will now be established with respect to three distinct sources of uncertainty: pseudo-randomness in complex, but determined systems, our main focus; fundamental randomness at the smallest scale, where quantum effects operate; and enigmas of human intentionality. Unfortunately for those who seek a tidy, quantified world, health processes typically involve combinations of all three types of uncertainty.

## PROBABILITY AND COMPLEXITY

Laplace famously argued, in the late eighteenth century (Hacking, 1975, p. 132), that chance plays no part in determined systems, the behaviour of which can, in theory, be predicted. (Systems which are not assumed to be determined will be considered below.) In practice, the behaviour of real, complex systems of cause and effect cannot be precisely predicted because of the non-linearity of their behaviour (Firth, 1991). In addition, real systems, however their boundaries are specified, cannot be causally isolated. Drastic changes can result from their interactions (e.g. a child panicking at a barking dog, running off a pavement and being knocked down by a car).

Cause–effect systems tend to non-linearity in three interacting ways. First, changes in one variable can affect another disproportionately. For example, moderate alcohol consumption may reduce mortality risk, while higher levels increase it, giving health educators a serious headache (Holman, 1996). Second, the effects of one variable may depend on how it combines with others, leading to statistical interaction effects. For instance, coffee consumption may significantly reduce the increase in risk of liver cirrhosis among heavy drinkers (Corrao *et al.*, 1994). The anti-oxidant beta carotene, found in fruit and vegetables, may protect non-smokers from cancer (although the evidence is inconclusive), but increases the risk for heavy smokers because the smoke converts beta carotene into a carcinogenic substance (Smigel, 1996). Third, multidirectional causal interplay produces complex relationships between initial states of a system and outcomes, through positive and negative feedback. For example, defining a poor pregnant woman as 'high risk', and thus as a problem, may lead to her avoiding maternity care, and so increase the level of risk (Handwerker, 1994). Such processes of reflexive recursion are further discussed below.

The behaviour of non-linear systems depends on combinations of variables. The number of calculations which we would have to make in order to predict the behaviour of such a system increases exponentially as the number of states of components of the system increases. The problem can be compared to the notorious one of attempting to fully analyse a game of chess. If, for simplicity, we assume that each player has 20 possible legal moves, and discount duplicate positions, then there are 20 possible positions one move ahead, 400 positions two moves ahead, 8000 positions three moves ahead, 160 000 positions by the fourth move, and so on. Faced with an unmanageable expansion of combinations, chess-players use simple heuristic rules to guide their decisions, for example attempting to gain a material advantage. However, such rules can only predict outcomes probabilistically, and good players recognise situations in which simple rules do not apply.

By attributing the probability of an outcome in a determined system to chance, we treat it as pseudo-random, accepting that its inherent complexity limits our predictive power. If we were able to predict perfectly, the probability of an event occurring would always be 0 or 1. Probabilities can arise in determined systems only from our ignorance, and are always epistemic (Thompson, 1986). As Winkler (1990, p. 153) puts it, chance and necessity are a 'dialectical couple'.

A thought example will demonstrate this point, and its strange implications. Imagine a town with a population of about 100 000, in which approximately 1500 people died each year. In the absence of additional information, the probability of an individual dying in the next year could be calculated, within a frequentist, inductive framework, as 1.5 per cent. However, we know that older people, men, smokers, those from lower socioeconomic groups and the socially isolated have a reduced average life expectancy. Thus, for instance, the probability of a person who had all the above attributes dying in the next year might be 10 per cent. Hence, a person's chances of dying are affected by how much we know about them!

If we could fully predict each person's age of death, their probability of dying during the year in question would be either 1 or 0. In the absence of such certain knowledge, a data set such as that for the age of death can be grouped in terms of a very large number of combinations of imperfectly predictive variables. Each will generate a different probability of dying in the next year for a given individual. Some groupings will fail empirically because they lack predictive power, for example differentiating groups on the basis of their surname beginning with an odd or an even letter. Some will be supported by theoretically plausible causal explanations, as in the case of the link between smoking and mortality. Nevertheless, faced with a cloudy, tangled spaghetti soup of causation, epidemiologists and other future managers must choose from a potentially huge set of combinations of predictor variables. An individual's 'risk' of a particular adverse outcome will depend upon which sub-group they are located in.

To give another example, a pregnant woman aged 35 may be told that her risk of having a fetus with Down's syndrome is about 1: 200. But, after a serum test, her risk, depending on the result, might double to 1: 100, or be reduced to about 1: 2000 (Cuckle, Wald and Thompson, 1987, p. 393). An individual woman's risk is changed by having the test, although the underlying population risk remains unaltered, and she may use her decision about being tested to control her level of risk (see Chapter 7).

The apparent strangeness of such results arises from a cognitive illusion. Risk statements about pseudo-random, complex systems refer to aggregates, and encode partial knowledge. Cigarette-smoking may dispose individuals towards lung cancer, high cholesterol levels increase the risk of CHD, or depression make people more likely to commit suicide. But most of those in the above high-risk groups will not suffer these consequences. Probabilistic knowledge provides a simplifying heuristic for predicting future states of such systems on the basis of induction from past averages.

Psychological research, discussed in Chapter 5, has investigated lay heuristics for simplifying probability problems. But probability is, itself, a heuristic as argued in the Introduction. Therefore, the devices which lay people draw on to simplify probabilistic reasoning have the epistemological status of heuristics about heuristics. Users of the probability heuristic have to pay a price for their partial, simplified glimpse of the future. They must accept the ecological fallacy: the assumption that individuals within a specified class will display its aggregate characteristics. This notion has become so deeply engrained in Western individualistic thought that it has become difficult to think of risk other than as a property of events. Thought demonstrations that the probability of the same adversity befalling the same person depends on how they are classified shatter the illusion that risk, in its frequentist derivation, appertains to individuals.

## The influence of social stereotypes on the use of the probability heuristic

Any social scientist would expect the specification of risk categories to be influenced by wider cultural attitudes and stereotypes as well as by scientific evidence. For example, Schiller, Crystal and Lewellen (1994) criticise the characterisation of male homosexuality as a risk indicator for HIV infection. At most, sexual orientation provides a crude proxy indicator for risky behaviour which individuals may or may not undertake. The idea of AIDS as a gay plague is explored in relation to risk imagery in Chapter 4. Although causally confused, the notion of a gay plague does have a stochastic basis if male homosexuals are more likely to behave in ways which increase the risk of infection. In the present 'indifference' phase of the epidemic (see Chapter 4; Weeks, 1991), some gay groups, ironically, are promoting themselves as a high-risk group. At a time of declining resources for HIV work, being identified as high risk does generate attention from the health-care system.

Bowler's (1993) work on UK health-professional perceptions of Asian women's birth patterns, discussed in Chapter 3, provides a critical example of the ways in which the risk heuristic and social stereotypes can mutually fuel each other. Bowler found that some midwives thought that Asian women tended to have shorter, easier labours, that they were attention-seeking, and that they had low pain thresholds. However, the belief that Asian women experienced shorter labour probably arose from their aggregate tendency, at this point in their social history, to have larger families, and so, on average, to be of greater parity. Since greater parity is associated with speed of labour, the prediction that Asian women would give birth more quickly was stochastically useful, although causally confused. The belief that they sought attention and could not tolerate pain may have been associated with the background assumption that Asian women underwent easier labour, and, therefore, had less cause for complaint. As shown in Chapter 3, this particular heuristic generated systematic error when a midwife expected an Asian woman delivering her first baby to experience a quick delivery.

It may be objected that midwives who reasoned in this way were simply mistaken, and in need of education. However, risk heuristics are employed, and the ecological fallacy accepted, because of causal and predictive uncertainty. In foggy temporal conditions, individuals will tend to detect the outlines of futures which their cultural background leads them to expect. They can then obtain probabilistic evidence which may support their position. Falsification depends on demonstration of the superiority of an alternative predictive grouping. Established risk heuristics may be difficult to dislodge because they work well enough with populations, and no probabilistic prediction, by definition, can anticipate individual outcomes with perfect accuracy.

## Limitations of the probability heuristic

The probability heuristic enables its users to obtain a view of the future which goes beyond the limits of their present causal knowledge. The price paid is stereotyping of individuals who are deemed to possess the characteristics of the category which the observer has created.

Professionals, attempting to manage risks for populations with limited resources, may respond to the characteristics of risk groupings, and, in consequence, become desensitised to warning signs in individual cases. For example, Scott notes, in Chapter 17, that numerous official inquiries into violent deaths caused by people with severe mental health problems have criticised health and social services for failing to respond to prior warnings given by family carers. Judgements made after an adverse event are influenced by hindsight effects (Chapter 5). Nevertheless, professionals may discount local information which could have enabled them to predict an oncoming disaster. They may attribute the known, low probability of members of the class of people diagnosed as severely mentally ill becoming violent to each individual within that category.

Official representations of risk factors may, in some cases, clearly distort known inductive probabilities for political ends. For example, social scientists frequently point out the tendency of policy-makers, e.g. the authors of *Health of the Nation* (DOH, 1992), and health professionals to talk up lifestyle risk factors deemed within the individual's control, and to ignore wider environmental dangers such as pollution and road traffic (Freeman, 1992; Roberts, Smith and Bryce, 1993). As pointed out in Chapter 16, child-protection agencies have traditionally focused on the family, while ignoring residential care as a source of risk, until confronted by unmistakable evidence of widespread abuse in the latter setting. Reed notes, in Chapter 12, that although elderly people are more likely to experience fatal accidents in residential care than in their own homes, the former are often regarded as a place of safety. Risk-selection processes will be illustrated below through the example of the treatment of maternal age as a risk factor for Down's syndrome.

Officially, the rational scientific approach to decision-making can be contrasted with lay reliance on rules of thumb.

> *The revolutionary idea that defines the boundary between modern times and the past is the mastery of risk: the notion that the future is more than the whim of the gods and that men and women are not passive before nature.* (Bernstein, 1996, p. 1)

A more critical approach compares scientific and lay heuristics concerning the future (Wynne, 1996) in terms of their implicit assumptions. Reframing probability as uncertainty about complexity allows values hidden in numerical probability ratios to be revealed. Observers can alter chance. This apparently magical power stems from a conjuring trick which depends on the culturally ingrained habit of externalising uncertainty.

## The externalisation of uncertainty

Returning to the first example of aleatory and epistemic probability given above, we would normally expect a competent member of our culture to be able to find their way around streets, through asking someone or buying a map. We would not normally expect someone to be able to predict the precise gyrations of a tossed coin, although a robot might well be able to do so (Thompson, 1986). Similarly, the editor's snooker cue ball occasionally ends up in an advantageous position because of luck, while a professional achieves the same position through skill. Players at all levels appreciate only too well the role of 'luck' in chess. Thus, in the dualistic account of probability, epistemic and aleatory probability refer to normatively 'easy' and 'hard' problems. However, what is judged easy or hard depends as much on the cultural beliefs, competencies and confidence, justified or misplaced, of the observer as on the inherent complexity of the problem.

Hacking (1975, p. 133) dismisses this point rather airily by noting that the calculation of probability is unaffected by its status as aleatory or epistemic. In doing so, he illustrates the common tendency, within a science-based culture, to try to solve a conceptual problem by quantifying it. However, for the social scientist interested in the ways in which social actors understand risks, the pseudo-distinction between lack of knowledge and chance raises an important question. Why are risks sometimes projected on to the world and seen as reflections of chance, but at other times reflected back on the perceiver and viewed as descriptions of uncertainty?

The distinction between chance and lack of knowledge turns not only on the complexity, relative to observers' resources, of the future which is being predicted, but, also, on their pragmatic concerns. Descriptions of the chance of something happening are generally intended to downplay ignorance, while accounts of lack of knowledge point attention to the need to learn more. A quantitative description of the chance of an event occurring asserts implicitly that we have learnt all we can about it. This form of description invites us to stop asking questions and to start acting, for example to reduce the amount of saturated fat in our diet, or to avoid unprotected sex with multiple partners.

Middleton and Curnock (1995) showed how consultants on a neonatal intensive care ward used risk discourse, paradoxically, to reduce uncertainty and legitimise their recommendations. One consultant asserted, in response to a query from a nurse manager, that there was '*no question*' that breast-fed babies were '*at greater risk*' of haemorrhagic diseases unless they were given a vitamin K supplement. In contrast, statements of lack of knowledge communicate a need to investigate the problem further. For example, the editor has noticed that applications to his local medical ethics committee to undertake random control trials sometimes use the language of uncertainty. Since the researchers seek to have their applications approved, they need to play-up the scientific community's ignorance.

When a spokesman from the British Dental Association was confronted, on television, with evidence that mercury amalgam from fillings had crossed the placenta (*Panorama*, 11/07/94), he responded that there was '*no evidence*' that mercury was dangerous to the fetus. This lack of evidence led him to conclude that mercury amalgam could be used safely. Ignorance, paradoxically, increased his certainty because it was projected on to the phenomenon in question. His implicit thinking can be glossed as, 'Mercury in the fetus has not been found to produce any dangerous effects. Therefore, it is safe.' The inescapable role of the observer's knowledge, and of decisions about what to investigate, in probability estimates is obscured in such accounts. Conclusions which meet the interests of a particular, powerful, group can be presented as objective, scientific descriptions of the world, rather than as statements about how much is known.

## Levels of predictive uncertainty

Three different levels of predictive uncertainty about the future occurrence of an event can be delineated: second order, first order and conditional. Continuous degrees of uncertainty between these three states can be identified. A fuller discussion of the debates surrounding higher order uncertainty can be found in a special section of the *IEEE Transactions on Systems, Man and Cybernetics* (Lehner, Laskey and Dubois, 1996).

**Second-order predictive uncertainty** occurs when the underlying future incidence of an event is completely unknown. In this limiting case, the 'probability' of the event occurring is 50%. It might or might not occur and we have no way of knowing which destiny, if any, is more likely. As noted in the Introduction, second-order uncertainty entails a double doubt, about the underlying incidence of an event, and about where it will occur (e.g. which individuals will succumb to a disease).

An example discussed by Bernstein (1996, pp. 17–18) illustrates reasoning based on full second-order uncertainty. Under Talmudic law, a man could not divorce his wife for premarital 'adultery' (i.e. sex with another man during the betrothal period). The Talmud justified this ruling through second-order probabilistic reasoning. Given that the bride came to the marital bed no longer a virgin, she might have had premarital sex either with her betrothed or with another man. If she had had sex with another man, it might or might not have involved rape. The Talmud further argued that each of these conditions (premarital sex with her betrothed versus another, and rape versus consent given premarital sex with another) had a 1 in 2 chance of occurring; and that, therefore, the probability that a betrothed woman had committed adultery was only 1 in 4 ($0.5 \times 0.5 = 0.25$), making it most likely (probability 0.75) that she was innocent.

This thinking must be placed in the context of additional devices for managing uncertainty. In Old Testament times (Deuteronomy, Chapter 22, Verses 13–29) a newly married woman accused of non-virginity had to display her bloodied garment to the city elders in order to prove her innocence. A woman could not be convicted of adultery where the sexual act took place in the fields, since she would have had no opportunity to cry out if she was being raped, but could not use the defence of rape in the city unless she could show that she had tried to obtain help. Thankfully, given that adulterers could be stoned to death, the presumption of innocence had been considerably strengthened by the time the Talmud was written (from around 100BC to 500AD).

Modern thinkers, in the unlikely event that they were troubled by the 'risk' of premarital infidelity, would seek to establish the underlying rates of the above events rather than treating them as equally unlikely. Nevertheless, this early example of statistical reasoning does illustrate the implication of second-order uncertainty, that alternative events are equally likely if their underlying incidence is totally unknown. One pregnant woman, interviewed for the research discussed in Chapter 7, reasoned in this way, arguing that her baby either had, or did not have Down's syndrome, and, therefore, that each outcome had a 50 per cent probability of occuring. In effect, she discounted the empirical evidence for specific, age-related frequencies of genetic disorders.

**First-order predictive uncertainty** occurs when the underlying incidence of an event within a population has been estimated through induction from observed frequencies. Such estimates may require an error term because of their limited accuracy. They depend on the assumption, inherent in inductive reasoning and sometimes problematic, that the past provides a sound basis for predicting the future. Therefore, the conceptual space between full second-order uncertainty (incidence unknown) and first-order uncertainty (incidence known) is filled with continuous gradations of doubt.

**Conditional predictive uncertainty** arises when the incidence of an event has been shown to vary within defined subpopulations. For example, the probability of a baby having Down's syndrome can be predicted in terms of its mother's age, an example considered in some detail below. The use of single or multiple conditional predictor variables reduces uncertainty which is transferred to subpopulations in which the estimated probability of an event becomes higher or lower than average. Again, different degrees of conditional predictive uncertainty must be postulated, depending on the extent to which the probability of an event can be more or less finely differentiated within subpopulations.

As argued in the Introduction, some combinations of conditional predictive factors will 'work' better predictively than others. However, an optimum predictive formula can never be unalterably established in conditions of uncertainty. Populations can be subdivided in an indefinitely large number of ways depending on the combination of predictive criteria selected. Many permutations of predictive factors will work well enough, reducing uncertainty to some extent. Their choice will be influenced by cultural, pragmatic and organisational factors. For example, it will be argued below that choice of maternal age as the main risk factor for genetic abnormalities, to the exclusion of others, has the advantage for health-service providers of limiting the number of pregnant women eligible for expensive genetic tests.

Predictive conditional uncertainty must be differentiated from **causal uncertainty.** The value of conditional predictors arises from the glimpses which they provide of the future, not from their causal status. For example, it has been recently shown that companies with better environmental standards earn a higher rate of return for investors. This finding leaves open the causal question of whether better run companies tend to be 'greener' or 'greening' is good for business. But, as fund manager Simon Baker pointed out,*All I need to know is that the companies on our list will show a better return'* (*Guardian* 05/05/97).

## PROBABILITY AND INDETERMINISM

The above discussion of the illusory duality of probability was confined to complex, determined systems. Statements about probabilities in such systems externalise knowledge limitations. We now need to extend the discussion to non-determined systems involving quantum effects and human action. Although these three sources of uncertainty will be differentiated analytically, the prediction of health outcomes requires their combination.

### Quantum effects

At the most microscopic level, randomness rules. Anything can happen, including the apparently impossible. For example, the tiny, but non-zero probability that electrons can 'tunnel' through a solid barrier produces a measurable effect because of nature's profligacy in electron production. Although averages can be foreseen, the behaviour of individual particles cannot, in principle, be predicted. Quantum effects generate irreducible ignorance.

Quantum effects may affect health processes, for example causing mutations at the molecular level which can lead to cancer if not corrected by the body's repair mechanisms (Cooper, 1993). They introduce an element of irreducible error which scientific progress in predicting the fate of individuals will never be able to remove.

### Probabilities involving human action

The concepts of probability and risk are usually used to predict the behaviour of complex physical or biological systems. We can distinguish between the behaviour of such systems, such as blood circulation, and human actions which are undertaken out of choice, for a purpose, and hence can be considered rational or irrational. A human being may act, successfully or unsuccessfully, in order to bring about a future state of affairs. Meaningful action can thus be explained by an anticipation of the future, while no intention is assumed in a physical or biological system. We can merely predict its future.

Our machinery for understanding probability, based on the separation of observer and observed, lumps together risks arising from human action with those caused by the behaviour of systems. For example, the risk of being burgled or murdered in a given location can be estimated through induction from past crime rates. Although such probabilities are based on large numbers of individual decisions, it has been known since the nineteenth century that national averages show consistency from year to year (Gigerenzer et al., 1990, p. 42), and that temporal comparisons can reveal historical trends or the cyclical impact of economic recessions.

Although risks arising from intentional human action can be treated probabilistically, the inductive leap from statistics about frequencies of past human actions to future risks is even more fragile than that needed for inductions about physical or biological systems. Aggregate human action depends on the vagaries of fashion, and on constantly shifting economic and cultural contexts. For example, lawyers in the USA estimated, in 1995, that British-born murderer Nick Ingram had a 10 per cent chance of succeeding in his final appeal against being sent to the electric chair. As so often in risk analysis, defence lawyers used this estimate pragmatically, to justify the decision to prolong his mental agony while they exhausted every avenue of appeal against an inhumane punishment. Their probability estimate, even if correct, depended on the unreformed working of a culturally and historically specific legal system.

In contrast, the number of recorded firework injuries in the UK leapt by almost 50 per cent between 1993 and 1994. This increase in health risk was probably caused by a government decision to deregulate imports in 1993 (Guardian, 4/11/96). Induction of the level of risk from the 1993 figures would give a flawed estimate of the future probability of being injured by a firework in 1994 because the sociopolitical context had changed.

The assessment of risk in individual cases raises even more problems with respect to intentional action than in relation to the behaviour of physical and biological systems. How do we know that a dependent patient, or one who 'has' a mental illness, will not be at high risk of harming themselves or others? Epidemiology can only provide predictions based on past aggregates and, in the case of intentional action, requires the assumption that intentions remain roughly constant. Yet, much health care, for example in psychiatry and child protection, depends on the claim to be able to predict behaviour in individual cases.

## COMBINATIONS OF RANDOMNESS, COMPLEXITY AND UNCERTAINTY ABOUT INTENTIONS

We have distinguished analytically between uncertainty arising from complexity, quantum effects and reasoned action. However, most health adversities involve combinations of two or more of these sources of uncertainty. For example, cancer may be triggered by damage to cells at the molecular level, perhaps involving quantum effects. But, in the vast majority of cases, potentially cancerous cells are quickly destroyed by the immune system through a chain of reactions which, because of its complexity, cannot be predicted in individual cases. However, the clinical outcome for a patient who does develop cancer may depend as much on their personal response, in its social context, as on physical treatment (Cunningham, 1996).

The mind/body problem and its relationship to risk analysis is taken up below with respect to the idea of reflexive recursion. In Chapter 18, Milner discusses the health-promotion paradox that encouraging people to worry about risks may, itself, damage their health. It will be argued that mind/body and reflexive recursion effects are systematically underestimated in a health care system which is still oriented, in practice, to treating bodies.

## AN EXERCISE IN DECISION-MAKING ABOUT PROBABILITIES

The reader is invited to make a decision in the two imaginary cases given below, before reading the commentary which follows.

---

**Case 1**

Just as you are about to book-up a last minute holiday, you hear that a coach has crashed taking tourists to the very resort you want to go to, and that 10 people were killed. The travel agent assures you that 1 000 000 tourists have visited the country in the last year, without road accident.

Do you change your hoiday destination, even though it provides exceptionally good value for money, and a relatively clean sea?

**Case 2**

Just as you are about to book-up a last minute holiday, you hear that local guerillas have attacked a coach taking tourists to the very resort you want to go to, and that 10 people have been killed. The travel agent assures you that 1 000 000 tourists have visited the country in the last year, without guerilla incident.

Do you change your holiday destination, even though it provides exceptionally good value for money, and a relatively clean sea?

---

*Source:* Adapted from Gigerenzer, 1991, p. 106.

**Figure 2.1**   An exercise in probabilistic judgement

Although the problems presented in Figure 2.1 do not have 'correct' answers, you might feel less anxious about continuing with your holiday in case 1, involving a coach crash, than in case 2, where the risk arises from guerilla activity. (The editor developed these examples after deciding to continue with his holiday in case 2, but in a state of considerable anxiety.)

Gigerenzer (1991) uses similar examples to demonstrate that probabilistic knowledge involves more than mechanical induction from observed frequencies. In each case, the observed frequency of an adverse event is the same, namely 1: 100 000. If probabilistic reasoning simply involved using observed frequencies to infer a future probability, then you should be equally willing or unwilling to risk holidaying in the two cases. A perceived difference between them arises because the events depicted give different clues about the future. You might feel, rightly or wrongly, that coach crashes can happen anywhere, so that the frequency presented provides a reasonable guide to the future risk of this event occurring in the resort you are considering. In contrast, guerilla activity tends to occur in spurts. The low observed incidence of tourist mortality within the **country** in question seems to tell us little about its future **local** prevalence.

The examples show that use of the probability heuristic to draw predictions from complexity requires 'local' knowledge of the particular phenomenon in question. Lay people can use claims to local knowledge in order to refute health professionals' probabilistic prognostications, as in the case of perceived HIV invulnerability, discussed previously; and in some of the examples about teenage unplanned pregnancy and genetic abnormalities considered in Chapters 6 and 7. The possibility for special pleading is built into the risk heuristic. Although subject to empirical falsification, such loopholes make health-risk reasoning problematic, and open the door to reality negotiations between professionals and clients. Their existence is part of the price paid for drawing on probability heuristics in order to reduce uncertainty about the future.

This Gigerenzerian approach to probability judgements derived from observed frequencies may be contrasted with that of Kahneman and Tversky (1972). Gigerezer argues that, in some circumstances, underlying base rates within a population may be rationally discounted. Kahneman and Tversky suggest that such discounting entails use of a simplifying, potentially distorting, heuristic. The reader is requested to carefully compose the exercise just presented with the case of the engineer versus the lawyer outlined by Dracup in chapter 5 (see the section on 'Representativeness').

## Attitudes to the future and cosmologies

Late modern, multicultural Western societies contain a wide range of belief systems about our relationships to the future. However, a secular, Darwinian mode of thinking predominates in the official health-care system. This approach is founded on the concept of probability, itself problematic, as shown above. Moreover, those who have internalised secular values, and understand health primarily in terms of risk, also employ other frames of thought. Even 'secular fundamentalism' sometimes slips at times of crisis. As Kingham argues, in Chapter 4, types of rationality which deviate from the official line are likely to be expressed in non-literal forms, for example in metaphors or images.

If the future is judged to express divine justice (personalism), deemed unalterable (fatalism) or fully discounted (hedonism) then questions of risk management do not arise.

These alternatives to risk analysis may appertain to cultures, individuals or mental states of the same person. Cultures encode their preferences in cosmological belief systems. Individuals may go against the grain of mainstream faith, for example, in our own society, by adopting fatalistic beliefs in the face of epidemiological conviction that individuals can control their probabilities of different personal futures through lifestyle choices. Finally, the same person may switch between implicit cosmologies in different circumstances or varying states of mind. Even the editor occasionally lapses into personalism when his bicycle tyres suffer a suspiciously high frequency of punctures.

## THE PERSONALISTIC UNIVERSE

Personalism involves the beliefs that the universe is morally ordered, and that futures express divine will. Adversity may be explained as a punishment for transgression, or as a test, the idea explored with some irony by Chaucer in the quotation at the beginning of this book. Douglas (1966) argued that preindustrial societies use personalistic cosmology to shore up a fragile social order with divine sanctions. Complex, highly specialised, industrial societies develop alternative regulatory mechanisms, such as police and legal systems. However, personalism coexists uneasily with scientific rationality in our current popular culture (Davison, Frankel and Davey Smith, 1992). Those who have adopted a predominantly secular attitude do not have available to them the response of the woman who cried out *'Where are you, God?'* (*Guardian*, 19/04/96) when a UN base in Lebanon was shelled by the Israeli army, causing scores of deaths and injuries among refugees sheltering there. (At the other extreme, of detached, probabilistic amoralism, the Israeli foreign minister, Ehud Barak, horrifyingly, described the incident as *'an unfortunate mistake'*.)

Personal experience of major health problems can strip away the veneer of scientific rationality. For example, one American study of parents of children with learning difficulties (Black, 1979) found that 40 per cent of parents responded to an initial diagnosis of mental retardation in their child with feelings of personal responsibility and guilt. One woman thought that she was being punished for hurting her parents by leaving home at the age of 15. Such beliefs only make sense within the framework of a personalistic, morally ordered universe, as opposed to one governed by 'blind' chance.

In a universe in which pseudo-randomness results from complexity, causally independent events cannot affect each other (although quantum events apparently can). As shown by Dracup in Chapter 5, this point is frequently misunderstood. For example, lay people commonly but mistakenly predict that a fair coin which has landed on heads several times in a row will be more likely to land tails up on the next toss. The laws of chance decree only that deviations from the average are likely to form a smaller proportion of the total data as more trials are carried out. Coin tosses do not 'remember' their predecessors. However, when vital and emotionally charged questions about health, life and death are raised, our departures from the principle of statistical independence may go beyond cognitive misconception, and implicitly invoke a personalistic universe.

In the Second World War film *The Longest Day*, a soldier, waiting for the invasion of France, wins $2500 in a dice game. At first he feels elated. But he then remembers that, after winning previously, he had broken his leg in a parachute drop, and returns to try to lose his winnings. Implicitly, he had been 'given' so much luck which he did not want to squander on gambling. Similarly, one of the pregnant women whose attitudes to risk are discussed in Chapter 7 suggested that families might be allotted only a fixed amount of genetic luck.

*My mam's got 14 grandchildren. There's nothing wrong with any of the 14. Are you pushing fate? ... And it was like, ee, you know, I've got three. I shouldn't go in for any more, because it is pushing fate, you know.*

If anything, the presence of 17 genetically normal close relatives indicated a reduced probability that her baby would inherit a health problem. Families are not awarded fair portions of good starts in life. Such sentiments coexist uneasily with science-based concepts of randomness and impersonal determinism.

In a personalistic universe, causally disassociated events can be magically connected. One women (see Chapter 11), whose life was devoted to caring for a husband with dementia asked *'Where have I gone wrong?'* when she compared herself with friends who could still enjoy activities together. Cohen (1993) notes that parents of very sick children may attempt to regain a sense of predictability and control by associating the outcome for their child to another event, for example the health of a plant. The blindness of chance becomes hard to accept for outcomes of vital personal importance (Clift and Stears, 1991). The editor must confess that, even while writing the first draft of these pages, and thinking about risk rationality, in 1996, he magically linked the footballing fate of Newcastle United with the electoral future of the then incumbent British government.

The magical nature of causal associations such as those made in these examples shows up clearly in the absence of a plausible causal connection. In other cases, science and magic seem to combine. Public attitudes towards the primary prevention of the feared killer diseases of the late twentieth century often incorporate the notion that individuals can control their own future health through lifestyle decisions. This position can easily slip into a personalistic model of the universe which treats ill health as individually deserved. For example, many young people who report having multiple sexual partners and not using condoms feel personally invulnerable to AIDS (Abrams *et al.*, 1990). More negative attitudes to condom use have been linked to both perceived invulnerability and a blaming attitude towards HIV (Clift and Stears, 1991). By implication, those who have not transgressed the moral order magically avoid dangers arising from random contingencies which they cannot otherwise control.

The concept of 'candidacy' has been used to depict a relatively benign tool, employed by the general public to predict and explain specific cases of coronary heart disease in terms of the occurrence of general risk factors such as obesity, lack of exercise, smoking, heavy alcohol consumption and family history (Davison, Davey Smith and Frankel, 1991). However, candidacy can be used to blame, and withhold sympathy from, those whose problems are judged to result from unhealthy choices. One older pregnant women, interviewed for our research, was told, without any explanation, that she needed a second scan. After *'a fortnight of hell'* worrying about what might be wrong with the baby, the radiographer said, according to this respondent:

> *Well, you know, we couldn't get a good enough picture. What do you expect with all that fat on you?*

Being fat has become a modern equivalent of embracing the Devil.

The belief that individuals can control their own health, at best a partial truth, provides a magical protection to those who, by way of contrast, do not make unhealthy choices and so do not 'deserve' to become ill. But risk factors, by definition, provide only a limited guide to the future in individual cases. Unlike the

Aztecs, who made a human sacrifice every day in order to ensure that the sun would continue to rise, most members of secular modern cultures assume that its motions, however convenient, are not affected by human actions. But the personalistic view of the universe is not confined to 'primitive' cultures which lack specialisation of labour and strong forces of social control, even if it does not receive official expression in science-based health-care systems.

Why has science failed, to date, to banish personalism despite overwhelming evidence against the argument that human beings were designed? Three explanations can be suggested. One involves historical time lags. The Darwinian idea that the complex biological structures could emerge out of chance processes only began to gain currency in the late nineteenth century. A lengthy psychohistorical period may be needed before such ideas are fully internalised and passed on through family socialisation even within the secular culture (Anders, 1994, p. 72). The finding of one study (Davison, Frankel and Davey Smith, 1992) that people aged 65 and over were more likely than those aged 18 to 31 to invoke luck or fate when thinking about health outcomes is consistent with this explanation.

A second candidate explanation draws on Piagetian developmental psychology. Piaget argued that young children 'naturally' view the world in a personalistic way, for example believing that a child who suffers a major accident as a result of transgressing is naughtier than a child who suffers a minor one (Piaget, 1932, p. 126). In vital matters of health, adults, lay and professional, may regress to an earlier stage of development. Dracup, in Chapter 5, discusses a study (Mitchell and Kalb, 1981) using fictitious vignettes which showed that nurses judged a hypothetical colleague more blameworthy for omitting to put a guard rail on a patient's bed if an accident occurred.

Third, many people find the theory of natural selection hard to accept emotionally because it consigns the human condition and major life contingencies to blind chance. Blaming individuals for health problems may simply reduce people's sense of vulnerability to random processes.

## FATALISM

Fatalism, which may or may not be associated with a personalistic cosmology, involves a belief that the future cannot be controlled. The concept of fatalism corresponds to the construct of external locus of control, used in an extensive body of quantitative research. Rotter (1990, p. 489) has defined external locus of control as the degree to which individuals expect that a personal outcome is *'a function of chance, luck or fate, is under the control of powerful others, or is simply unpredictable'*. However, the status of fatalism as a cultural norm, for example among the poor in Bangladesh (Bhaduri, 1992), and as a counternormative psychological 'syndrome' in Western, individualistic societies, must be distinguished. Fatalism only stands out as a psychological problem against a cultural background of faith in the efficacy of individual action.

The official view, encoded in the ideology and practice of prevention (Freeman, 1992), maintains that future health outcomes can be predicted probabilistically in terms of conditional risk factors, and that individuals can at least partially control their future health through rational decision-making based on knowledge of these factors (not smoking, moderate alcohol consumption, exercise, etc.). Relative to this norm, the attitude to the future described in Rotter's well-known definition appears deviant (Davison, Frankel and Davey Smith, 1992). The most popular explanation of fatalism in the social psychological literature views it as a response to the experience of powerlessness among socially disadvantaged groups (Lefcourt, 1992). Hill and Machin, in Chapter 3, cite evidence that Asians and Africo-Carribeans living in the UK are more likely than Whites to explain health outcomes fatalistically (Howlett, Ahmad and Murray, 1992). But they suggest that this difference may reflect a greater prevalence of health disadvantage among the former two groups rather than cultural variation.

This explanatory model excuses fatalism, as a response to social injustice, while taking for granted its pathological, irrational status. However, by definition, future outcomes involving risk cannot be predicted perfectly. Space for chance is built into the idea of risk reduction, giving rise to a popular residual category of luck or fate which complements rather than contradicts belief in individual control over personal health outcomes (Davison, Davey Smith and Frankel, 1991).

This pattern of beliefs about the future, based on residual fatalism, can be contrasted with a more pervasively fatalistic personal response to the experience of powerlessness. Three of the adults with learning difficulties studied in depth by Heyman et al. (1997) had adopted generally fatalistic attitudes to the world after experiencing severely adverse events which they could not prevent, for example, exclusion from the parental family. Fatalism, for them, both reflected their experience of social powerlessness, and provided compensation, through an attitude of philosophical acceptance and enjoyment of present time.

## Positive fatalism

Even those who criticise the categorisation of fatalism as a form of pathology (Crawford, 1977; Davison, Frankel and Davey Smith, 1992; Freeman, 1992) tend to consider negative fates, and to implicitly exclude positive destinies. This bias neatly parallels that often pointed out in the risk literature, towards concern with the probability of negative outcomes. But research into lay accounts of health behaviour shows that individuals may view their fate positively, developing a sense of personal invulnerability. For example, pregnant women may reject amniocentesis because they feel convinced that their baby will be genetically normal (Rothman, 1988). Some young people do not use condoms because they feel invulnerable to AIDS (Woodcock, Stenner and Ingham, 1992), as noted above.

Positive fatalism, like its negative counterpart, can be grounded in induction from previous experience. Most younger people in Western societies will have experienced a lifetime of good health, will not have encountered premature death, and will have been distanced from serious illness and death in older relatives. The inference of invulnerability suffers from no more than the fault inherent in all forms of inductive risk analysis: that the experienced past provides only a flawed guide to the future.

## HEDONISM

While personalism involves belief in divine agency, and fatalism the view that events cannot be controlled, hedonism discounts time at a high rate, preferencing present benefits over future costs. As one young pregnant women (see Chapter 6) said: '*I would rather have a short life, when you enjoy yourself.*' Another youngish woman, newly diagnosed as having diabetes (see Chapter 8), stated that she was '*not particularly worried about the future. It doesn't prey on my mind.*' She, thus, balanced the needs of the present against the demands of the future by discounting time heavily, and so could justify a relaxed stance towards the rigorous requirements of insulin control.

Some carers of people with dementia (see Chapter 11) were determined to resist thinking about the future or accepting the trajectory of inevitable decline put forward by professionals. Faced with the unpreventable loss of a loved relative, they made the best of a precarious present. Health professionals sometimes failed to understand the logic of this form of coping, and were determined to challenge relatives' unrealistic optimism, as they saw it.

Health promoters cannot logically refute hedonistic arguments even in the deadly case of tobacco, because individuals or groups can discount time at any rate they choose. They can display celebrities dying of lung cancer who express regret that they did not heed health-education warnings at a younger age. However, the determined hedonist can discount the risk of such regrets in later life as part of the price to be paid for present enjoyment.

## Describing probabilities

The representation of probabilities, and their use in negotiated decision-making, are central themes in late modern, risk-oriented, health management. Descriptions of probability rest on implicit, taken-for-granted decisions about what to count as an event, which event classes to predict, and what risk factors to include in the probabilistic equation. The present section considers the communication of probabilities within contexts in which health entities, their consequences and predictors have been selected.

It might be supposed that the communication of numerical probabilities requires only a simple process of converting a known numerator/denominator relationship, established by induction, into a percentage or ratio, and explaining it to clients. However, this apparently simple translation process requires a number of choices: between qualitative and quantitative encoding of probabilities; between a positive or a negative orientation; and about how to deal with second-order uncertainty.

### QUALITATIVE REPRESENTATIONS OF PROBABILITIES

Probabilities can be described in three ways: quantitatively (e.g. 1: 100, 1 per cent); qualitatively (e.g. low, high); or in ways which incorporate a value judgement about whether a hazard should be accepted (e.g. safe, dangerous). These three types of description contain embedded in them progressively more information about the speaker's attitude to the probability in question. A probability of 1: 100 might or might not be judged high. High risks should, *ceteris paribus*, be avoided, but can sometimes be justified, for example, as the only means of saving a life. However, 'danger' should be avoided, while we should not worry about possible hazards which have been deemed 'safe'. Hence, these latter terms contain prescriptions.

As Dracup points out in Chapter 5, qualitative descriptions of probability were used long before quantitative representations were developed (Zimmer, 1983). The UK Chief Medical Officer, Kenneth Calman, has recently called for standardised mapping of quantitative probabilities on to qualitative terminology. He has suggested that, for example, a probability of >1: 100 should be described as high and one of 1: 000–1: 10 000 as low. This call illustrates the tyranny of numbers, since the meaning of probabilities depends on expectations, and on the nature of the benefit and risked adversity in question (Weber and Hilton, 1990), as noted in Chapter 5. For example, few people would consider a probability of 1: 100 of dying as a result of a tooth extraction as 'low', or the same probability of dying after a heart transplant as 'high'.

Repeated government insistence, during the BSE crisis of 1996, that British beef was 'safe' translated into the assertion that the allegedly low probability of humans catching CJD from their traditional Sunday dinner **ought** not to prevent the public from eating it. This coupling of probabilistic description and judgement about its acceptability provides an authoritarian device which can be used by those who seek to prevent people from deciding for themselves how to respond to a given probability of an adverse event.

UK government attitudes towards BSE can be instructively contrasted with the official health-education line which distinguishes '*safer*' sex, with a condom, from '*high-risk*' '*unprotected forms*' (Health Education Authority, 1992). This use of language suggests, somewhat impractically for the future of the human race, that all 'unprotected' interchanges of sexual fluids should, ideally, be avoided, regardless of the social context. Differences in the probability of infection, for example in monogamous relationships and in paid sex, which might have been represented numerically, are obscured. However, despite the comparatively high prevalence of HIV in the USA, the probability of an American in the 'general population' becoming HIV infected has been estimated at 1: 5 000 000 per heterosexual act of intercourse without a condom, and 1: 5 000 000,000 for such an act using a condom (Chapman, 1992). Individuals are more likely to die in a passenger aeroplane crash than to become HIV infected through heterosexual intercourse without a condom.

Strong arguments can be put forward in favour of sexual practices which reduce the rate of HIV transmission, and so prevent its prevalence from increasing in the future. But accounts of condomless sex as 'unsafe', and of British beef as 'safe', incorporate value judgements about risk management which cannot be justified in terms of probability estimates, themselves problematic. Political ingredients have been added.

## QUANTITATIVE REPRESENTATIONS OF PROBABILITIES

Qualitative representations of probabilities come prepackaged. In contrast, medical risks, such as those associated with surgical outcomes and genetic abnormalities, are often presented statistically. However, these statistics always include more than neutral description. Comparisons across health-care sectors raise the question of why probabilities are presented qualitatively in some sectors, and quantitatively in others. Genetic counsellors, as was shown in Chapter 1, in the section on the 'liberal' concept of expertise, emphasise that the different options open to pregnant women – to have amniocentesis or serum-screening – have different advantages and disadvantages. Comparison of the representation of probability in genetic counselling and in HIV prevention suggests that professionals will be more likely to cite numerical probabilities if they believe that medical choices involve multiple costs and benefits, and that, therefore, a clearly best buy cannot be identified. The complexities associated with the deceptively simple task of communicating probabilities to clients will be explored below with respect to the example of the presentation of genetic-testing information to pregnant women.

### Communication of probabilities in prenatal genetic counselling

The communication of numerical probabilities from professionals to clients, where it does occur, itself involves choices, including the level of precision and the direction in which the probability is presented. Rapp (1988b) observed a form of linguistic code-switching in the ways that genetic counsellors in the USA described probabilities to pregnant women. The code chosen depended on the counsellor's implicit assumption, based on the woman's social background, about her level of understanding. Probabilities could be represented in a simplified, rounded verbal form (e.g. 1 in 100); as more precise numerical ratios accompanied by explanation, suggesting that the woman did not understand complex statistics, but was capable of learning; or as an exact ratio without explanation, implying that the woman would understand it without needing further explanation. Tapes of genetic-counselling sessions in an English hospital, obtained for the research discussed in Chapter 7, showed that consultants and registrars often rounded probability estimates. However, one woman, a research midwife aged 36, married to a university lecturer, had been told that her probability of having a child with Down's syndrome was 1: 311, an impressive but spurious display of accuracy.

The probabilities of adverse events can be represented as the odds of an event either happening or not happening. Dracup, in Chapter 5, cites evidence (Tversky and Kahneman, 1981, p. 251) from psychological studies that decision-making is affected by the direction in which a probability is presented. For example, a woman may be told either that she has a probability of 1: 100 of having a miscarriage through amniocentesis, or a probability of 99: 100 of not suffering this adversity. Professionals may use the latter, more optimistic, descriptive device in order to encourage risk acceptance. Although we do not have direct evidence to support this hypothesis, the following example from our maternity research illustrates the tactical significance of the choice of probability direction:

> At the end of the day, even if you say, well, the risk of miscarriage [from amniocentesis test] is 2 in 100, then 98 in 100 don't. It is all a numbers game. It's all just getting the balance. (Registrar, giving genetic counselling to pregnant woman aged 36)

The same counsellor had earlier represented this woman's 'background risk' of having a baby with a genetic abnormality as 1: 90, but had not pointed out that she therefore had a chance of 89: 90 of a normal baby. Since she was predisposed towards amniocentesis, this example illustrates the use of probability direction to support a negotiated consensus, rather than medical oppression.

In a science-based culture, numerical probability statements carry with them an in-built implication of precision. As Lupton (1993, p. 425) puts it:

> In its original usage, 'risk' is neutral, referring to probability, or the mathematical likelihood of an event occurring.

However, the apparent accuracy of quantitative probability estimates can give a misleading impression of expert ability to predict the future. Registrars and consultants were observed, in our research, to give substantially varying estimates of the maternal, age-related risk of having a child with Down's syndrome. For example, women aged 36 received estimates of this probability which ranged between 1: 175 and 1: 400. Such discrepancies may be explained, in part, by the steepness of the age-related risk increase for older women. In consequence, risk levels depend on how precisely the woman's age is calculated, and on whether her age at conception or her current age is considered. One woman was told that her risk was 1: 310 at age 36 but 1: 240 at age 37. Such second-order uncertainty about the risk estimate itself was rarely communicated.

Another complexity involves the question of whether Down's syndrome alone, or serious genetic abnormalities of all kinds, are considered. The doctor who quoted the highest level of Down's syndrome risk (1: 175) at age 36, also told the woman that her risk of the child having any abnormality was 1: 90. The combined probability of a large number of relatively rare abnormalities may outweigh the odds of the baby having the single most common problem: namely Down's syndrome. But these other syndromes were not mentioned by other genetic counsellors. Thus, depending on the way in which age was calculated and the range of conditions under consideration, a 36-year-old women could be quoted a risk of genetic abnormality ranging from 1: 90 to 1: 400.

Although the consultants and registrars took great pains to present information to women as carefully as possible, occasional errors were instructive. For example, the women faced a difficult choice between the limited accuracy of serum-screening (AFP) and the risk of a spontaneous abortion from amniocentesis. One doctor, advising a woman who was leaning towards amniocentesis, said:

> If it [maternal serum-screening] comes back a risk of 1 in 20, then you panic even more and think, 'A quarter of these babies are going to be abnormal.'

The doctor should have said that 5 per cent of the babies would be abnormal. The problem is not so much that '*the ordinary lay person, the man in the street, is weak on probabilistic thinking*' (Douglas, 1994, p. 50), but that the complexities of probabilistic reasoning can confuse even experts paid to communicate them on a daily basis. Mistakes may not occur randomly, and may support the negotiated consensus built up during the counselling session.

## Conditional probabilities

It was argued, in the first part of this chapter, that a science-based culture, which seeks to separate the subjective and objective, and to treat probability as part of the natural background, misrepresents the relational character of probabilistic knowledge. Probability statements refer to the accuracy with which an observer can predict a particular class of events. They depend on a specification of the numerator and denominator in the frequency ratio which is influenced by its cultural, political and organisational context. A population can be subdivided in an indefinite number of ways, many of which will work well enough predictively, as they will differentiate aggregate groups with higher and lower probabilities of experiencing a given future event. The influence of cultural and organisational factors on the selective specification of such conditional risk factors is illustrated below with respect to the example of the relationship between maternal age and the risk of carrying a fetus with Down's syndrome.

### DOWN'S SYNDROME AND THE '*TERRIBLE AGE PROBLEM*'

The management of the genetic risk of Down's syndrome provides a good illustration of processes of selection of risk factors in health management. The hospital site for our research, like many others, had adopted a financially driven policy of offering genetic testing only to older women. Because of the link to testing, age became a major concern for both younger and older women whose pregnancies were managed by the hospital. Consultants and registrars often defined the agenda of genetic counselling in terms of maternal, age-related risks. As one said, '*Get yourself ready, and we'll have a chat about age-related risks*', while another referred to '*this terrible age problem*'.

However, the probability of producing a fetus with Down's syndrome is associated with a number of other factors, including family history (Mikkelsen *et al.*, 1995); maternal exposure to abdominal X-rays (Rose, 1994), and low-level environmental radiation (Bound, Francis and Harvey, 1995); conceiving in the winter months (Puri and Singh, 1995); and paternal factors, since, in 8 per cent of cases, the third chromosome which causes Down's syndrome comes from the father (Mikkelsen *et al.*, 1995). Maternal age predicts the probability of a fetus having Down's syndrome more powerfully than any of the other individual factors mentioned, but the latter still have substantial predictive power. The incidence of Down's syndrome is approximately doubled both among women who have had four abdominal X-rays (Rose, 1994), and among those who conceive in the winter months (Puri and

Singh, 1995). By way of comparison, women aged 35 or over are about 6.5 times more likely than younger women to conceive a fetus with Down's syndrome (Lopez, Stoner and Gilmour, 1995). The odds ratios obtained will depend on the precise way in which the numerator and denominator are defined. Nevertheless, the above rough comparison suggests that screening could be targeted much more accurately if additional risk factors were taken into account.

We have found no published research which has probed the causal status of the association between maternal age and Down's syndrome, using standard multivariate techniques. Since most older women have genetically normal babies, this association must be mediated by other factors which might be identifiable, enhancing prediction, or even modifiable, opening up possibilities for prevention. The collective, unreflexive decision not to undertake such research makes maternal age an apparent bedrock risk factor.

The selection of maternal age as the main indicator for screening intensifies the 'terrible age problem' for older pregnant women, as can be seen in Chapter 7. However, this selection reflects economic constraints, organisational requirements and cultural attitudes as well as biomedical contingencies. A consideration of the economics of screening suggests that a 'good' screening criterion, from the viewpoint of those who have to allocate resources, both selects those at highest risk, and excludes a large part of the potential population from being tested. Maternal age meets these requirements, since the incidence of births tails off in older age groups. Paradoxically, two-thirds of babies with Down's syndrome are born to women aged under 35 (Crandall, Lebherz and Tabsh, 1986). Selection of additional criteria would increase the number of women qualified for routine screening, most markedly in the case of season of birth, and multiply organisational complexities.

Social attitudes may also influence the amount of selective attention given to risk factors. The data discussed in Chapter 7 will show that many older pregnant women feel stigmatised on account of their age. Conversely, the use of exposure to maternal X-rays as a criterion for screening might not be too well received by the medical profession because of the questions about iatrogenesis which would be raised. As noted in Chapter 1, the US National Academy of Science (cited in Rose, 1994, p. 150) argued that constitutional factors might lead women both to need more X-rays, because of poorer health, and to be at greater risk of congenital abnormalities. The causal status of the relationship between maternal age and Down's syndrome has not been subjected to similar probing.

## CONDITIONAL PROBABILITY, DIFFERENTIATION AND GENERALISATION

The unlimited possibilities for specifying combinations of conditional factors enable both professionals and lay people to manipulate probabilities through the use of differentiation and generalisation. Risk differentiation involves as much separation as possible of the conditions which generate lower and higher probabilities of an adverse event. Conversely, risks can be maximally generalised by aggregating the probability of an adverse event over as many conditions as possible.

These tactical options arise from the shaky epistemological status of probability as a heuristic device based on acceptance of the ecological fallacy that the aggregate properties of a specified category can be attributed to the individuals within it. As maintained above, populations can be grouped in many ways, for inductive purposes, which work 'well enough', and which generate different probabilities. This argument is now being taken a stage further through the proposition that individuals, groups or vested interests can partially control probabilities via their decisions about how to group events for predictive purposes. Sadly, you cannot directly change disease processes in this way, but you can modify the best prediction. (You might also be able to modify the disease process indirectly by altering expectations, through processes of reflexive recursion, as will be argued below.)

The tactical uses of differentiation and generalisation to maximise or minimise the acceptability of a line of action the desirability of which has been predetermined, for example on financial grounds, are outlined in Table 2.1.

## Examples of differentiation and generalisation

Strategic use of differentiation and generalisation can be clearly seen in responses to public health panics. As long as health concerns about BSE could be officially discounted, the UK government encouraged sales of as many animal parts as possible. The public were told, for example, that veal brains could be safely eaten because calves were too young to develop signs of the disease (implying that the asymptomatic cannot infect). In effect, the risk was 'spread' across all the body parts of the entire cattle population.

After the admission, in March 1996, that human cases of CJD had probably been caused by the consumption of beef products, their acceptability temporarily plummeted in the UK. The government then adopted a strategy of differentiating unsafe food products, such as meat from the oldest animals, spinal cord, brains. Differentiation enabled a case for the safety of the remainder to be sustained, since the most dangerous elements had been removed from the food chain. Similarly, public debate about gun control, in response to the Dunblane massacre of children in March 1996, can be understood in terms of generalisation and differentiation. Gun opponents generalised that any legally held gun could, potentially, be used to murder. Defenders, who had previously resisted additional restrictions, differentiated

Table 2.1   Tactical use of risk differentiation and generalisation

|  | | Strategic aim | |
|---|---|---|---|
|  | | To maximise risk acceptability | To minimise risk acceptability |
| Assessment of current risk acceptability | Currently acceptable | Generalise | Differentiate |
|  | Currently unacceptable | Differentiate | Generalise |

between guns locked up safely in clubs and those kept in private homes, which, they now conceded, might be banned.

Differentiation and generalisation can be used equally well in the micro-management of health risks, as the following example illustrates. The health authority justified its decision, in March 1995, to refuse a second round of treatment for leukaemia to Jaymee Bowen on the grounds that she had only a 2 per cent chance of surviving painful further treatment. Commentators felt that the health authority was also influenced by its cost (£75 000).

The use of a quantified probability, presented as highly accurate, supported the decision not to offer treatment. Jaymee Bowen was eventually treated through a charitable donation. The private doctor who took the case considered that the girl had a survival chance of about 1 per cent, but believed that further treatment was justified in order to see whether she belonged to a group with a good or bad prognosis. He was, in effect, saying that if the relevant class of leukaemias was differentiated further, then the probability of survival associated with each subclass might be higher or lower than the average 1 per cent. By admitting to a degree of uncertainty, he could justify his decision to continue with the case. Following private experimental treatment, her chances of survival were, in October 1995, put at 30 per cent. The initial probability estimate, as always, provided a global average, used in this case to justify non-intervention. Obtaining more information allowed this probability to be differentiated into a set of subcategories associated with either a higher or lower chance of survival. The initial probability was presented as an unalterable scientific fact. But, on closer examination, it dissolved. The decision about how far to look was based on pragmatic grounds. Sadly, Jaymee Bowen died on 22 May 1996, widely admired for her courage in the face of adversity.

Examples of differentiation and generalisation will be found in two of the chapters in this book. An older pregnant women, discussed in Chapter 7, did not wish to terminate her pregnancy in any circumstances. She decided to refuse serum-screening because she felt that a positive result would increase the probability of her having a baby with a genetic abnormality, and lay her open to moral censure from those who disapproved of deliberately giving life to a disabled child. By not having a test, she averaged the lower and higher probability of having an abnormal baby which would have followed from a negative or positive result. However, such reasoning varies, and can only be uncovered through qualitative, idiographic research. Another woman in this study, who had also decided not to terminate her pregnancy in any circumstances, chose to accept serum-screening because she felt intuitively certain of obtaining a negative, reassuring result.

Heyman and Huckle (see Chapter 9) found that family carers used differentiation and generalisation to manage risks associated with the problematic issue of freedom of the locality for adults with learning difficulties. Family carers who felt that their relative could not roam freely without incurring unacceptable dangers used 'horror stories' to justify this restriction on their autonomy, generalising from specific anecdotes. For example, one story concerned a middle-aged adult wandering off on her bicycle as a child, and having to be looked for by the police. Another story involved a second-hand account of an adult with learning difficulties falling asleep on a bus, and ending up 40 miles away from her home.

Some of the sample did have freedom of the locality, but, in most cases, at the cost of considerable anxiety for family carers and the adults themselves. They managed this risky situation by differentiating sharply acceptable and unacceptable risks. One man with learning difficulties was allowed to go to local pubs, but not night clubs, and a woman went out in the daytime by herself, but not after dark. By differentiating circumstances in which the probability of an adverse event was judged higher or lower, adults with learning difficulties and family carers could create a zone in which the adult could have some autonomy, with beneficial effects for their quality of life.

## Reflexive recursion and risk escalators

### ARE DUCKS AND CRAYFISH RISK EXPERTS?

Even in the greenhouse world, the north-east of England occasionally experiences severe winter weather. In such conditions, the editor likes to perform the following transaction with the local semi-wild ducks, who are eventually well rewarded for their participation. If he throws bread some distance, the hungry birds will gobble it up without hesitation. If he places bread close to his feet, most ducks will ignore it, presumably because they are not prepared to accept the perceived risk of being attacked. However, for some birds, a border zone can be found in which they will visibly hesitate for some time before either snatching the bread or moving out of the subjective danger area. These border zones vary in distance for individuals, but move closer to the source of apparent danger in proportion to the severity of the weather, and the resulting hunger of the birds.

Recent research (discussed by Motluk, 1997) suggests that other animals carry out complex cost-benefit calculations involving risk. Injections of the neurotransmitter serotonin stimulate an aggressive tailflip reflex in crayfish who have successfully fought-off competitors, but inhibit this reflex in animals who have lost a series of fights. The reflex is affected by the pattern of experiences, rather than single successes or failures, demonstrating its sensitivity to probabilistic information. (However, crayfish respond more readily to success than failure, suggesting that humans are not the only species who indulge in 'unrealistic optimism', as discussed in Chapter 5.)

Are ducks and crayfish 'risk experts', like toddlers making their first steps, as described by Adams (1995, p. 1)? Their decisions involve a sophisticated computation and balancing of costs and benefits, weighted by their probabilities. Similarly, each can outperform any Nobel Prize-winning biochemist in their manufacture of enzymes and other biologically active chemicals. In another sense, involving reflexive awareness, ducks, crayfish and toddlers cannot be credited with the status either of risk experts or world-class chemists. It all depends on how risk is defined.

Adams' own illuminating discussion of risk homeostasis illustrates the need to incorporate reflexive awareness into the analysis of future management. Risk homeostasis involves actions designed to maintain a selected optimum level of risk in response to changing circumstances. People may drive less cautiously when wearing seatbelts, or cross dangerous roads more carefully. As Milner points out in Chapter 18, they may defeat the risk-reducing objective of using sunblocks by exposing themselves for longer periods (McCregor and Young, 1996). Homeostasis may occur because people enjoy a given level of risk for its own sake, or because they have worked out an implicit trade-off between perceived benefits and the probability of costs, for instance between the enjoyment of sunbathing and the risk of skin cancer.

Ducks and toddlers cannot respond to a horror story, or to yet another report of a newly discovered risk. And the concept of homeostasis leads to circularity because the optimum 'homeostatic' level can only be defined by observing what individuals do. For example, drivers who behave less cautiously when wearing seatbelts can be held to be increasing their levels of risk to a putative optimum level, while those who do not change their driving behaviour can be seen as using seatbelts to reduce their levels of risk from a previous excessive level. The concept of reflexive recursion will be preferred to that of homeostasis, because the former focuses on symbolic processes, and reminds us that their impact can only be identified idiographically. Adams' important insight, that probabilities are changed by our responses to them, will now be applied to the analysis of health management.

## OVERVIEW OF THE CONCEPTS OF REFLEXIVE RECURSION AND RISK ESCALATOR

The last sections of Chapter 2 will develop the concept of risk escalators which may be driven by reflexive recursion. A brief overview is offered below of the inter-related set of ideas which will then be considered in more detail.

The term 'reflexive recursion' will be used to refer to changes in behaviour which, first, result from thinking about the probability of an adverse event, and which, second, alter that probability. The concept of 'risk escalator' denotes a graded system of treatment states of lower and higher perceived intensity, aimed at achieving a given therapeutic aim, which an individual may move through. For example, a patient may receive progressively higher or lower doses of a particular drug. A person with mental health problems may be treated by their GP; by a community psychiatric nurse, or by a psychiatrist, as an outpatient; as a voluntary inpatient; or as an involuntary inpatient. Other examples of risk escalators will be given below. In general, the treatment stages of higher intensity entail more radical interference with the client's physical body and/or personhood, and reflect a shift in the balance of safety/dependency versus risk/autonomy towards the former.

Our notion of stages of treatment intensity does not entail the assumption that treatment levels can be calibrated objectively, just that a given observer ranks them as more or less intense. Similarly, our concept of 'therapeutic', in this context, implies only that an observer judges that a given system of care promotes, or fails to promote, a valued therapeutic aim, for example, to restore a client's mental health, or to ensure that a baby is delivered safely. Riak escalators may be more or less 'driven' up or down by the processes of reflexive recursion involving positive feedback. For instance, a medical treatment might inadvertently exacerbate the problem it was designed to tackle, leading to worse symptoms and stronger application of the treatment, and so on. Conversely, acceptance of the risk entailed by giving a vulnerable client group a small increase in autonomy might enable them to develop personal competencies which, in turn, enable them to manage still greater degrees of autonomy more safely.

Observers may disagree about whether a given risk escalator should be judged therapeutic or anti-therapeutic. It will be argued below (see Table 2.2) that these judgements are linked to an observer's view of the nature of the positive feedback effects driving up and down risk escalators. In brief, up escalators seen as subject to strong positive feedback will be judged to generate therapeutic over-reactions (as in the argument that prison breeds criminals, or that hospital births produce Caesareans). On the other hand, down escalators which are believed to be based on weak positive feedback will be seen as neglectfully under-reactive (as in current critiques of UK community care).

## Dimensions of relexive recursion

A series of dimensions, outlined in Table 2.2, and discussed below, provide a starting point for analysing processes of reflexive recursion.

### EMOTIONALITY AND CALCULATION VECTORS FOR REFLEXIVE RECURSION

Vector refers to the hypothesised causal mechanism underlying reflexive recursion, and may involve a direct emotional response, a reasoned action, or a combination of the two.

**Table 2.2**  Dimensions of reflexive recursion on health risks

| Dimension | Pole one | Pole two |
| --- | --- | --- |
| Emotionality vector | High | Low |
| Calculation vector | High | Low |
| Perceived effect direction | Health-enhancing | Health-damaging |
| System openness | Closed (circular) | Open (spiral) |
| Second-order reflection and communication | Present | Absent |

As an example of the former, players of competitive sports, notoriously, risk tensing up when close to victory. Lane (1995) argues that the management of pregnancy as a high-risk health problem can give rise to 'cascades' of intervention. Medical procedures designed to reduce risk cause the woman anxiety, affecting indicators of the progress of the pregnancy which justify further interventions leading to even higher anxiety, until the system escalates out of the woman's control, and has to be managed through a Caesarean section. Mansfield (1988) cites evidence from animal studies that experimental maternal stress induction, for example through the use of bright lights and noise, increases birth-related risks, for example of spontaneous abortions.

In contrast, women receiving chemotherapy for breast cancer may become emotionally distressed at its cessation because its very unpleasantness reinforces their sense that the medical system is actively fighting the disease (Ward *et al.*, 1992). This distress might, in turn, reduce patients' ability to recover from the disease. Emotional responses depend on interpretative frameworks.

The calculation vector for reflexive recursion affects risk management through a reasoning process. For example, Woodcock, Stenner and Ingham (1992) found that many young people in rural districts believed that they did not need to use condoms because of the low prevalence of HIV in such areas. This finding opens up the possibility that the prevalence of HIV will increase more rapidly in rural districts just because people taking sexual decisions consider themselves not at risk. In contrast, the incidence of HIV dropped rapidly, if temporarily, among male homosexuals after they were identified as a high-risk group (Law *et al.*, 1996).

In many cases, reflexive recursion will result from the combined effect of emotional and calculative responses to risk. Moran and Barker, in Chapter 16, discuss the example of a child whose school found out that he had been beaten by his father, and called in the child-protection agency. The parents responded angrily to this referral, exacerbating the risk in the view of the agency. As a result, the child was removed from his home. Escalation in this case involved transmission along a chain of calculated and emotional responses by different parties, leading to an emergent outcome which the initiator of protection – the school – did not anticipate.

The following quotation illustrates a similar process over a short time frame. The respondent worked at a day centre for people with learning difficulties, and the data was collected for the research discussed in Chapter 9.

> *Sometimes I think it [information about service-users] can be quite detrimental to a person ... And I remember a woman coming in to do the night shift ... And this other member of staff who had been on the day shift gave her this life history of this bloke, on how 10 years ago he had attacked somebody in a lift, and he done this and this. By the time he had finished, this woman was terrified, and it was the case that he went to one side of the table, she went to the other.* **And he picked up on that immediately.**
> (Author's emphasis)

This quotation neatly illustrates the risk-management dilemma arising out of reflexive recursion. Symbolic communication about a risk can amplify it through recursive processes, in the above case because the client might have responded aggressively to the care worker's fear. Conversely, if a hazard is not identified, then preventative efforts are precluded.

Evidence that reflexive processes affect longer-term health outcomes is considered in the next section.

## REFLEXIVE RECURSION AND EFFECT DIRECTION

Reflexive recursion may damage health through positive feedback. Conversely, thinking optimistically about the future can bring about a self-fulfilling prophecy in which adverse outcomes are delayed or averted.

Experimental studies suggest that psychosocial interventions can benefit health in many different ways. The ubiquitous power of placebos to ameliorate virtually any medical condition is long established (Lundh, 1987). If warts can be cured through visualisation plus faith (Spanos, Stenstrom and Johnston, 1988), then so, perhaps, can more serious maladies. However, the finding from a well-known and respected random control trial (Spiegel *et al.*, 1989) that women with metastatic breast cancer who received psychotherapy lived on average about twice as long (36.6 months) as a control group (18.9 months) has sparked remarkably little research interest. A recent meta-analysis (Meyer and Mark, 1995) identified only five random control trials which had investigated the medical effects of psychotherapy on cancer patients. Field experiments (Schulz, 1976; Rodin and Langer, 1977) found that apparently superficial interventions designed to enhance elderly people's sense of autonomy – a lecture and being encouraged to water their own plants – improved their health, and significantly reduced future mortality (from 30 per cent to 15 per cent over 18 months in the latter study). A drug with such effects would have won its discoverers the Nobel Prize, but these findings have stimulated little research interest.

Correlational research suggests that mental processes have pervasive health effects (Martin, 1997), although such research cannot unambiguously establish causal direction. Being diagnosed as hypertensive increases the rate of work absenteeism regardless of whether treatment is given or not (Hayes *et al.*, 1978), leading these researchers to recommend a revision of treatment philosophy. Johnston (1986) concluded from a research review that prior anxiety and lack of perceived control predicted poorer operative outcomes. Prospective studies show that mental health consistently predicts future longevity over a period of decades even when known risk factors such as smoking, alcohol consumption and socioeconomic background are controlled (Singer *et al.*, 1976; Martin *et al.*, 1995). Girls, but not boys, who suffer high levels of anxiety, end up, on average, five centimetres shorter than those who do not (Pine, Cohen and Brook, 1996). This finding suggests that the relationship between anxiety and growth may be mediated by a gender-specific hormonal process. Activities which promote a sense of wellbeing, such as attending cultural events (Bygren, Konlaan and Johansson, 1996) and pet ownership (Beck and Meyers, 1996) may prolong life. The editor's household cat has experienced a substantial increase in attention since the latter finding was publicised.

The present form of science-based culture significantly underestimates reflexive recursion, which embarrassingly invokes the unresolved mind–body problem, cuts across the culturally and academically split categories of the mental and the physical, and challenges unidirectional models of causation.

## REFLEXIVE RECURSION AND SYSTEM OPENNESS

In a closed system, reflexive recursion feeds back on to the response under appraisal, while, in an open system, it activates new kinds of response.

According to the European Headache Federation (Day, 1996), up to one-third of chronic headaches in European countries are caused by the regular overuse of analgesics such as aspirin and paracetamol, and can be cured simply by not taking them. The act of taking analgesics may reinforce people's definitions of themselves as chronically ill, and so result in increased tension, and a greater incidence of headaches – leading, in turn, to a further use of analgesics. Although speculative, this explanatory model provides a good example of circular reactions within a closed system of reflexive recursion. Similarly, according to Kaplan (1995, p. 142), overstrong prescriptions exacerbate myopia, thus creating a need for ever-stronger lenses.

Closed systems of reflexive recursion can be visualised as circular. Open systems, in contrast, can be represented as spirals in which a series of staged responses are brought into play as danger signs become more or less intense, depending on the direction up or down the spiral of perceived risk in which the person is travelling. Both types of system can also be thought of as risk escalators (Heyman, 1995a, p. 31), in so far as the response to perceived risk itself increases or lowers the probability of the adverse event the response is designed to avoid.

In 'cascades' of intervention (Lane, 1995), discussed above, intensive monitoring invokes an anxious response from the woman in labour, provoking more active medical intervention, and further anxiety, until a medical emergency is precipitated. On a longer time scale, putting a child on an at-risk register may itself harm the child emotionally by damaging family relationships (Jackson, Sanders and Thomas, 1995). If the child then develops 'behaviour problems', societal responses such as expulsion from school, legal sanctions and eventual imprisonment may each in turn increase the probability of a more Draconian response. Such possibilities are considered by Moran and Barker in Chapter 16.

As well as going up, escalators can come down, and therapeutic properties may be attributed to descending motion. For example, a large hospital in north-east England processes offenders with learning difficulties through a medium security unit, rehabilitation wards and rehabilitation houses (although individual pathways will vary). As patients progress through this system, they are offered, at each stage, increasing amounts of autonomy, trust and risk acceptance. Thus, the medium security unit, where offenders start their careers at this hospital, contains four subunits in which control of patients' behaviour is progressively loosened. For example, they are only allowed to use the kitchen without staff supervision when they graduate to the third subunit. Patients whom staff regard as failing to cope with the demands of each level may be sent back to one which offers less autonomy. While working their passage through the hospital system, patients may be allowed home on supervised visits, short unsupervised home visits or longer periods of home leave. Eventually, most will be released, usually to community-care homes. However, many patients leave the area, and continuity in the operation of the downward therapeutic escalator can be lost. Where such systems work as intended, each progressively lower level of intervention allows increased autonomy, building on successful experience at easier levels, but provides reduced protection for the individual and the community.

The question of the extent to which specific kinds of health risk are affected by recursive processes raises considerable contention, and has become highly politicised. This issue will be taken up below.

## SECOND ORDER REFLEXIVE RECURSION AND RISK COMMUNICATION

Second-order reflexive recursion and communication involve reflection on, and communication about, reflexive recursion itself. Since the vectors in question involve thoughts and feelings, the introduction of second-order considerations can be expected to have a dramatic effect on circles or spirals of risk. For example, the dynamic of 'cascades' of intervention (Lane, 1995) discussed above, depends on the absence of recognition by health professionals, and the woman giving birth, of the emotional impact of risk-assessment measures. The King's advice to the Hatter in *Alice's Adventures in Wonderland* (Carroll, 1988, p. 101, first published 1865) similarly suggests a lack of awareness of reflexive recursion:

> Give your evidence, and don't be nervous, or I'll have you executed on the spot.

The suspicion that risk-alarm bells are triggered by professionals' own actions fundamentally undermines the therapeutic legitimacy of a system of care based on escalating responses to higher levels of risk. For this reason, analgesic manufacturers have been reluctant to fund studies of their overuse as a cause of chronic headaches (Day, 1996). Reflection about reflexive recursion has a critical, analytic quality lacking in reflex-like first-order processes (Beck, 1996, p. 28).

## Risk escalator dynamics and perceived therapeutic quality

Table 2.3 on page 101 maps some possible relationships between the perceived therapeutic quality of a health-care system and the direction of intensity of different stages of intervention. It focuses on an observer's belief, typified in the rows, about the efficacy of an intervention relative to given therapeutic objectives. The two columns represent the directions, upwards and downwards, in which a client may move through a closed or open therapeutic system, with the gradient defined by differences in perceived intervention intensity.

Table 2.3    Second-order reflexive recursion and critical analysis of the management of risk in health care

|  | Interventions of increasing intensity (Upward escalator) | Interventions of declining intensity (Downward escalator) |
| --- | --- | --- |
| Intervention system judged therapeutic | Minimisation of positive feedback | Maximisation of positive feedback |
| Intervention system judged non-therapeutic | Maximisation of positive feedback | Minimisation of positive feedback |

Observers will not necessarily agree about the calibration of the intensity of qualitatively different therapeutic interventions. For example, staff in one day centre (Swain, Heyman and Gillman, 1996) operated a highly regulated system for managing the 'challenging' behaviour of adults with learning difficulties. This system, previously, had involved the following steps in ascending order of intensity: being confined to a 'time out' chair, but not isolated; being isolated in a safe room; and being subject to physical constraint. Day centre staff had recently reversed the order of the last two stages, in order to make their system consistent with that operated in residential care. However, in practice, they did not physically constrain service-users. Since the change had been implemented, isolation in a safe room was no longer used because this response could only be reached, in the new system, if physical constraint proved ineffective. The new standardised gradation of responses to challenging behaviour appeared to deviate from the one held intuitively by day centre staff.

## THE THERAPEUTIC LEGITIMACY OF SYSTEMS OF INCREASING INTENSITY

Whether a system of increasing or decreasing intensity of care is seen as therapeutic depends upon the observer's opinion about the strength of feedback effects. Therapeutic systems of increasing intensity suffer from a potential tendency towards upward escalation through positive feedback. As argued above, those who wish to maintain the legitimacy of such a system have to deny the validity of positive feedback effects: that instrumental monitoring affects physical indicators (Lane, 1995); that institutionalisation damages the health of the elderly (Chapter 12); that child-protection orders increase family stress, and so the risk of abuse (Chapter 16); that low scores on performance indicators damage schools; or that prison trains criminals.

Those who fear the dynamics of upwards escalators may take steps to prevent them from starting. As a diabetic patient, quoted in Chapter 8, said, '*If you worry about things sometimes it just makes it more of problem.*' A community psychiatric nurse, quoted in Chapter 11, '*all along the line … tried to tell [family carer of person with dementia] the next possible step*' regardless of the latter's expressed wish '*not to know*'. Since the medical trajectory for dementia descends inescapably downwards, family carers may wish to postpone contemplating the future so as to preserve an atmosphere of normality for as long as possible. Teenage pregnant women (Chapter 6) felt that teachers minimised contraceptive education because '*They don't like to say to teenagers you can have sex.*' The teachers, according to their pupils, appeared to be trying to avoid starting up sexual escalators. Concern not to send permissive messages may also have motivated the government to tone down the first safer sex advertising campaigns in the mid-1980s (see Chapter 4).

Heyman and Huckle (1995a, p. 146) found that carers of adults with learning difficulties prohibited activities which they saw as safe in themselves, in case they led the adult into danger. One parent, asked if she had any worries about her grown-up son's relationship with his girlfriend, said:

> *Yes. At one time we had to stop them cuddling … Because, after all, if they start kissing, where does this lead to?*

Similarly, some argue that the legalisation of prohibited substances would merely recognise social reality, while others oppose this move on the grounds that it would send a permissive 'message' to potential users. Proponents of 'zero tolerance' policing maintain that suppression of petty crime and public nuisance prevents those involved from moving on to more serious offences, while its critics argue that this policy merely punishes the victims of failed economic and welfare policies.

Professionals may seek to avoid the dysfunctional potential of positive escalators. The following quotation (Swain, Heyman and Gillman, 1996), obtained from a staff member at a day centre catering for people with learning difficulties, unusually, locates 'challenging behaviour' in an interpersonal context which includes the professional response.

> *This [formal sanctions, e.g. 'time-out', 'chair'] exacerbates the situation, because that person if they do it [challenging behaviour] because they don't like crowds or whatever, or they think that somebody is annoyed elsewhere in the room, the fact that they are being responded to in that way makes their behaviour escalate. And so you end up with something that could have been avoided, if it were caught first thing.*

Professional efforts to avoid anti-therapeutic upward escalators can have unintended consequences. A woman receiving adjuvant therapy for breast cancer, interviewed by Cowley (1996), was told that she needed the treatment only as an insurance policy. Believing herself cured, the patient decided to go on holiday. She was then advised by a second doctor that she required adjuvant therapy urgently. The first doctor had, presumably, minimised the risk of the cancer recurring in order to reduce the patient's level of anxiety, but had inadvertently affected her motivation to continue with treatment.

## THE THERAPEUTIC LEGITIMACY OF SYSTEMS OF DECREASING INTENSITY

Health-care systems of decreasing intensity suffer from the potential weakness that they may leave clients with insufficient support for a given level of dependency, a standard criticism of current British approaches to community care for vulnerable people. Those who wish to defend the therapeutic nature of such systems have to emphasise their potential for positive feedback, with lower intensity support producing increased competence, and reduced risk, allowing a progressively reducing level of intervention. In contrast, those who criticise such tapering-off systems will minimise the potential for positive feedback, arguing that levels of dependency are not readily altered.

This analysis sheds light on some of the concerns of carers of people with learning difficulties, discussed in Chapter 9. Family carers frequently argued that their child had achieved their potential, and that little could be gained by giving further training, for example in road-safety skills, or sex education. Professionals believed that family carer over-protectiveness denied adults learning opportunities, in effect magnifying their disability.

Since systems of declining intensity involve progressive reductions in care inputs, those who promote them risk being charged with using a therapeutic rationale to justify resource savings, as illustrated by the following quotation from the research discussed in Chapter 9.

> They wanted him [son with learning difficulties] to go to the [mixed disability] centre so that he could make room for someone else ... I said no ... Some of his friends went there and later got married and got jobs ... They [people who moved to the mixed centre] are more advanced than [son].

Resource constraints may, paradoxically, prevent downward escalation, as service-users cling on to caring resources such as day centre places which they would not be able to regain if needed in the future (Heyman and Huckle, 1995a); or may stimulate upward escalation, as when elderly people seek institutional care prophylactically, in case it should be unavailable if needed in the future (Davison and Reed, 1995). Moran and Barker (Chapter 16) have detected a recent trend, driven by financial constraint, for child-protection agencies to avoid informal meetings. Professionals have to call formal case conferences in order to obtain support for families even if they judge that the level of risk does not warrant a child-protection order. In such cases, resource constraints, perversely, lead to higher intensity, more protective, and more expensive responses.

## Conclusion

Chapter 2 has focused on the probability component in risk analysis, and has followed on from the analysis of values in Chapter 1. Probabilistic reasoning has become a standard mode of thought in Western societies only since the seventeenth century, and its emergence is bound up with the linked developments of science, capitalism and secular belief systems. The average, a fundamental, taken-for-granted concept in late modern societies, has been firmly established as a basic tool for thinking about the future only since the second half of the nineteenth century.

The official model of probability presumes the randomness of events, as when The Royal Society (1992, p. 2) asserts that 'risk obeys all the formal laws of combining probabilities'. This chapter has attempted to demote the status of probability in risk analysis to that of a heuristic. Treating complex events as if they contain a random element provides predictive glimpses of the future which go beyond the existing state of knowledge. But such glimpses are obtained at the price, as with any form of simplification, of systematic error.

Users of the probability heuristic have to commit the ecological fallacy, attributing properties of groups defined for predictive purposes to individuals within those groups. The groupings which probabilistic prediction based on induction from observed frequencies has to draw on cannot, themselves, be defined unambiguously. Their boundaries can be influenced by empirical evidence, since an optimal grouping will differentiate the observed frequencies of an adverse event between sub-groups as much as possible. Nevertheless, many less than optimal groupings will have some predictive value, and the best predictive grouping can only be established in the special case where perfect prediction can be achieved. In this case, probabilistic reasoning, and risk analysis become redundant.

Understanding probability in risk analysis as a simplifying heuristic enables a number of important insights into lay and professional health-risk management to be developed. First, the probability heuristics established by psychologists can be seen as simplifications of simplifications. For example, medical staff group pregnant women by maternal age in order to establish their individual probability of carrying a fetus with Down's syndrome. This method of grouping has powerful predictive value, but simplifies since most women in the 'high risk' groups will not be carrying such a baby, and because a number of other known predictive factors, including season of conception, maternal X-rays and paternal factors, are not entered into the risk equation. Women may then simplify the risk equation based on maternal age still further, for instance by using the availability heuristic (Tversky and Kahneman, 1973) and reasoning from their own personal experience of a small number of cases (see Chapter 7). Alternatively, they may avoid both heuristics by drawing on detailed beliefs about an individual case. Such thinking has its own problems, which the probability heuristic was designed to rectify, for example reliance on unverifiable intuition. Health professionals need to appreciate the tension between nomothetic and idiographic risk-reasoning, and to avoid exaggerating the predictive power of the former.

A second important implication of treating probability as a heuristic is that the specification of risk-groupings can be seen as susceptible to strategic and political as well as empirical influences. Risk-groupings may express implicit cultural values, and even prejudices, for example homophobia or racism. Individuals and social groups may construct probability groupings so as sway the answers obtained from risk investigation in predetermined directions. For instance, patients may avoid seeking diagnostic information which would either increase or decrease their probability of having a particular health problem, thus maintaining their risk at an intermediate level. Lay people and policy-makers may generalise or differentiate risk-groupings in order to maximise or minimise risk acceptability. For example, parents of people with learning difficulties have been observed, variously, to generalise danger from isolated incidents in order to justify a protective policy, or to localise risk with a high degree of specificity in order to limit a relative's autonomy as little as possible.

Once symbolically established, risk concerns become real in their consequences. Some of the processes involved can be understood by considering health-care systems as risk escalators more or less driven by processes of reflexive recursion. A system of this kind contains a series of qualitative or quantitative steps, not always entirely consensually ordered, each of which entails a shift in the balance of autonomy versus safety. Individuals may move 'up' such a system, towards safety at the price of autonomy, as their clinical need becomes more serious. Alternatively, they may be driven up such a system by reflexive recursion, as in the 'cascades' of maternal intervention discussed by Lane (1995).

Movement down risk escalators may result, beneficially, from processes of reflexive recursion, for example when people with disabilities learn from modest risk-taking, and are enabled to cope with more hazardous situations. Critics of such downward-moving systems may contest the power of reflexive recursion, for instance the potential of a relative with learning difficulties to learn from experience. In general, 'up' risk escalators will be viewed as therapeutic if they are believed not to be susceptible to positive feedback involving reflexive recursion, while 'down' escalators need such feedback to make them therapeutic. This framework can be used to understand debates between professionals, and between professionals and service-users, about the value of a wide range of therapeutic systems, such as child protection, maternity and mental health care.

In Chapters 1 and 2, a series of arguments about the value and probabilistic aspects of health risks have been outlined and illustrated with qualitative examples. Both value and probability have been considered not as properties of events, but of the ways in which individuals and groups look at events. Probability and value should not be regarded as purely subjective, but a range of differing viable perspectives needs to be acknowledged. Simplistic appeals to the authority of science or for 'evidence-based' practice gloss over the rough and ready status of risk-reasoning.

The chapters that follow have resulted from extensive dialogue between authors: an advantage of preparing an edited book in one location. The remainder of Part One considers risk-reasoning and management from different social science perspectives. Parts Two and Three explore the issues raised in Part One in particular spheres of health and social care activity.

MERTHYR TYDFIL COLLEGE
LIBRARY

# 3 'Race', health and risk

## Mick Hill and Tony Machin

## Introduction

This chapter explores relationships between risk discourse and ideas about ethnicity, in the health field. It is argued that this discourse becomes ethnically bound, and is perpetuated through research practices. Examples of the ways in which notions of ethnically specific risk permeate the practice of health care are considered, and alternative approaches, based on cultural insider perspectives, are discussed.

### HISTORICAL AND CONTEXTUAL BACKGROUND

The practice of attributing specific health-risk factors to 'races', or, latterly, culturally defined ethnic groups, largely originated in the revolutionary period of the Enlightenment. As such, it is essentially a modernist project in which a number of distinctive but generally related processes can be seen to have been operating. These include the development of the discourse of Western superiority, the foundation of biomedical and human science, and the emergence of the idea that humans can attain mastery over the 'natural' environment.

Hall (1992) suggests that the 'West' represents an historical rather than a geographical construct. Deployment of the term 'Western' now signifies a type of society that is urbanised, capitalist, secular and modern. The concept of the 'West' is not neutral, and its usage allows the classification of societies into a Western versus non-Western opposition which provides a standard model for comparison. Such comparison inevitably contains evaluative elements. The West (and by proxy, all things Western) are seen as good, desirable and developed. Conversely, non-Western equates with notions of underdevelopment, inferiority and undesirability. However, the West, as well as gaining a historic hegemony over 'the Rest', has a long legacy of excluding its own internal others, for example Gypsies and Jews. The term 'Western' can thus be seen as a part of a language system which allows its users to stereotypically collapse a number of variables into one picture. Being non-Western equates with being non-industrial, rural and underdeveloped. Hall suggests that the discourse of the 'Rest and the West' still continues to shape public perceptions and attitudes. This discourse frames Western biomedical repudiation of non-Western systems of healing.

Said (1978, p. 3), in his influential critique of Eurocentric ideology describes Orientalism as a discourse whereby *'European culture was able to manage and even produce the Orient politically, sociologically, militarily, ideologically, and imaginatively.'* The doctrine of Orientalism thus places Western thought in a whole series of possible relationships with the Orient, while maintaining the upper hand. The 'Orient' came to be seen as a legitimate object of academic attention for the anthropologist, historian, sociologist, linguist and others. The common feature of the discourse of Orientalism (Said, 1978, p. 41) was a set of ideas which *'supplied Orientals with a mentality, a genealogy, an atmosphere; most important, they allowed Europeans to deal with and even to see Orientals as a phenomenon possessing **regular characteristics'** (our emphasis).

Orientalist thought has left an enduring, if unrecognised, legacy to both medicine and the social sciences. The attribution of risk to various subpopulations hinges on the assumption of cultural homogeneity. Lupton (1993) has argued that we can discern two broad forms of risk discourse. One is founded in ecological concerns about risk at the environmental level. The second is concerned with 'lifestyle', and individualises strategies of risk management. This type of discourse can readily be dovetailed with the assumption of homogeneity, that members of a particular reference group ascribe to a uniform set of cultural practices and values. The professional construction of risk within minority ethnic groups (MEGs) frequently takes this form. In contrast to this epidemiological approach toward risk assessment, a body of anthropological work critically examines the culturally dependent nature of risk, and provides valuable insights into lay strategies of risk assessment and management. Douglas (1994) argues that although the idea of danger may be found in all cultures, the concept of risk is culturally specific. Furthermore, Douglas contends that culturally dependent strategies of risk management arise in response to contradictory experiences and moral confusion. Which factors are defined as 'risky' depends on the dominant cultural orientation at particular times and places. Risk-management strategies usually involve the proscription of certain practices, foods, religious rites, etc. within a particular belief system. Culturally bound forms of risk assessment and management, therefore, become associated with the defence of specific lifestyles, and cultural markers of distinction in themselves.

The foundation of the subdiscipline of tropical medicine can be seen as a manifestation of Orientalism, as a Western construction of the risky other. The aspirations of tropical medicine to be a benevolent enterprise can be redefined as indicators of a thoroughgoing colonialist, paternalist attitude

(Doyal, 1979). The expansionist instincts of Western biomedicine were also in play, and underpinned the tendency of Western medicine to pathologise entire populations. The historical, pseudo-Darwinian origins of biomedical categories still in use are often overlooked. For example, Gould (1980), discusses a paper 'Observations on the ethnic classification of idiots', written by Dr Down in 1886. This paper argued that 'Caucasian idiots' could be classified in terms of the degree to which they approximated African, Malay, American–Indian, and Oriental peoples. The prevailing orthodoxy of the time held that stages of human evolution had produced, ultimately, the White European 'race'. In this scheme, 'Orientals' were represented as lower human races, and 'idiot' individuals within 'higher human races' classified as 'atavisms', or throwbacks to lower stages in the evolutionary process. The issue of ethnically bound medical risk needs to be understood in this historical context. Sheldon and Parker (1992) suggest that the failure to adequately conceptualise ethnic difference is a persisting feature of medical research in this arena.

## 'Race', ethnicity and health

### CONCEPTS OF 'RACE' AND ETHNICITY

Smaje (1996) argues that social and health research are bedevilled by entrenched contradictions in their conceptualisations of ethnicity. He suggests that concepts of ethnicity can be divided into two kinds. First, ethnicity can be considered as a form of cultural self-identification and lived experience. Ethnicity in this sense enables a set of people to create and maintain a sense of group identity and solidarity, and to distinguish themselves from others (Mason, 1990).

Second, ethnicity can refer to an externally constructed and imposed set of arbitrary categories, which members of such categories do not necessarily accept. Smaje (1996) argues that this latter approach entails accepting ethnicity as an explanatory category *sui generis*, or as an object for analysis. Smaje describes the latter approach as primordialist. Ethnicity, in this sense, is defined independently of an individual's world view and refers to a purportedly fixed characteristic. The former approach, in contrast, is instrumentalist. Ethnic identity is viewed as one resource among many, which can be mobilised when needed in order to assert collective political or economic interests. Its deployment will, therefore, vary considerably across contexts. Jenkins (1986) neatly summarises these two approaches, by suggesting that the former view provides 'Us' statements, through claims to identity, while the latter involve 'Them' statements which are rooted in the cultural hegemony of Western societies.

### THEORISING ETHNIC DISTINCTION

Health researchers have, in practice, homed in on arbitrarily selected indicators of possible ethnic difference. Smaje (1996, p. 142) argues that *'Ethnic ascription [in this sense] is thus a profoundly social process, in which the obvious facts of human variation act as raw material for the construction of ethnic categories.'* In the UK, ethnic distinction has largely been ascribed in terms of phenotypic differences in appearance, geographical origin and religious belief. For example, Bhatt and Dickinson (1992), in a consideration of health-education material aimed towards MEGs, suggest that the provision of health advice could be considerably enhanced if language, rather than skin colour, religion, or country of origin was seen as the key source of human variation.

Health research which latches on to empirical indicators fails to provide theoretical underpinnings for notions of ethnicity. The social sciences provide a variety of explanatory schema which are heatedly contested, as might be expected. For example, Marxists (e.g. Miles, 1984) have argued that ethnicity represents a reified feature of class relations. In this conceptualisation, ethnic groups are seen as racialised class fractions, and issues of race and racism are subordinated to the socioeconomic class (Smaje, 1996). 'Race' is therefore explained in terms of its deployment in the service of the perpetuation of capitalism.

Postmodern approaches to ethnicity reject any notion of clear-cut ethnic identity, In Smaje's (1996, p. 146) terms, ethnicity *'shades almost into a rootless local pluralism'*. Postmodern conceptualisations of ethnicity avoid the persistent binary opposition of primordial and instrumentalist approaches. There are as many ethnic identities, on this view, as there are people to live them. However, such a rejection of ethnic categories leaves the postmodern approach open to the charge of relativism. Such an anti-essentialist claim, that ethnic categories do not exist at any level of generality, may serve to obscure important cultural anchorpoints of individual identity, as well as power relationships between ethnic groups.

Within the remainder of this chapter, it is argued that ethnic health status, and professional assessments of ethnically bound risk, are framed by Western forms of thought which are themselves products of recent colonial history. Professional risk assessment shows almost complete disregard for the perspectives of MEG members.

## Western rationality and the construction of ethnic health risk

Even a cursory examination of online search facilities reveals that research into race, ethnicity, and health outcomes continues to be a substantial enterprise. However, the quality of much of this work has been criticised (Sheldon and Parker, 1992; Ahmad, 1993). Ahmad argues that this research has failed to enhance an understanding of the principal health threats afflicting MEGs, or to offer any prescription for health improvement at a practical level. He suggests that much of the work has been empiricist, treating ethnicity as a natural state marked by indicators, and has been culturally reductionist, presupposing the homogeneity of ethnic groups. Reductionism and empiricism decontextualise MEG health experience, including culturally specific risk-management strategies, and favour predictive categories of ethnicity and medically defined risk. In seeking to expand on the 'racially biased' nature of health-care research, Ahmad (1993, p. 11) suggests that proper account must be taken of the *status of interplay between two constructs: Namely those of 'race' and bio-medicine, and their potential(s) for social control'*.

Ahmad notes the following areas of commonality between Western medicine, and Western approaches towards 'Oriental' others:

- Expansionist tendencies are central to both Western imperialism, and Western biomedicine.
- Both Western imperialism and biomedicine can be viewed as forms of social control, and both appear preoccupied with normative modes of conduct.
- Both Western imperialism and biomedicine have seldom been successfully challenged by those subjected to their regimes.
- Both Western imperialism and biomedicine offer 'technical fixes' to what has been constructed as a problem. For example, the former was founded on a doctrine of civilisation, while the latter remains preoccupied with allopathic approaches to disease.
- Both enterprises are underpinned by the Eurocentric rationality of the Enlightenment. Just as non-Western nations are judged inferior by Western yardsticks, non-Western means of risk assessment and management, and the systems of health care which generate them, are dismissed as superstition and quackery within the dominant discourse of biomedicine. Both Western imperialism and biomedicine have incorporated the threat of outside challenge in order to maintain effective domination.

Just as European colonialism expanded globally, employing the concept of 'race' in order to justify its conquests, so medicine has extended itself into areas of life over which it previously held no sway (Armstrong, 1987a). However, the capacity to territorialise new areas, whether geographical or intellectual, requires the effective exercise of power. While history books provide stark examples of the power of coercive brutality, evident in the enforcement of imperialism, the exercise of medical power is most often explained in ideological, cultural, and discursive terms. One strategy for the maintenance of effective dominance appears to pervade both Western industrialised societies generally, and medicine more specifically. Armstrong (1987b) has argued that incorporating and marginalising outside threats as means of neutralising their potential challenge has been one of biomedicine's most effective means of defending its power base. For example, 'alternative therapies' have been recast as 'complementary therapies' and incorporated into medicine, as have the social sciences through the development of biopsychosocial medicine. Similarly, instances of tokenism in the selective appointment of Black people to prominent positions, and the founding of palliative social institutions, litter the history of Black people's civil rights, both in the UK and the USA.

The main territory on which Western imperialism and medicine converged, at a practical level, was the subdiscipline of tropical medicine. However, Ahmad (1993) has argued that several areas of current medical practice continue to reflect dominant Western ideologies. Such ideologies continue to frame professional assessments of risk, which are then discursively deployed on to MEG populations. At the level of policy, institutionalised racism can be identified in administrative practices. For example, the Commission for Racial Equality (1992) criticises health authorities for failing to provide adequate information about their services in appropriate media, thus placing people from MEGs at a considerable disadvantage in terms of their access to services. Current professional ideologies are perpetuated by medical research into the health of MEGs, and are reflected in day-to-day professional practice.

The term 'racialisation' was first employed by Fanon (1978), in his seminal paper *Medicine and Colonialism*, to describe the ways in which Western science uses a racial taxonomy to categorise whole populations. Such taxonomies are often based on phenotypic differences which arise out of interactions with our environment, rather than on hereditary, genotypic differences. Cashmore (1988) has argued that racialisation privileges biological and pseudo-biological over social concerns. 'Race', phenotypically assigned, is ascribed the status of a natural and value-free means of determining difference. This form of determinism assumes that behavioural differences between 'races' have biological roots. The health experiences of MEGs are then conceptualised primarily in terms of a restricted set of exotic diseases, such as rickets, tuberculosis and sickle-cell disease, and broader health considerations are ignored.

The consequences of this approach towards attributing medically defined risk are twofold. First, it may lead to a cultural group being blamed for particular types of medical pathology. For example, Ahmad (1989) discusses the creation of the category of 'Asian rickets', which was explained in terms of un-British eating habits and lifestyle, as well as possible genetic differences in vitamin D metabolism. Second, concern with exotic diseases may take medical attention away from a more general consideration of MEG health. Sheldon and Parker (1992) argue that, in consequence, health-planners refer to the special needs of groups rather than considering whether services adequately meet the health needs of the population at large. Bhatt and Dickinson (1992, p. 76), in an examination of health-education literature aimed at MEGs, note *'apparent gaps, anomalies, over-emphases and unequal attention to both topics and to groups within the minority communities'*.

## THE PERPETUATION OF ETHNIC RISK

Ahmad (1993) suggests that social research into the health needs of MEGs has been conducted in a climate of intellectual apartheid. Medical and health research have mostly constructed the problems which they investigate in exclusively Western terms. The areas selected for attention reflect the interests and dominant ideologies of those with the power to define the agenda. Ahmad (1989) notes that research into the health of ethnic groups is heavily clinically biased, and has tended to pathologise MEGs. He argues that the readiness to challenge the fundamental precepts of biomedicine which can be seen in the sociology of health and illness has not been so evident in the study of ethnicity and health.

Sheldon and Parker (1992) detect an increased tendency for ethnic groupings and 'race' to be used as independent variables in medical research. There appears to be a diachronic element evident in much of this research. Once constructed, ethnic categories are assumed to possess an unchanging character. How the results of the studies are supposed to relate to the improvement of MEG health is seldom discussed. Sheldon and Parker (1992) argue that the inclusion of the race/ethnic variable on a routine basis can in itself encourage researchers and professionals to link levels of health risk to racial differences. As a result, specific ethnic health problems can be conflated with the effects of more general disadvantage, for example resulting from poverty (Benzeval, Judge and Smaje, 1995). Studies are often too weak to differentiate the actuarial risks associated with 'race' from those connected to other factors such as social class and gender.

The concept of ethnicity is often used euphemistically and interchangeably with that of race in the research literature. Specific ethnic and racial categories are not used consistently. Racial/ethnic markers may be used in correlational studies without critical consideration of their meaning. Census data, a readily accessible resource, may be used without consideration of the limits to usefulness of secondary data (Bulmer, 1980). Sheldon and Parker (1992, p. 107) suggest that *'There is nothing so powerful as a large and available data set for encouraging the suspension of disbelief.'*

Uncritical acceptance of ethnic distinctions results in ethnicity being accorded the status of a 'natural' category. Sheldon and Parker (1992) suggest that, as a result of the reification of the concept of ethnicity, ethnic variations are accepted as bedrock causes of health risks with which they are associated, and, therefore, do not prompt a search for further explanation. Smaje (1996) argues that, although epidemiologists and clinicians have provided an impressive set of findings about ethnic differences, they have been less concerned to fully consider the social significance of their findings. Explicit consideration of race/ethnic variables in the interpretation of results is hampered by the methodological limitations outlined above. Biological reductionist and/or culturalist explanations of ethnic variations in health status are accepted uncritically.

Sheldon and Parker (1992) argue that 'culture' is often inadequately operationalised in health research, and is reduced stereotypically to issues such as diet, religious practice, mourning rituals and contraceptive practice, etc. The work of Qureshi (1989, p. 4) illustrates this tendency when he asserts that *'Muslims, Jews, and Buddhists (Chinese) do not practise a social class or caste system.'* Cultural stereotyping continues to be evident within medical literature. For instance Gartrad (1994, p. 170) claims, of Muslims, that *'Their commitment to religion is deep rooted and adherence is taken seriously,'* and that *'Generally, the birth of a boy is welcomed much more than that of a girl, as boys tend to remain with their parents and carry on the business in the family name'* (Gartrad, 1994, p. 171). This last quotation offers three stereotypes for the price of one, based around ethnicity, gender and economic activity. In summary, Sheldon and Parker (1992, p. 104) suggest that:

*Health research appears to be reflecting the process of racialisation ... whereby the idea of race or ethnicity is increasingly being introduced to help define or give meaning to the population.*

The rest of this chapter considers health professional practice with respect to ethnicity and risk, and explores alternative, cultural insider perspectives. It is contended that the racialisation of risk results not only from methodological drift towards the use of racial indicators, but also pervades the day-to-day realities of professional practice.

## Responses of health-care professions to ethnic diversity

### VICTIM-BLAMING, CULTURAL STEREOTYPES AND RISK ATTRIBUTION

The charge of victim-blaming for health problems among certain ethnic groups has often been levelled. Donovan (1984) cites various examples of the ways in which 'minority ethnic' individuals or their cultures have been blamed for poor health outcomes. Donovan suggested, at that time, that research had largely ignored the views of ethnic populations, and had been mainly preoccupied with conditions believed to affect specific ethnic groups, like sickle-cell anaemia in relation to African-Caribbeans, or rickets in relation to people of Asian descent, as already noted. Donovan argued that this victim-blaming approach isolated ethnic individuals and groups, framing them as problematic. Proffered solutions ethnocentrically require individuals to change their behaviour so as to conform to the norms of the White European majority. More recent research illustrates this process of assigning responsibility to individuals or groups.

Bowler (1993) conducted a small-scale ethnographic study investigating South Asian women's maternity experiences in a British hospital, and midwives' stereotypes of the women. An important theme which emerged from the data was that of communication difficulties. Professionals often held the women responsible for such problems. For example, one midwife (Bowler, 1993, p. 160) felt that it was *'disgusting not to speak English after so long in Britain'.* Another important theme was lack of compliance with care, for example poor attendance to antenatal and parent-craft appointments. At least some of this 'poor attendance' could be attributed to communication difficulties, including the women's names being read out wrongly in outpatient departments.

The same study provides a highly instructive example of risk calculation based on stereotypes. The women in the study were often labelled as attention-seeking, and as having low pain thresholds, which professionals saw at odds with the often short labours the women experienced. However, shorter labour times are associated with high parity (number of previous deliveries). Bowler points out that Asian women are, currently, more fertile than other ethnic groups, and so more likely to experience rapid labour because of their higher average parity. Health professionals may confound parity with ethnicity, and see rapid delivery as a 'racial' characteristic of Asian women. Bowler (1993, p. 168) cites a midwife in the study as saying, of an Asian women who had been taken to the delivery suite:   *'Oh, she'll be back in an hour, they're always quick.'*

However, this woman was having her first baby and the birth had been induced, both indicators of the longer labour which actually took place. As argued in Chapter 2, such risk-reasoning entails the ecological fallacy since characteristics of a population – higher average parity and lower delivery time – were attributed to an individual. Although causally erroneous, such reasoning is actuarially justified because, on average, Asian women will, currently, experience the lower risk of an extended labour. The midwife's grouping of Asian women, rather than women of low parity, for predictive purposes had clearly racist undertones.

## Lay cultural approaches to health risks

### LAY CULTURAL PERCEPTION OF HEALTH RISK

Several studies have explored the perceptions of members of ethnic groups about health and health beliefs. Howlett, Ahmad and Murray (1992) utilised a secondary data set from *The Health and Lifestyle Survey* (Blaxter, 1990) in an exploratory study. Asian and African-Caribbean cases were identified from the data, and matched controls selected from White European respondents. Analysis focused on concepts of health and illness, and illness causation. Comparisons suggested that, in terms of their health concepts, White respondents were more likely than Asians to emphasise physical energy, while Asians gave functional definitions of health more frequently. African-Caribbeans were more likely than Whites to mention physical energy and strength, but less likely to focus on functional issues.

Asians and African-Caribbeans more frequently explained health outcomes in terms of luck or fatalism than did Whites. Howlett, Ahmad and Murray (1992) argue that this difference, also found by Donovan (1986), might reflect greater experience of powerlessness among socially disadvantaged groups, rather than directly cultural differences. Howlett, Ahmad and Murray (1992) concluded that, in general, similarities between ethnic groups outweighed differences. They also noted that health-promotion messages about specific problems, for example smoking, were not having as much impact on the Asian and African-Caribbean communities as on Whites, perhaps because of communication problems.

### LAY CULTURAL MANAGEMENT OF HEALTH RISK

Specific ways of understanding health problems are related to particular ways of managing them, for example through the often cited, and complex, system of beliefs concerning 'hot' and 'cold' foods and medicines (Manderson, 1987) which may be used to correct a perceived imbalance, ameliorate discomfort, or treat an illness. As noted in Chapter 18, Ayuverdic medicine, unlike its Western counterpart, attempts to heal the mind and the spirit, as well as the body.

Bhopal (1986) examined the interrelationship between 'traditional' and Western medicine in an Asian community in Glasgow. A sample of Asians were interviewed, and samples of GPs and health-visitors completed a questionnaire. The study aimed to establish the role of traditional medicine in the Asian community, and to assess professional understanding of Asian medicine. Asians showed a high level of knowledge about herbal remedies, the Asian Healer and the theory of hot and cold foods. Culinary ingredients were frequently used to treat, for example, abdominal discomfort, earache and toothache. Asian respondents regarded the medicinal use of culinary ingredients as convenient, safe, inexpensive and effective.

Bhopal (1986) found little awareness or knowledge of Asian medicines, beliefs and practices among health professionals. He identified a number of barriers to the take-up of Asian medicine by Asians in a British context, such as the lack of availability of medicinal ingredients, and health-establishment disapproval. On the other hand, interest in alternative therapies is increasing in the wider community, waiting-lists create a barrier preventing the use of conventional health care, and well-established Asian communities can offer a stock of knowledge about traditional remedies.

The perspectives of members of ethnic groups need to be considered in relation to the dynamics of relationships between first generation immigrants and those that follow. Ahmad (1992) has suggested that a 'gradient' of cultural health beliefs and practices may exist between first and subsequent generations of immigrant settlers. The process of integration may create problems of survival for ethnic cultures. Anwar (1986) has argued that children of Asian parents born or brought up in Britain are caught between two cultures: that of the home, dominated by their parents' culture, and that of work, school and neighbourhood. Anwar suggests that stress and conflict, with their associated health risks, are inevitable, given the potential for social and psychological gaps over such issues as the family, religion, dress, marriage and personal freedom.

Two methodological difficulties arise in research concerned with 'alternative' health philosophy and practice. First, researchers may be seen as representatives of the dominant Western system, and so as implicitly or explicitly disapproving. Underreporting of health activities which do not conform to the tenets of Western medicine may result. Researchers who are not immersed in the philosophy underlying such practices may even lack the ontological underpinnings needed to understand them. Second, ethnic communities have been examined in a fragmented way, making replication difficult. However, it should not be assumed that non-Western health practices are stagnant. The work of Bhopal (1986), Anwar (1986) and Ahmad (1992) points towards a degree of intergenerational flux as well as cultural exchanges with the wider society.

## ALTERNATIVE CULTURAL PRACTITIONERS AND ALTERNATIVE CATEGORISATION SYSTEMS

### The Hakim

Ahmad (1992) discusses what he sees as Western medicine's hegemony over definitions of health and disease, in relation to a particular type of Asian healer, the Hakim. A Hakim is known within his own culture as a scholarly and wise healer. The Hakim go beyond pathology and psychology, to encompass familial, societal and religio-spiritual aspects of the individual. The Hakim's diagnostic procedures may seem 'low tech' from a Western perspective, as they are based on pulse, urine, examination of faeces, etc., and place a strong emphasis on case history. Ahmad argues that the hot and cold concepts (Manderson, 1987) which the Hakim draws upon, are not entirely alien to White British populations, though they remain largely unacknowledged contemporary medical wisdom.

Little research has been done on the use of Hakims in the UK, but there may be some resident Hakims in the UK. Visiting Hakims are consulted here, and individuals see them when visiting India and Pakistan. Ahmad discusses criticisms of the Hakim's practice from the perspective of Western medicine, particularly the use of lead and arsenic, and concern that coinvolvement of Hakim and general practitioner might engender conflict and danger. However, Ahmad points out that Western medicine can be criticised as a form of social control which is patriarchal, capitalist/exploitative and imperialistic. He argues that scientific evaluation of the Hakim's practice is difficult, given the more holistic nature of its focus, and the impossibility of assessing its value through random control trials. Ahmad concludes that a more workable interface between Western and alternative therapies, which would not marginalise or demonise the practice of Hakims as healers, could be developed.

## THE SINKING HEART

An interesting case example of a health disorder defined within a minority ethnic community is provided by Krause (1989), who discusses the concept of the sinking heart which he found in use among the Punjabi community in Bedford. This condition involves an illness in which physical sensations in the heart or the chest are experienced. These symptoms are believed to result from excessive heat, exhaustion, worry or social failure. Krause compares this concept with Western notions of depression, medical models of heart distress and type A behaviour patterns related to stress. He argues that sinking heart does not match any of these notions. It compares most closely to psychosocial explanatory models of stress, but only in form rather than content.

One problem in equating the Western notion of depression with sinking heart is that the concept of hopelessness does not have the same meaning for first-generation Punjabis as for Westerners. The Punjabi notion links such feelings explicitly to the heart. Diagnosing depression is likely to be counterproductive with this group, since Punjabis associate depression with self-centredness. Similarly, a diagnosis of heart disorder ignores the emotional aspects of sinking heart. This condition, as understood by Punjabis, thus falls between Western categories, and differs from them qualitatively.

## POTENTIAL CONFLICTS IN PHILOSOPHIES UNDERPINNING PRACTICE

Anderson, Elfert and Lai (1989) explored the tension between health-care ideologies and ethnic belief systems. They compared the impact of chronic illness in children on Chinese and Anglo-Canadian families. They argue that the ideology of normalisation which underpins Western health-care practices for people with disabilities may not be shared in other cultures.

The quotations given below (Anderson, Elfert and Lai, 1989, pp. 252–3) illustrate the difference in perspective between the above ethnic groups.

*He is to us now a normal child ... We just treat him normally. This is the best way to look at it ... because if you are going to worry about it I think you can cause harm to the child, and that is not good for the child.* (Anglo-Canadian mother)

*A lot of parents as a general rule don't accept that the child is not normal, and they try hard to make the child normal, but eventually they are going to have to accept the fact that they aren't.* (Chinese mother)

Anderson, Elfert and Lai (1989, p. 269) argue that divergence in understanding disability may result from historical, socioeconomic and political differences rather than culture *per se*.

*What may be regarded as due to cultural differences, then, may not be a function of culture as much as the economic situation of the family, their immigrant status and feeling of uncertainty about the future, and their concern with survival in a new country.*

The Chinese concept of normalisation is based on the idea that a normal child has the capacity to earn a living, and thus sustain a future. In consequence, Chinese families may be less interested in striving for normality through physical rehabilitation, and less motivated to participate in therapy. The Chinese concept of normality may be at odds with the prevalent ideology of normalisation, with the result that the professionals view the family as non-compliant.

## Discussion

This chapter has explored some fundamental mismatches between the health-related rationalities of different cultures. Anderson, Elfert and Lai (1989) show how the ideologies which underpin Western professional practice can be at odds with those of minority client groups. Krause (1989), in exploring the Punjabi concept of sinking heart, illustrates the way in which Western categorisation systems can fail to encompass conditions which are taken for granted within a specific cultural group. It has been argued here that these mismatches in risk assessment and management are underpinned at the most fundamental ontological level. Much of the research reviewed shows how differing world views can generate intercultural incomprehension. In many instances, cultural mismatch appears to result in victim-blaming practices, with MEGs discursively constructed by professionals as fundamentally responsible for their own health disadvantages. Ethnic and racial categories provide all-too-convenient groupings for probabilistic inference, a heuristic device which requires acceptance of the ecological fallacy, through attribution of the characteristics of a category of people to individuals.

The treatment of particular MEGs as homogenous discounts differences within them (Sheldon and Parker, 1992). Cultural groups within late modern societies are synchronic and permeable, in states of constant transition fuelled by intergenerational changes in practices and the cross-cultural exchange of ideas. Howlett, Ahmad and Murray (1992) concluded that, although differences in health attitudes and beliefs between ethnic groups can be identified, similarities were more noticeable. Some apparently cultural differences may result from socioeconomic differences. For example, fatalistic attitudes may be fuelled by poverty-related experiences of social powerlessness. Similarly, institutional responses towards ethnically bound health risks are unlikely to remain static, given the degree of institutional reflexivity present in late modern societies.

Smaje (1996) argues that health-care professionals who seek to become more ethnically sensitive could begin to address the methodological difficulties involved in researching ethnicity, health and risk. Much research into minority cultures occurs in geographically isolated subpopulations (Bhopal, 1986; Donovan, 1986; Krause, 1989). Findings cannot be generalised to other ethnic groups. Researchers who are seen as representing the dominant professional system may find it difficult to access insider perspectives from within other cultural groups. Their members are likely to have experienced disapproval of health-related practices which do not fit with the prevailing medical approach (Ahmad, 1992; Bhopal, 1986). Social desirability effects and the underreporting of such practices can be expected. Smaje (1996) identifies three critical issues of methodology. First, the validity of ethnic categories can be questioned, since the fluidity of a multicultural society makes any classification scheme problematic. Second, as already noted, ethnic differences may be confounded with other sources of variation, for example in socioeconomic status. Third, Smaje emphasises the value of ethnographic research approaches to the investigation of ethnicity and health.

Given the changing situation of ethnic groups in the UK, research conclusions about the relationships between health and ethnicity must be treated with caution. Findings will need to be subjected to constant revision. This chapter has suggested that current UK health-care approaches to attributing health risks to people from MEGs, and responses to their own health-belief systems, incorporate wider discriminatory attitudes and negative stereotypes.

# Risk imagery and the AIDS epidemic

## Mike Kingham

## Introduction

Every health risk has an associated range of cultural and historical symbolic representations. In this chapter, a number of theoretical problems will be pursued with respect to the translation of risk into visual analogues and metaphor systems (Sontag, 1984, 1989; Chaplin 1994). Throughout, the term 'image' will be used as shorthand for the non-literal encoding of a health risk in visual and/or verbal form. The term will, thus, encompass cartoons, jokes, dramas, symbols and artefacts.

To understand a health risk, we need to be able to decode the various means through which it is made culturally visible. In the modern world, lay and professional people construct images, and transmit them through cultural artefacts, such as stories, jokes, photographs, graphics, artwork, poster campaigns, badges, television and film. This chapter examines the history of jokes and cartoons associated with the AIDS epidemic. It is argued that members of a social group understand risk through powerful, culturally created images. This approach counterbalances a quantitative 'science' of risk which implicitly devalues the emotional and the aesthetic.

Health-related risks other than AIDS, equally, have their own associated imagery. For example, driving safety campaigns provide powerful, graphic depictions of the carnage, mutilation and suffering caused by various forms of road accident. Their risk messages are usually encoded in a dramatic form, based on real incidents, and accompanied by a jarring soundtrack. The make-up and special effect artists employed to bring 'realism' to these campaigns, have often, ironically, worked on the production of commercial horror films.

Newspapers, television media and billboard sites are used for large-scale campaigns concerned with advising the public how to manage an assortment of health-related risks, such as smoking, drinking and driving, and safe sex. Citizens in the 'Risk Society' (Beck, 1992) live in an iconographic landscape of risk imagery. Safety is maintained and policed by 'the world's largest industry' (Adams, 1995, p. 31), which includes the army, police, fire and ambulance services and those who define and enforce building and transport regulations. Increasingly, the work of health and social service personnel is concerned with risk management, for example in child protection (Chapter 16), health promotion (Chapter 18) and nursing (Chapters 13–15).

Adams (1995) estimates that the risk industry employs 1.5 million people in Britain alone. The professional groups concerned with safety produce sales brochures, advice leaflets and poster campaigns. All lobby for government and public attention, using carefully designed promotional and media material which employ pictures and graphics at least as much as text. Powerful and provocatively constructed imagery, manufactured by the public relations industry, draw our attention to potential risks.

The chapter addresses the following questions through historical analysis of images, primarily jokes and cartoons, produced in response to the AIDS crisis. Who constructs risk imagery and for what purposes? What are the social and psychological functions of the imagery? Are there patterns and sequences in risk imagery?

## Subcultures and the production of imagery

In analysing risk imagery, it is important to locate its genesis. Who produces the imagery, and why? As a social phenomenon, AIDS illuminates the symbolic boundaries used to differentiate human beings from one another. 'They' have AIDS. 'We' do not. AIDS is regarded as a disease of this or that group: for example gay men, intravenous drug-users, people of colour, and their involvement with this or that behaviour, such as the injection of illicit substances or deviant sexual practices.

Since the mid-1980s, social groups have organised in response to the symbolic boundaries erected to marginalise the AIDS-afflicted. Some have used cultural objects which possess shared meanings as tools with which to dramatise, challenge and transform the stigma of AIDS. For example, one of the most visible American groups, AIDS Coalition to Unleash Power (ACT UP), has annexed the pink triangle: the symbol used initially by the Nazis to identify interned homosexuals, and later taken up by the international gay rights movement as a marker of solidarity.

Attention must also be paid to images produced by expert professionals, assisted by advertising and public relations specialists, often on behalf of the government. The status and power of a particular expert group may enable them to identify and frame the nature of a risk, and thus influence the information and imagery that is produced 'in the public interest'.

AIDS health-information campaigns initiated by activist and government agencies have differed markedly. The Terrence Higgins Trust, a charitable organisation which worked initially on behalf of the gay community, decided that AIDS-information leaflets should be colloquial, blunt, direct and uncompromising about safe sex. One of their earliest safe sex leaflets 'illustrated' aspects of safe sex with pictures of condoms, lubricants and sexual toys. The leaflet talked explicitly of *'sucking and fucking'*. In contrast, government agencies were concerned not only with communicating 'technical' information about AIDS-risk factors, but with the question of how to inform without creating public offence, or appearing to encourage 'immoral' behaviour. The earliest government campaigns described sexual activities in technical jargon. Full-page campaigns in national newspapers were produced in black and white text, and without graphics. The information given was complex and detailed.

A political dimension surrounded the first national TV campaigns, *'Iceberg'* and *'Don't die of ignorance'*, which ran in 1987. When the first cuts of the films were shown to Norman Fowler, Secretary of State at the Department of Health and Social Security, he objected to both their content and their style. The films were recut and then presented to the Whitelaw Committee, which was co-ordinating the government's AIDS strategy. The copy was simplified, a drill sequence altered to avoid any suggestion of innuendo, and references to condoms were removed. This toning-down of the campaign attracted criticism. An advertising executive, Romola Christopherson, commented that the copy for the *'Don't die of ignorance'* campaign *'smacked of being a product of a concerned bureaucracy'* (*Body Positive Newsletter*, 30/07/89). The Conservative government faced the political dilemma that they could not use vivid imagery to hammer home the AIDS safety message without, in their own terms, appearing to endorse behaviour which challenged their notions of family values. In relation to the ideas discussed in Chapter 2, the government sought to avoid inadvertently switching on a sexual risk escalator.

In contrast, subsequent anti-drugs/AIDS campaigns had a stronger visual impact. Press and poster campaigns used street language, such as 'smack' and 'fix', showed bloody needles, scarred arms and the dirt, grime and general seediness associated with the drug culture. War photographers Don McCullin and Clive Arrowsmith produced powerfully realistic visual images. The slogan accompanying this 1988 campaign stated *'It only takes one prick to give you AIDS.'* In spite of the strength of the imagery and the irony of this slogan (an alternative reading of the slang 'prick' in relation to the sexual transmission of AIDS), the Whitelaw Committee allowed the campaign to proceed.

Whether the communication of health risks is undertaken by street-level activists, newspaper journalists, or expert groups working officially, they all have to communicate their messages powerfully and effectively. For any given campaign the audience will reflect, in retrospect, on the information and imagery that were used. An interesting research question concerns the alternative campaigns that were considered. A hidden history of censorship, editorial license and alternative decision-making underlies any creative enterprise. What imagery and information were left on the cutting-room floor? Who left it there, and why?

# Risk imagery and the AIDS epidemic

This section examines the imagery that has come to be associated with the AIDS epidemic in more detail. Dreuilhe (1987, p. 20) encapsulates the fear triggered by the AIDS epidemic.

> The Earth quaked, and the shock waves of AIDS awakened monsters from the depths of our collective imagination, monsters of a species we had long thought extinct. This plague has attracted the inevitable swarm of AIDS researchers, officials, businessmen, and journalists, and they are the ones who have monopolised the media. We people with AIDS, who devote every waking moment to our own survival, have been unable to prevent those loquacious experts from stealing our thunder and robbing us of the only thing we have left: our illness.

Why should AIDS awake monsters from the depths of our collective imagination? Western, science-based, societies have not experienced the full impact of 'plague' for many centuries. Before the epidemic, they had become confident that high living standards, the development of public health schemes and advances in medical technology had banished mass killer infectious diseases permanently. However, our historical imagination conjures up powerful images of the plagues of old, of rats, pestilence, pockmarked bodies, and strictly enforced quarantines.

The AIDS epidemic arrived at a moment in history when sex was thought to be relatively safe, liberated through the sexual revolution of the 1960s, and the political battles fought by feminist and gay activists. But, at the same time, many people continued to be morally concerned about sexual behaviour. As a senior civil servant, quoted in the *Sunday Times Magazine* in 1987, commented on the Thatcher Cabinet *'What is the point in talking about AIDS to people who don't believe in sex anyway?'* With sex and fear as key ingredients, AIDS became a battleground for the competing views of the state, scientists, activists, self-help groups and the general public.

An epidemic caused by a new and deadly virus, with an identified set of risk factors and risk groups, emerged at the same time as powerful new media, such as satellite and the internet. AIDS has received more scientific, media and popular attention than any other disease in history. Heightened social, political and media concern, in the 1980s, led to the generation of an extraordinarily rich and complex set of AIDS imagery. The rest of this section briefly reviews some of this material, providing a context for the historical analysis of AIDS humour which follows.

## SYMBOLS AND SYMBOLIC ACTION

AIDS campaigners have used a range of symbolic devices to enhance social awareness of the disease. The red AIDS ribbon offers a remembrance of those who have died, and those still suffering. The ribbon provides a warning symbol and a reminder of the need to practise safe sex. It is used on National AIDS day (another symbolic marker), and has a strong cultural resonance with the Red Poppy used to commemorate the war dead. The ribbons and metal badges are sold throughout Britain.

Numerous AIDS action and support groups have created their own symbols by using T-shirts with special messages about HIV risks. The messages range from simple information about using condoms to the provocative defence of sexual preferences and sexual rights, such as 'You call it sodomy, we call it fabulous.' In the 1980s the Body Positive group created its own badge which said simply 'I am Body positive.' The badges allowed individuals to acknowledge their HIV status, and maintain a positive group identity in the face of public prejudice.

Mueller (1995) discusses the symbolic importance of the 'Quilt Campaign'. Gay rights activist, Cleve Jones, joined other marchers in tacking placards adorned with the names of persons who had died of AIDS on to the wall of a Federal building. From a distance, Jones was reminded of a patchwork quilt which evoked 'such warm old memories of comfort' (Mueller, 1995, p. 6). Inspired by a Biblical passage, 'Take care of a good name, for this shall continue with thee, more than a thousand treasures precious and great' (Ecclesiastes, 41), Jones created the NAMES Project Quilt.

Mueller observes that Jones constructed the first NAMES quilt panel to honour the memory of his best friend, Marvin Feldman. She notes that it was designed to represent the two defining statuses of his friend's life: his Jewishness and his homosexuality. Feldman's name was displayed against a background of triangles, the Nazi symbol for homosexuality, and the Star of David. Reflecting on the experience of fabricating a quilt panel for his friend, Jones felt that his 'grief had been replaced by a sense of resolution and completion' (Ruskin, 1987, p. 18). Jones recognised that, by including the range of people who had been affected by AIDS, the NAMES quilt could serve to not only relieve personal grief, but to transform prejudices between gays and straights.

Panels in the quilt memorialise people of all ages, genders, ethnicities, races and sexual orientations. By 1992 the quilt had grown to 20 064 panels. It is now exhibited all over the world. Mueller observes 'that the quilt was able to marshal the aesthetics of the mourning quilt as an expression of personal grief and an artistic rendering of deceased individuals and expand it to that of a national political symbol of deviance disavowal and the universality of AIDS' (Mueller, 1995, p. 9).

## AIDS AND THE MASS MEDIA

### News reporting

Television and newspaper reporting of health risks are far from neutral. In the early years of the epidemic, AIDS information and imagery were carefully selected for maximum public impact, and helped to shape some of the homophobic and prejudicial attitudes that surround the disease. Early imagery concentrated on the fear surrounding different ways of contracting the virus. (In this period, the means of transmission were not firmly established.) Pictures and stories portrayed a vicar wiping the chalice during communion, the Football Association banning kissing and cuddling on the pitch, the emergency services worrying over giving the kiss of life, and moves to ban gay blood-donors.

Television news depends more on striking visual images than do the print media (Chapman and Lupton, 1994). A story will rarely make the television news unless accompanied by visually compelling images. Although the print media do not rely quite so much on images, many news stories, particularly those on the front page, include visual images. News magazines use colourful photographs, graphs, or other visual representations to illustrate their stories.

Chapman and Lupton (1994) argue that, in the analysis of media coverage, attention should be paid to the choice of visual images and the messages they communicate. Headlines, a specific genre of news-writing, eschew the conventions of the orthodox sentence by presenting the crux of the new story in as few words as possible in an attempt to attract readers' attention. The careful selection of nouns and verbs, rhetorical devices such as alliteration, punning, metaphors, references to other discourses, and the creative use of a restricted lexicon make headlines a fascinating element of news language.

The imperatives of journalism rest on drama, controversy, conflict, human interest and brevity. As a result the complexities of medical research or health risks are often simplified, trivialised or distorted. AIDS headlines, such as 'AIDS is a potential Holocaust' (Sunday Mail, 22 March 1987) and 'AIDS came in on Skytrain' (Sun, 23 April 1985), powerfully combine myth with sensationalism. Even an advertising group used AIDS imagery in promotional campaigns for their products. The controversial Benetton clothing advertisement showed the skeletal picture of a young man dying from AIDS and being cradled by his father.

## Film and theatre drama

The cinema and theatre have always played an important part in engaging the public in 'sickness dramas'. Television plays like *Casualty* bring the everyday life of hospitals into the homes of millions of viewers. Film drama has explored mental illness (*One Flew Over the Cuckoo's Nest*), disability (*My Left Foot*), terminal illness (*Whose Life is it Anyway?*) and many other conditions.

A distinctive genre of AIDS dramas have been produced for cinema and TV. They have dealt with the problems of living with a stigmatised condition, and examined the social and emotional consequences of AIDS in a powerful way. Films like *'The Normal Heart'* and *'The Lie'* have explored both homosexual and heterosexual responses to becoming HIV positive. In 1993, Tom Hanks was awarded an Oscar for his portrayal of an AIDS victim in the film *Philadelphia*. The content and imagery of these films attract the attention of a mass audience, and provide another important vehicle for defining the cultural meaning of AIDS.

## Stars

An important element of media-reporting has been the attention given to celebrities who contracted the HIV virus. Gossip about the homes, love affairs and lifestyles of the rich and famous sells newspapers and magazines. AIDS has claimed, among others, Liberace, Rock Hudson, Arthur Ashe, Rudolph Nureyev and Freddie Mercury. Their illnesses and deaths have ensured that other celebrities have taken up the AIDS cause. Elizabeth Taylor has raised funds for AIDS research, and the Hollywood film industry has set up many charity benefits. Some celebrities have denied their HIV status, and tried to withdraw from the media gaze. Others, however, have spoken publicly at press conferences, thus helping to fight prejudice.

### The virus as an image

The virus itself has become an icon of the 1980s, a cultural marker of the history of the human race in the last 15 years. Language and imagery associated with classifications of the virus and its manifestations, for example, HIV, T-Helper Cells, immune reaction, Kaposi's Sarcoma, has emerged. An image of the virus has been frequently used in health-promotion literature, and has often appeared as a graphic in the background of news bulletins. In the allegedly therapeutic process of visualisation, people with HIV are helped to visualise their virus, to see their T-helper cells, and to think positively about their condition.

Political battles have raged over the 'discovery' of the virus, and the rights to patent antibody tests. International pharmaceutical companies and scientific groups have sought funding for research into the virus, and the WHO has its own international AIDS division. Images of the virus are locked into our consciousness in a way associated with few other diseases.

## METAPHORICAL UNDERSTANDING OF THE AIDS EPIDEMIC

Our thinking about AIDS risks is strongly influenced by metaphorical imagery embedded in the language we use. Sontag (1989) commented on the use of military, science-fiction, Biblical, invasion, assault, plague and punishment metaphors to give AIDS meaning. Ross (1989) analysed AIDS-reporting in the American press during the early 1980s, and identified six main metaphors: AIDS as a plague; AIDS as death; AIDS as a punishment for sin; AIDS as a crime; the battle against AIDS; and the AIDS sufferer as unknown stranger. Lupton (1994b) notes the way in which the Australian press linked AIDS with homosexuality, through notions like the 'gay plague' and the 'gay killer germ'.

Watney (1989, pp. 64–73) distinguished between two types of AIDS imagery. In the 'terrorist model', HIV is conceptualised as an 'external invader, an illegal immigrant shinning up the white cliffs of Dover'. This model condones the use of HIV antibody-testing as a means of identifying the unseen invader before it can enter and destroy. The 'missionary model' treats HIV infection as a 'heathen entity, strange and exotic, thriving on immorality, bestiality, unnatural acts and ungodly practices'. Watney argues that this model invites a return to Judaeo-Christian values and their attendant institutions: Church, marriage and the family.

Media accounts of AIDS have frequently invoked the metaphorical discourses of discrimination, prurience, racism and stigmatisation, with an associated imagery of plague, sin, deviance, divine retribution, apocalypse and holocaust. All these images served to create a sense of panic, and incite vilification of people with, or deemed at high risk of, HIV infection. Kroker and

Kroker (1988) draw parallels between the fear of AIDS and a generalised fear of the breakdown of immunological systems. They also note a striking resemblance between the medical discourse surrounding AIDS and military rhetoric.

In the early years (1981–86) of AIDS-reporting, risk, in Western societies at least, was seen as centring around a specific and contained threat to reviled deviant outgroups. When the epidemiology began to suggest a threat to heterosexual populations, national AIDS-information campaigns were mobilised in a discourse which extended potential risk wholesale to every individual, regardless of their sexual proclivities.

In 1987, the British government launched its 'Iceberg' campaign, metaphorically indicating that, like an iceberg, the AIDS threat to the population was two-thirds hidden under the water. Also in 1987, the Australian government launched its 'Grim Reaper' campaign. Lupton (1994b, p. 52) notes that this campaign:

> drew heavily upon medieval and horror movie imagery, portraying the grim reaper, a horrifyingly skeletal and skull-headed figure swathed in a black hood carrying a scythe and (incongruously) a bowling ball. Instead of ten pins, a collection of stereotypes representing the diversity of 'ordinary' Australians were knocked down (killed) by the huge bowling ball aimed by the figure of death. The intention was to render the abstract notions of death, danger and risk more familiar and to demonstrate that people are like ten-pins before AIDS, vulnerable and powerless to protect themselves.

The period since 1991, which has been characterised by a lack of media concern with the disease, and by an associated decline of metaphor, is considered at the end of the chapter.

To summarise, metaphor allows us not only to convey meaning verbally, but to conceptualise the world (Lakoff and Johnson, 1981). Metaphors operate systematically, invoking related categories. They work through association, with objects or concepts joined by their similarities rather than their differences. The establishment of such associations relies on shared knowledge and belief systems. Metaphor, therefore, does not manifest itself at the level of the word, but at the level of discourse. Metaphorical activity, like that surrounding AIDS, occurs around sites of difference. It is used in power struggles which involve ideological contention between competing value systems.

## AIDS risk imagery in jokes and humour: A case study

The risk imagery to be examined in more detail below is drawn from AIDS jokes and cartoons. Theoretical studies have shown that jokes are a serious business. We make jokes about the things that threaten us. In a classic paper, Radcliffe-Brown (1965) demonstrated that jokes are to be found at the tension points in human relationships. Jokes about 'Blacks', the Irish, women and homosexuals are concerned with categories of human being who potentially threaten a prevailing social order. Homosexuals, for example, challenge naturalistic assumptions about sexual relationships. The joke provides a form of social control, a put-down used to keep people in their place. The old adage that *'sticks and stones may break my bones, but words will never hurt me'* does not stand up to close inspection.

An extensive 'sick humour' genre can be found in Western cultures. Jokes have been made about cripples, leprosy, venereal disease, spastics, thalidomide and death itself. By joking, we seek to make light of our fears. The AIDS epidemic has produced an extensive range of jokes and humour. The author has systematically collected examples for the period between 1982 and 1990. The material came from oral street humour, graffiti, cartoons in newspapers and magazines, and the jokes of professional comedians.

More than 600 oral jokes and cartoons were obtained for this study. Only a small sample will be used in the text, as illustrative examples. Each piece of humour was dated, where possible, and chronologically filed. A content analysis of the risk imagery in the material was undertaken, and a grounded theory technique (Strauss and Corbin, 1990) used to examine changes in the pattern of the humour over time. This analysis of a 'historical sequence' of AIDS risks as represented in humour has been heavily influenced by Obrdlik's (1942) study of humour in the Polish response to the Nazi occupation of their country

## AIDS RISK IMAGERY IN HUMOUR: A FOUR-STAGE HISTORICAL MODEL

Table 4.1 identifies four chronologically distinct stages of societal reaction to the AIDS epidemic. These reactions are linked to, but analytically distinct from, shifting epidemiological assessments both of the incidence of the disease, and of its modes of transmission.

### Stage 1: The isolation stage (1981–1983)

In this early phase, the 'known' epidemiology for AIDS was firmly associated with 'deviant' groups. Jokes were targeted against heroin addicts, homosexuals, haemophiliacs and Haitians. This early period is characterised by oral humour and street-level jokes in the form of vicious one-line barbs. They functioned as a boundary marker between the normal healthy heterosexual and the diseased deviant. Common in our culture, they circulate in pubs, clubs and playgrounds, and are used by 'stand-up' comedians (see Figure 4.1). Similar types of jokes have been made about thalidomide and polio victims.

**Table 4.1**  AIDS humour: A four-stage historical model

| Stage | Period | Target | Joke type |
| --- | --- | --- | --- |
| Isolation | 1981–1983 | Them (deviants) | Outsiders |
| Transition | 1983–1987 | Possibly us | Relationships |
| Strategic response | 1987–1991 | Us (heterosexuals) | Policy |
| Indifference | 1991– | The distant threat | The jokes stop |

Gay = Got Aids Yet

Aids = Wogs (Wrath of God Syndrome)

Gay rights = AIDS

**Question:** How do you get AIDS?
Answer:   One poof and you're dead.

**Question:** What's the hardest thing about getting AIDS?
Answer:   Trying to convince your parents and friends that you're Haitian.

**Question:** What kind of pricks give you AIDS?
Answer:   Needle pricks.

**Question:** What's the medical definition of AIDS?
Answer:   A disease that turns fruits into vegetables.

**Figure 4.1**   Examples of street jokes and graffiti

In most cases, the jokes operate via linguistic devices such as punning, spoonerisms and paraphasia. The answer to the question *'How do you get AIDS?'* relies on the hearer of the joke making a number of connections: that POOF (a slang word for homosexual) sounds like PUFF (smoking a ciga-rette); and that AIDS is associated with homosexuality in the same way that smoking is linked to lung cancer. The 'pricks' joke fuses attack on sexual licence and intravenous drug-taking, thus connecting the two kinds of deviance presumed to have caused the epidemic. Other forms of joke oper-ate by drawing attention to problematic or ambiguous forms of identity. For example, the answer to the question *'What's the hardest thing about getting AIDS?'* suggests that being a heterosexual Haitian is less stigmatising than being homosexual.

The acronym examples which head the list in Figure 4.1, e.g. AIDS=Wogs, often originated in 'writing on the wall', sprayed as a form of graffiti-like social comment. These acronyms are particularly insidious. In the example above, AIDS is simultaneously associated with people of colour (wog being a racist epithet) and punishment from God for 'deviant' sexual behaviour. This acronym reflects the *'missionary metaphor'* identified by Watney (1989) and discussed above.

These early jokes, though simple in form, contained powerful and cruel put-downs, targeted at deviant outsiders. They served the social function of distancing AIDS victims from the rest of civil society. The jokes operate on the imagination by conjuring up and reinforcing conventional prejudices. They do not invite any rational, critical or sympathetic response from the listener, and close-down the possibility of a measured and informed understanding of AIDS risks. The jokes themselves do not come out of a social vacuum, but draw on the myths and prejudices encapsulated in the early reporting of the epidemic by tabloid news-papers. This early reporting itself contributed to the homophobic panic reaction to AIDS.

## Stage 2: The transition stage (1983–1987)

In this period, the virus was perceived to be spreading from deviant groups, and to be threatening the heterosexual population. Jokes and imagery centred on specific risk factors and problematic relationships, rather than on risk groups. The science of the virus was at an early stage. Modes of transmission were not firmly established, and explanatory schema centred on the risks associated with the exchange of body fluids such as semen, saliva and blood.

These fears and anxieties were amplified by the tabloid press. The news media were saturated with picture-based stories of risk contexts. On 25 November 1986, for example, Pendennis reported in the *Guardian* that the Labour MP Harry Cohen had tabled a question in Parliament about the safety of French kissing in the light of all the AIDS scares. The Table Office in the House of Commons would not allow the use of the expression French kissing, and substituted the technical phrase *'oral osculation'*. Inevitably, numerous jokes about 'osculating' in public were soon circulating.

A similar range of pictures and stories were used to dramatise contact with infected blood. It was well known, at this stage, that haemophiliacs had contracted the virus from contaminated blood-plasma products. Pictures and stories covered the possible everyday risk of infection associated with hospital injections, dentistry, acupuncture, tattooing, ear-piercing, and contact with accident victims. One story raised the possibility that a visit to the hairdressers entailed risk. On 5 October 1986, the *Observer* carried a story with the headline *'The Unkindest Cut'* about a barber in Tewkesbury who asked customers to stick their heads in a dustbin full of disinfectant before entering his shop. He was responding to a story in the *Gloustershire Echo* which revealed that health officials wanted to enforce regulations to halt the spread of AIDS through the use of barbers' infected scissors.

With respect to the risk of being infected from semen, images, stories and jokes about safe sex became more common during this period. The humble condom's move from relative obscurity can be seen in the *Financial Review's* account (17 February 1987) of the *'extraordinary metamorphosis of the condom into an object imbued by the medical profession with medical significance on a par with the discovery of penicillin'*.

In this period the tabloid media had a field day. Almost any risk factor could be turned into a dramatic, picture-based story. In 1986 the spoof memorandum (source unknown) displayed in Figure 4.2 was circulating. It encapsulates in joke form a range of the common fears that had come to be culturally associated with AIDS transmission.

In this period, jokes about AIDS risks were formalised in cartoon form. Using satire, ridicule, fantasy, apocryphal stories and plain exaggeration, cartoonists made fun of prevailing fears surrounding the transmission of the virus. Leading cartoonists, working for mainstream British newspapers, contributed in graphic form to the development of the AIDS cartoon genre. An example, by Steve Bell, is shown in Figure 4.3 on page 130.

Bell used talking dogs, with powerful effect, to ridicule common prejudices surrounding the transmission of the virus. In another strip, he has two

---

MEMORANDUM

To: All Members of staff
From: The Management
Date: 18 February 1986
Subject: Medical coverage of AIDS

--------------------------------------------------------------------------------

Following recent government guidelines, the management feel it prudent to offer the following advice and instructions to be implemented as office policy.

1   It will now be your responsibility to ensure that all staff in your section *do not share needles*.
2   All internal mail can only be licked by registered blood donors who have not changed partners for the last four years.
3   Any person sharing a cup or telephone will have to wear a condom.
4   All toilet seats are to be burned after use.
5   Any person caught sitting in another person's chair, not wearing a condom, will be severely reprimanded.
6   Should any member of staff require medical attention, it is imperative that the person administering the treatment uses a condom.
7   All ignorant persons are encouraged to seek employment elsewhere.
8   In the unlikely event of any person dying on the premises, you should arrange for a forklift truck to remove the corpse to the accounts department where it is expected that the incident will not be noticed until pay day.

---

**Figure 4.2**   A spoof memorandum about the spread of AIDS

lorry drivers (*Guardian*, 15 December 1986), Sid and Alexis, discussing a spoof *Sun* headline: *'I Had Sex with East-Enders Dog.'*

On the basis of this news headline Sid is so overcome with fear that he decides to kill himself. The telling point of the strip is contained in the billboard which displays the advertisement shown in Figure 4.4 on page 131.

Whereas Bell directed frontal assaults on the hypocrisy and misinformation contained in popular press-reporting on AIDS risks, Posy Simmonds deals with moral dilemmas and problem relationships. In *'Thinking of you at Christmastide'* (*Guardian* 15 December 1986), she has Stanhope (a businessman) going down with a dose of flu at Christmas, and agonising over whether or not these AIDS-like symptoms had resulted from his affairs with female office staff. In the brilliant cartoon strip shown on page 132 in Figure

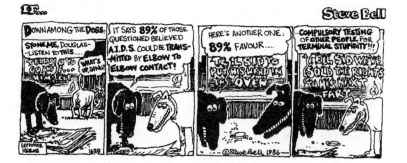

**Figure 4.3**   IF Cartoon. Steve Bell, *Guardian*, 25 November 1986.

---

Newspapers: Don't die of ignorance

Gay or straight, male or female, anyone can get thick from reading lies. So the more lies you read the greater the risk. Protect yourself, read the condom.

*Source:* Guardian, 15/12/86

**Figure 4.4**    Advertising poster represented in Steve Bell cartoon

4.5, Simmonds captures the smugness and complacency of those who feel safe from the AIDS virus.

In this period, almost every type of AIDS risk was imaged in a cartoon frame. Even the Department of Health and Social Security made AIDS jokes. Its 1986 Christmas card showed a street-vendor trying to sell mistletoe at Christmas. The caption underneath the cartoon says *'I just can't seem to shift it, what with all this AIDS about'* (*Observer*, 28 December 1986). The newspaper found this joke, from an official health body, *'terribly sick'*. Its existence reflects the extent to which HIV transmission had become a source of cultural unease, and, therefore, a joking matter.

Griffin (*Mirror*, 7 January 1987) nicely captured the problems of running a safe blood-donation service. He depicted a blood-donor clinic attended by an assorted cast of characters who should definitely not give blood (a heroin addict, promiscuous couples and a vampire). A spoof set of BMA guidelines for blood-donors is displayed on the clinic wall. They suggest that you should not give blood if you are a homosexual, have been to Africa or the USA, have had sex in the last four years, are a bit of a lad, etc.

Edwina Currie MP was quoted as saying, in February 1987: *'My message to the businessmen of this country, when they go abroad, is that there is one thing, above all, that they can take with them, to stop them catching AIDS and that is their wife.'* Jak immortalised Edwina's advice in the cartoon shown in Figure 4.6.

Two kinds of idea are found in these cartoons. Most drew on normative press-reporting of AIDS risks, and upheld conservative values. This humour reinforced prevailing prejudices, and functioned in a way similar to the early, street-level jokes previously identified in relation to the isolation stage. These jokes defines risk at the level of individual deviant behaviour, and reduced complex, multicausal explanations for transmission to simplified, unicausal explanations. The same explanatory position can be identified in many newspaper cartoons of this period. In contrast, the cartoons of Steve Bell and Posy Simmonds opened up more serious debate about the complex issues surrounding HIV transmission. Their jokes cast doubt on the received wisdom being paraded as fact by the majority of the tabloid press.

**Stage 3: The strategic response stage (1987–1991)**

In January 1987, *Marxism Today* carried a cartoon by Nick Newman which captured the prevailing mood and fears of the UK at this time. The cartoon depicts a librarian deciding to move the bestselling *Joy of Sex* book from the health section of the library to the horror section. In five years, 'normal sex' itself had been reclassified. With rising concern that the incidence of HIV was

132

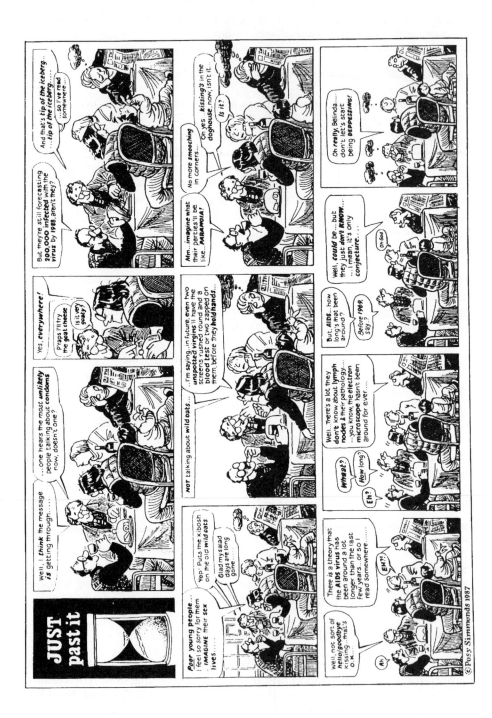

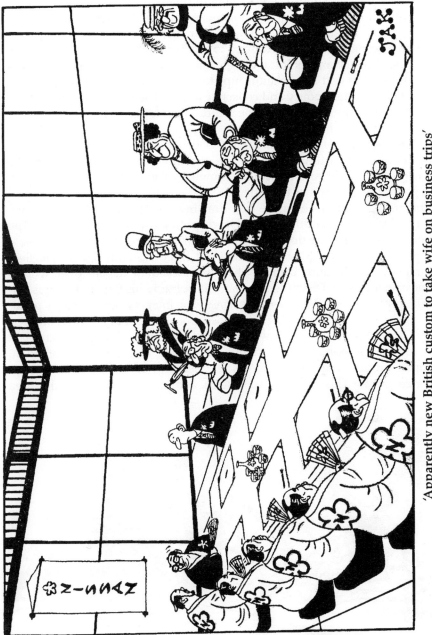

'Apparently new British custom to take wife on business trips'

**Figure 4.6** Jak Cartoon. *Mail on Sunday,* 15 February 1987.

about to rise exponentially, and that heterosexuals were now at risk, a new stage in the history of the epidemic began.

In this period, it was no longer the deviant other who was seen as at risk, but, potentially, everyone. The government finally tried to develop an AIDS policy and strategy, and major national campaigns, *'The Iceberg'*, and *'Don't Die of Ignorance'*, mentioned above, were launched. Jokes and risk imagery of the period recognised that a strategy to combat AIDS must include behavioural, social policy and political dimensions. A shift can be seen from jokes about risk factors and risk relationships to cynical humour about the inadequacy of government policy and collective action. The luxury of joking about someone else's misfortune could be afforded no longer. The joke had now turned into gallows humour.

Just as the national AIDS campaign was being launched, political cartoonists were already casting doubt on the eleventh-hour intervention by the government. Les Gibbard's cartoon, shown in Figure 4.7, graphically portrays government action as too little, too late.

Similarly, Garland (see Figure 4.8), drawing on Rembrandt's famous picture of physicians standing around a corpse, substitutes members of the Thatcher Cabinet for the doctors, while the corpse represents AIDS victims.

Sophie (*Guardian*, 5 May 1987) depicted three skeleton figures labelled, 'ignorance', 'death' and 'blame'. They are locked in debate over who is responsible for the AIDS epidemic. Blame is pointing his finger at homosexuals. The caption reads *'Nice teamwork blame'*. The imagery here suggests political impotence and scapegoating. The most apocalyptic imagery was conjured up by Gerald Scarfe, and is shown in Figure 4.9. In the full-page colour plate used for the cartoon, Adam and Eve are buried in the Garden of Eden. Wrapped around the tree of life is the serpent, represented as a giant poisoned penis. This imagery represents a dramatic shift from the idea

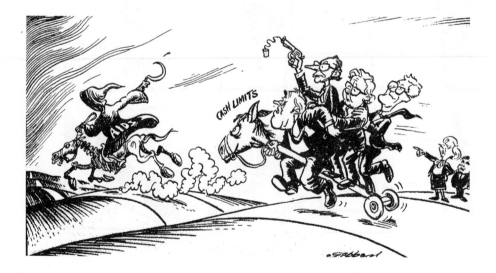

**Figure 4.7**    The Posse Sets off. Les Gibbard Cartoon. *Guardian*, 4 November 1986.

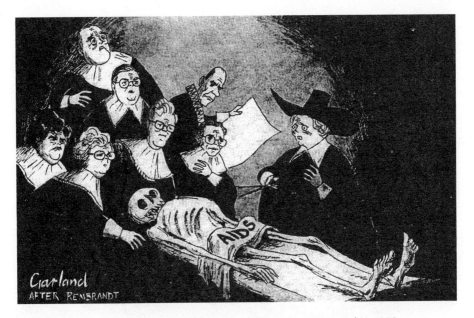

**Figure 4.8**    After Rembrandt. Gerland Cartoon. *Independent*, 4 November 1986.

that a small number of deviants had been infected, to a view that the virus now held the whole of humanity in its deadly embrace.

This period sees a marked shift in AIDS imagery, from an earlier micro-focus on risk relationships to a macro-concern with policy failures. Jokes about the politics of AIDS surfaced for the first time, and punctured the polite government fiction that all was well.

## Stage 4: The indifference stage, 1991–

In the 1990s, the AIDS epidemic has come to be generally regarded as on the wane in America and northern Europe. The *Sunday Times* criticised the view of AIDS as a threat to the heterosexual population. Deviant groups became redefined, in the light of prevailing epidemiological and scientific evidence, as not threatening the wider 'normal' population.

Now, concern focused on the global spread of the disease. For example, the headline *'Third World Faces Atomic Bomb Effect of AIDS'* (*Australian Advertiser*, 25 June 1990) linked the destructive power of HIV to the nightmare of nuclear war. Similarly, other papers headlined the Third World threat in graphic terms, as in *'Africa's Grim Reaper: AIDS is running rampant'* (*Sunday Mail*, 22 April 1990) and *'Asia is AIDS latest target'* (*Sun Herald*, 29 July 1990).

Lupton (1994b, p. 116) argues that, in the 1990s, AIDS is losing its shock value, and has become a stale subject for the news media. The urgency surrounding the AIDS crisis has ebbed, and the state is beginning to withdraw funding from, and commitment to, the fight against AIDS. In these circumstances, she observes that *'there is now a paucity of metaphors for AIDS ... the articles that are now being written are more prosaic. Instead of being the target for metaphors, AIDS is now used as an adjective e.g., AIDS fear, AIDS girl, AIDS issue, AIDS drugs.'*

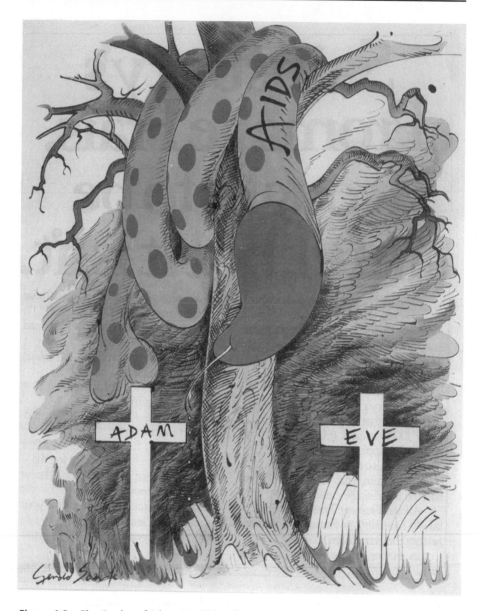

**Figure 4.9**   The Garden of Eden. Gerald Scarfe Cartoon. *Sunday Times,* 21 June 1987.

This most recent period has been characterised as a *'crisis of indifference'* (Weeks, 1991) and a *'period of routinisation'* (Strong, 1990). The disease, in Western societies, has reached either a temporary plateau or a self-limiting stage in terms of the incidence of new cases. Different strains of the HIV virus have been identified, and their future trajectories are unknown. The disease may fade away, grow slowly but inexorably, or take-off again. Although European and American societies now display a degree of indifference to the 'threat from within', developing countries face a risk explosion. However, this apparently distant danger can be kept at arms length, a problem for the foreign 'other'. Homophobia at the national level has been replaced by indifference to the AIDS-afflicted lives of people in distant, non-Western countries.

In this period, joking about AIDS risks has stopped. As argued earlier, jokes arise from threats and social tensions. They provide an unobtrusive indicator of how seriously a given problem is taken. The AIDS example may possibly illustrate a more general 'humour cycle', marked, at one end, by the birth of a joke genre, and, at the other, by its decline and death.

## Discussion: Historical sequences and patterns in risk imagery

This chapter has explored a number of ideas about the nature of risk imagery. The literatures on risk and imagery are both extensive. However, little work has been done on linking these two intellectual domains, and there is, currently, a paucity of critical material exploring the empirical detail, dynamics and functions of risk imagery for different health-related concerns.

The chapter began by asking 'Who constructs risk imagery, and for what purpose?' Various agencies have been identified, including government, scientists, the risk industry, the media, anxious or bored citizens, and marginalised minorities. In the case of the AIDS epidemic, all these groups have tried to articulate their fears and concerns, using many different channels of communication.

No single 'correct' or 'objective' account of the unfolding of a period of history can be identified. If we want to understand the creation and fashioning of AIDS-risk images, we need to define whose history of AIDS is being reconstructed, and the value position of the narrator. Medical (Connor and Kingman, 1988), gay activist (Altman, 1988), and feminist (Richardson, 1987) histories of the epidemic look quite different. This chapter explores the epidemic from the perspective of the cultural/media response, and argues that this response went through four qualitatively distinct stages. The identification of historical stages can always be questioned, since the old is never fully discarded, and anomalies and temporal overlaps usually occur. However, the stages identified, and their chronology, match those described by other researchers (Weeks, 1991; Strong, 1990; Altman, 1988).

Broadening the focus raises the question of whether different epidemics share a common history of types of cultural response. Strong (1990) has written of the 'epidemic psychology' which can be manifested in the face of a major outbreak of disease. He suggests that, like wars and revolutions, epidemics can create an atmosphere of lack of control, catching societies up in an 'emotional maelstrom' which evokes strong feelings of fear, suspicion, moralisation, irrationality and panic, and brings forth a need to take strong actions. Only a detailed study of the history of different epidemics will show whether or not common sequences of 'epidemic psychology' can be identified.

Porter (1986, pp. 11–13) examines the epidemics of the Black Death, syphilis and cholera and identifies social responses to the fear associated with these disease outbreaks. Commenting on the Black Death, he says that *'medieval preachers doled out dooms and damnations with no more inhibitions than the Sun. Living in the shadow of death, late medieval man reacted with a culture of terror, dominated by the charnel house images of skulls and skeletons, the dance of death, a rampant Satan and a punitive God.'* Similarly, Porter observes that *'the coming of Syphilis (brought back by Columbus some said, and then spread by the foul French, the Spanish and the Italians, or some other filthy foreigners) fired that disgust for the corruption of the flesh which haunted Shakespeare and his contemporaries, and, so D.H. Lawrence claimed, trapped the nation in life denying Puritanism for the next three centuries.'* In all these cases, as with AIDS, political 'establishments' manipulated strong imagery, catalysed by fear. Porter argues that the exploitation of this fear generates new dangers which must be countered through co-operation between the medical profession, the government and the public.

Risk perceptions are influenced not only by expert scientific and technical information, but by their metaphorical representation. In the late modern world, global mass media play a crucial role in symbolising risk, although the relationship between media activities and public opinion is a complex one. News and dramatised stories, with their associated imagery, play on our emotions and fears, and embed themselves in our collective psyche. They move us towards a socially mediated ideology of risk, which is fuelled by our human emotions and the certain knowledge of our own mortality. They address the vital cultural question, beyond the scope of science, of what a health risk means.

The challenge to sociologists, Davis (1991) suggests, is to highlight the ambiguous elements of symbolic meaning, and to describe the ways in which, out of crises, their negotiation and resolution, actors create novel forms of symbolic meaning from material which is both familiar and indeterminate.

# Reasoning about probabilities

## Chris Dracup

## Introduction

Although problematic, the definition of risk as the probability of an adverse event does highlight the importance of the concepts of probability and value in the analysis of health risks. This chapter is concerned mainly with the first of these concepts, probability, but looks briefly at the complicating question of whether probability and value are independent.

In Chapter 2, the history of the concept of probability was reviewed. Measured against the history of mathematics, probability theory developed relatively recently, in the seventeenth century (Hacking, 1975). Mathematicians still disagree about the status of the concept of probability, and the assignment of probabilities to events still gives rise to problems except in contrived situations, such as games of chance. In such games, shuffling decks of cards, casting fair dice, turning a roulette wheel, etc., are used to ensure that all simple events have the same probability of occurrence.

Greater difficulties arise when we try to assign probabilities to more everyday events, for example the probability that a birth will result in a male child. Here, we have no *a priori* grounds for believing that males and females are equally likely. Probability is often estimated in such situations by reasoning backwards on the basis that the relative frequency of an event tends towards its probability as the number of observations increases. In consequence, we often equate the observed relative frequency of an event with its probability. However, relative frequency and probability are only guaranteed to be equal for an infinite number of observations. The accuracy of estimates of probabilities based on smaller samples can always be questioned. Defining the population of interest (e.g. all births ever, all live births, all births in a particular country) raises further problems. This frequentist approach has particular difficulties with events which only occur rarely, such as the first manned space flight, and must assume that past frequencies will hold true in the future (see Chapter 2).

Bayesian statisticians take a very different approach to assigning probabilities. According to them, probability describes a personal or subjective opinion. Therefore, an event can have as many different probabilities as there are people judging it. Bayesian statisticians update their subjective probabilities as relevant data are accumulated, using the prescriptions of Bayes Theorem. Application of this theorem ensures that two people who initially hold different views about the probability of an event will come to closer agreement as more and more relevant data are accumulated. Frequentists find this approach too subjective. For them, it seems to exert too little restriction over the appropriateness of initial values for the probability of an event.

Given the difficulties associated with the concept for mathematicians, it would be surprising if lay people had a perfect grasp of probability, its evaluation, manipulation and interpretation. Research from many different fields, over the last few decades, would appear to support the conclusion that our grasp of the concept is fragile, and its use sometimes inappropriate.

Psychologists have attempted to cast light on a number of basic issues. How do people assign probabilities to events? How accurate are these assignments? How closely do people's manipulations of probabilities agree with the algebraic rules for combining probabilities? How do adjectival descriptions such as 'likely' and 'certain' map on to numerical values? Are people's assessments of probabilities independent of the value of the events to which they refer? I will not attempt to exhaustively review the research on each of these issues, but to demonstrate their relevance to health-risk analysis, providing the interested reader with an entry point into the literature.

## Rules of thumb – heuristics

Until the early 1970s, psychologists working in this field tended to subscribe to a Bayesian view of probability. Much research effort (Phillips and Edwards, 1966; Pitz, 1968) was expended comparing the ways in which humans changed their opinions about the probability of an event in the light of new information with the predictions of Bayes Theorem. Researchers interpreted the results of their studies as showing that humans were flawed Bayesians. They responded to the Bayesian properties of the experimental tasks, but to a lesser degree than Bayes Theorem specified. However, the revelation (Marks and Clarkson, 1972, 1973) that people were using a very simple non-Bayesian strategy to generate their responses coincided with other findings that humans might employ simple rules of thumb in assessing probabilities in many situations, and led to the demise of the Bayesian approach.

Tversky and Kahneman (1974) identified three rules of thumb, or heuristics, discussed below, which can account for a wide range of judgemental tendencies which appear inconsistent with probability theory, for example, the well-known Gambler's Fallacy. After a long run of heads resulting from the toss of a fair coin, people become increasingly willing to bet on tails (Stewart, 1995). As Tversky and Kahneman stressed, these rules of thumb can sometimes generate approximately correct solutions. However, heuristics work through simplification, and so will lead to inappropriate conclusions in some conditions. Tversky and Kahneman generated examples of such conditions in order to demonstrate the existence of the heuristic mechanisms, and the biases which could result if they were over-relied on.

## REPRESENTATIVENESS

Use of the representativeness heuristic involves making probability judgements on the basis of similarity. For example, if people are asked to estimate the probability of a person described in a thumbnail sketch being a librarian, they will tend to give higher estimates to the extent that the description agrees with their expectations about librarians. This seems a reasonable approach. In general, people belonging to a particular profession can be expected to be similar to one another. Problems arise when other factors which should be taken into account are neglected because of a reliance on representativeness.

Kahneman and Tversky (1972, p. 443) used the following problem to demonstrate that too heavy a reliance on representativeness could lead to the neglect of sample-size information. The figures in brackets represent the number of people who endorsed each possible answer.

*A certain town is served by two hospitals. In the larger hospital about 45 babies are born each day, and in the smaller hospital about 15 babies are born each day. As you know, about 50 per cent of all babies are boys. The exact percentage varies from day to day. Sometimes it may be higher than 50 per cent, sometimes lower.*

*For a period of one year, each hospital recorded the days on which more than 60 per cent of the babies born were boys. Which hospital do you think recorded more such days?*

>*The larger hospital (12)*
>*The smaller hospital (10)*
>*About the same (that is, within 5 per cent of each other) (28)*

The modal response, 'About the same', fits with the representativeness heuristic, as more than 60 per cent boys equally represents the 50 per cent boys expected at each hospital. However, this response disregards sample size. The variability in the percentage of boys born is much higher in a hospital where only 15 births take place each day than in one where 45 births take place each day. The smaller hospital, then, can be expected to have more days on which more than 60 per cent of those born are boys.

The example can easily be developed to give it some practical importance. Assume that each hospital needs to screen all male infants for a particular syndrome, but that the screening procedure is costly and the materials short-lived. How many testing kits will each hospital require, and which hospital risks wasting more kits which have passed their use-by date?

In Chapter 2, the relevance of overall probabilities to individual cases was questioned. The example given below (Kahneman and Tversky, 1973, p. 241) shows that a reliance on the representativeness heuristic leads us to give too much weight to individuating information, and to disregard population data which contains useful information.

*A panel of psychologists have interviewed and administered personality tests to 30 engineers and 70 lawyers, all successful in their respective fields. On the basis of this information, thumbnail descriptions of the 30 engineers and 70 lawyers have been written. You will find on your forms five descriptions, chosen at random from the 100 available descriptions. For each description, please indicate your probability that the person described is an engineer, on a scale from 0 to 100.*

One of the descriptions read:

*Jack is a 45-year-old man. He is married and has four children. He is generally conservative, careful, and ambitious. He shows no interest in political and social issues and spends most of his free time on his many hobbies which include home carpentry, sailing, and mathematical puzzles.*

> *The probability that Jack is one of the 30 engineers in the sample is* _____ *per cent.*

Jack was designed to be rather representative of an engineer, and fairly unrepresentative of a lawyer. Participants duly rated the probability of him being an engineer as rather high. However, a second group of participants were given a version of the task in which the proportions of engineers and lawyers were reversed. Their ratings of the probability that Jack was an engineer differed little from those of the first group. The two different proportions, or base rates, provide useful evidence. If Jack's description was drawn at random from 30 engineers and 70 lawyers, then, without reading the description, the probability of Jack being an engineer would be only 30 per cent. But if the proportions were reversed, this probability (again without reading the description) would be 70 per cent. The base rate provides useful information even when the description of Jack has been read, but an over-reliance on representativeness leads to it being given little or no weight.

The above example demonstrates the strength of the influence of information about an individual on our judgements of probabilities of events associated with that person. Given individuating information, we tend to give insufficient weight to relative frequencies in the population as a whole. This illustration comes from a situation where the relevance of the population probability cannot be denied. Much greater discounting of underlying frequencies might be anticipated where the relevance of the population information can be questioned because, for example, of non-random sampling from the population.

Most of Tversky and Kahneman's examples require fairly large groups of participants (the hospital example) or two groups of participants treated in different ways (the engineer/lawyer example) to demonstrate the importance of heuristics. The following example often yields interesting results at an individual level. The reader is encouraged to attempt the example before continuing with the chapter.

> Bill is 34 years old. He is intelligent, but unimaginative, compulsive, and generally life-less. In school, he was strong in mathematics but weak in social studies and humanities. Please rank order the following statements by their probability, using 1 for the most probable and 8 for the least probable.

> > Bill is a physician who plays poker for a hobby.
> > Bill is an architect.
> > Bill is an accountant.
> > Bill plays jazz for a hobby.
> > Bill surfs for a hobby.
> > Bill is a reporter.
> > Bill is an accountant who plays jazz for a hobby.
> > Bill climbs mountains for a hobby.

Tversky and Kahneman (1983, p. 297) constructed the description of Bill so that he represented an accountant (A), but was unrepresentative of someone who plays jazz for a hobby (J). However, Bill should appear neither too representa-tive nor unrepresentative of an accountant who plays jazz for a hobby (A and J). They predicted that the representativeness heuristic would lead people to regard A as most probable, A and J as next most probable, and J as least proba-ble. This ordering was shown by 87 per cent of experimental participants.

However, in order to be an accountant who plays jazz for a hobby, Bill must play jazz for a hobby. Therefore, the probability that he plays jazz for a hobby must be at least as high as the probability that he is an accountant who plays jazz for a hobby. A and J is a subset of J and its probability cannot be greater than that of J. Tversky and Kahneman named this violation of probability theory the conjunction fallacy. Similar effects would be expected if a patient were described as having a particular illness, and ratings were made of the probabilities that the patient would show a common symptom, a rare symptom, and both the common and rare symptom.

A further confusion about the probabilities of symptoms can be traced back to the representativeness heuristic. Eddy (1982) found evidence, in physicians' journal articles and letters, that many confused two different conditional probabilities, equating, for example, the probability that a woman had breast cancer, given a positive X-ray, with the probability of a positive X-ray, given that she had breast cancer. (For example, if the X-rays generated a high proportion of false positives, then the probability of having breast cancer, given a positive X-ray, would be quite low. At the same time, the probability of a woman with breast cancer having a positive X-ray could still be high, if the test produced a low rate of false negatives.) Heller, Saltzstein and Caspe (1992) found evidence of the same confusion among paediatric residents, and a similar fallacy has even turned up in elementary statistics textbooks (Dracup, 1995). A real life example, and its management by the health-care system (the high rate of false positives which results from prenatal serum-screening for genetic defects) is discussed in Chapter 7, in the section on 'Intuition'.

Dawes et al. (1993) attributed such confusions to base-rate neglect, caused by reliance on representativeness. The representativeness heuristic lacks direction. The extent to which Bill has the features of a jazz-playing accountant remains the same, regardless of which of the two conditional probabilities we are required to estimate. So, if we base our estimates on representativeness, we are likely to give the same estimate for the two different conditional probabilities.

## AVAILABILITY

When people derive estimates of the probability of an event on the basis of availability, they rely on the ease with which they can remember, or generate, examples of the event. More available events tend to be judged more probable. Once again, this heuristic can be useful in many situations. However, other factors than frequency affect the availability of examples. When frequency and availability diverge, probability assessments may show considerable bias.

Consider the issue of the probability of a subset of some greater set (as illustrated in the discussion of the conjunction fallacy above). Tversky and Kahneman (1983, p. 295) asked people to estimate the number of seven letter words of the form ----*ing* in four pages of a novel. In a second version of the question, they were asked to estimate the frequency of -----*n*- words (seven letter words whose penultimate letter was '*n*'). The median estimates for ----*ing* was 13.4, but for -----*n*- words, it was only 4.7. Of course, ----*ing* is a proper subset of the set -----*n*-. That is, -----*n*- contains all the ----*ing* words as well as others such as ----*ent*, ----*end*. However, ----*ing* type words can be generated very easily. They require only that a four-letter verb be found, to which '*ing*' can be added. On the other hand, words of the type -----*n*- are less easy to generate (unless we realise that they include ----*ing* words) but occur more frequently!

A factor which might affect availability, but be independent of probability, is vividness. Certain causes of death are much more vivid than others, for example murder, accidents and some illnesses. Reliance on the availability heuristic would lead to overestimation of the frequency of such deaths, and this does, indeed, occur. Slovic, Fischhoff and Lichtenstein (1982) compared people's estimates of the frequency of death from various causes with the actual numbers of deaths attributable to each. Accidental deaths were judged about as frequent as deaths from diseases, although diseases actually claim about 16 times as many lives. Homicides were incorrectly judged about as frequent as deaths from stroke, but strokes claim about 11 times as many lives even in the USA. The authors also report the results of a follow-up study, in which a strong positive correlation between newspaper coverage of deaths from various causes and people's estimates of frequency was found (once the actual frequency had been partialled-out statistically).

## ANCHORING AND ADJUSTMENT

According to this heuristic, participants will anchor their probability estimates on an initial value, if available. They will not make adequate adjustments in the light of their knowledge. Judgements can become anchored to initial estimates which have little validity. Tversky and Kahneman (1974) span a wheel of fortune containing the numbers 0 to 100 in the presence of experimental participants, and asked them whether the resulting number accurately reflected the proportion of African countries belonging to the UN. If participants rejected the number, they were asked to give their own estimate for the true proportion. A group given an initial value of 10 produced consistently lower estimates than did a group who had been provided with an initial value of 65. The initial values influenced these estimates, despite their irrelevance. Unlike representativeness and availability, anchoring and adjustment does not relate to another psychological process such as memory or judgements of similarity. The term seems rather to provide a simple naming of a frequently observed phenomenon, but offers little by way of explanation as to why it should occur.

## CHALLENGES TO THE HEURISTICS APPROACH

The heuristics approach has generated research in a wide range of applied settings, and provided explanations of many of the phenomena with which the remainder of this chapter is concerned. Some researchers worry that it has had too strong an influence, and has not progressed very far theoretically in the 20 or more years since its origins. Some have maintained that the fallacies and biases identified by Tversky and Kahneman result from their adoption of just one of the many alternative views of probability (Cohen, 1979; Gigerenzer, 1991).

Gigerenzer (1991) argued that the Bayesian basis of many of Tversky and Kahneman's demonstrations, which require participants to assign probabilities to one-off events, would be rejected by most statisticians who adopt a frequentist approach to probability. When Gigerenzer reformulated a number of the problems in frequentist terms, much less participant bias was found. Recently, Jones, Jones and Frisch (1995) have attempted to reconcile the differing views, presenting evidence that greater representativeness effects are obtained with single-case judgements, while availability plays a stronger role in frequency judgements. However, reconciliation cannot be detected in the most recent published positions of either Kahneman and Tversky (1996) or Gigerenzer (1996).

## Hindsight bias

Hindsight bias concerns the way in which outcome knowledge affects people's subjective expectations that events will happen. Fischhoff (1975) gave five versions of the same historical passage to different groups of experimental participants. The passage discussed the conflict between the British and the Gurkhas of Nepal. After reading the passage, participants were required to give their subjective probabilities, on the basis of the information provided, for each of four possible outcomes to the conflict, for example British victory, Gurkha victory. The control group of participants was simply asked to assign probabilities to each outcome on the basis of the information in the passage. The four experimental groups were also told, incidentally, that one of the outcomes had actually occurred. Each of the experimental groups assigned a higher subjective probability to the 'known' outcome than that given by the control group. Judgements with the benefit of hindsight could not be equated with those made in foresight. Neither warning participants of the hindsight effect, nor exhorting them to work harder, appeared to counteract such effects (Fischhoff, 1977).

Arkes *et al.* (1981) studied the hindsight effect in the diagnoses of practising physicians. A case history was presented to each doctor, along with four possible diagnoses, whose probabilities they were asked to estimate. A foresight group carried out this task without outcome knowledge. Each of the four hindsight groups was told that the case illustrated one of the four possible diagnoses. A hindsight effect was found overall, but was mainly confined to the group who had been told that the case suffered from a disease which the foresight group had judged rather unlikely. Arkes *et al.* argue that the effect may have been attenuated because of the physicians' appreciation of the unreliability of diagnoses. They may not have fully believed the outcome information. Nonetheless, the finding of a hindsight effect leads us to question the value of a second opinion made with knowledge of the first.

Mitchell and Kalb (1981) asked nurses to adopt the role of a supervisor required to evaluate a subordinate's performance. One of the behaviours investigated involved the failure of a nurse to replace a bed rail. Experimental participants who were told that the nurse's lapse had resulted in injury to the patient rated this outcome as more likely, and saw the subordinate as more responsible for the behaviour, than did those who were not told about the accident. Knowledge of the outcome, again, influenced the way in which an action was judged.

Hindsight effects have been demonstrated for women's estimates of their probability of being pregnant (Pennington *et al.*, 1980), judgements about the outcome of a presidential election (Leary, 1982), examination-marking (Murphy, 1979), property-pricing (Northcraft and Neale, 1987) and auditing (Kinney and Uecker, 1982). Anchoring and adjustment, and availability, have both been offered as explanations of the effect. Participants 'know' that the true probability of one particular outcome is 1, and cannot adjust enough for their real uncertainty before the outcome. They also find it easier to retrieve information consistent with the 'known' outcome, and so tend to overestimate its probability.

Attempts to implicate motivational factors have failed. For example, Leary (1982) could not demonstrate self-esteem and self-presentation effects in his study of predictions of the outcome of the 1980 presidential election, although hindsight distortions were found. Attempts to mitigate the bias have typically required participants to consider the reasons why outcomes other than the 'known' one might have occurred. Such instructions tend to decrease the effect. However, few authors would claim that they remove it entirely (but see Arkes *et al.*, 1988).

In a meta-analysis of hindsight bias research, Christensen-Szalanski and Willham (1991) concluded that the overall magnitude of the effect was quite small. Nonetheless, they argued that even these small effects might have important consequences for practitioners in some situations. Recently, Stahlberg *et al.* (1995) found slightly attenuated hindsight effects with groups. However, groups do have a clear advantage when the effect is studied by asking the group to remember their previous probability estimate, rather than by comparing the estimates of groups with and without outcome knowledge.

Taken together, these findings have particular relevance for inquiries into infrequent events such as accidents, child abuse, and killings by patients with mental health problems. The research suggests that investigators who possess full outcome knowledge will frequently make inaccurate judgements of what responsible agencies should have been able to foresee. What an inquiry might, with hindsight, identify as flashing amber lights may, justifiably, have been treated as nothing more than random noise by those handling the matter on a day-to-day basis.

Conduct of the inquiry by a panel or tribunal, rather than an individual, would not seem to offer any remedy according to the findings of Stahlberg *et al.* (1995). A discussion of the effects of hindsight is included in the official report into the death of the abused child Jasmine Beckford (London Borough of Brent, 1985). Unfortunately, this discussion does not refer to psychological research. The panel's belief *'that hindsight is of assistance to us in our task, being no more than reasonable foresight, with the additional benefit of knowledge of what has actually occurred'* (p. 33), seems inconsistent with research findings.

## Unrealistic optimism

Weinstein (1980) found that, for a large range of life events, people judged positive outcomes, such as living past 80, as more likely to happen to them than to other members of the population, and negative events, such as lung cancer, as less likely. The optimism shown by an individual cannot be labelled 'unrealistic' as that person may have a lower probability of suffering a particular negative life event. However, when most people hold such a belief, some must be unrealistically optimistic.

Svenson (1981) showed that 87.5 per cent of his US student participants rated themselves as above the median for driving safety. The median is defined as that value above which 50 per cent of the members of a group score. For 87.5 per cent to believe themselves better than the median, some must have underestimated their accident potential. Zakay (1983), who also detected unrealistic optimism, attributed the effect partly to motivational factors, and partly to the availability heuristic. He argued that, because of press coverage etc., individuals can retrieve examples of negative events happening to others more easily, while positive events happening to oneself can also be accessed easily.

Weinstein and Klein (1995) drew attention to the implications of this bias (and the relative lack of success of manipulations designed to reduce it) for media-based health-promotion campaigns. For example, people may accept that smoking causes lung cancer. But if they judge this outcome less likely for themselves than for other smokers (McKenna, Warburton and Winwood,

1993), they will not see a need to change their own behaviour. In contrast, it has been proposed that positive illusions, including unrealistic optimism, may foster mental health, helping people to cope in a dangerous world (Taylor and Brown, 1988). However, Colvin and Block (1994) concluded, from a review of the evidence, that the relationship remained unproven.

## Verbal expressions of probability

Zimmer (1983) noted that, historically, verbal expressions of uncertainty were used long before the development of mathematical probability theory. Even today, people tend to prefer to give information about certainty, employing terms like likely or doubtful, than to use numbers (Erev and Cohen, 1990; Wallsten *et al.*, 1993). People seem to see verbal expressions as more consistent with the vagueness which typically accompanies their feelings of (un)certainty. In contrast, people tend to prefer to receive probabilistic information in numerical form. The issue of the correspondence between these two forms, therefore, takes on considerable significance. What should a patient understand from a doctor's statement that she probably has breast cancer?

Methods of mapping the meaning of probabilistic terms on to numbers were developed by Wallsten *et al.*, 1986. These show, for example, that the word 'likely' implies a probability around 0.8, but stretches as low as 0.5 and as high as 0.99. This variability gives plenty of room for misunderstanding. Moreover, numerical evaluations depend on the base rate of the event in question (Wallsten, Fillenbaum and Cox, 1986). The sentence 'Rain is likely' has very different implications if Manchester, rather than Las Vegas, is being discussed. Weber and Hilton (1990) showed that the interpretation of such terms as a 'slight chance' varied not just with base rate, but also with the severity of the event under consideration. A slight chance was interpreted as implying a higher probability for a more severe condition – skin cancer – than for gastric disturbance.

This demonstration of the lack of independence between the meaning of probability terms and the value of the outcomes they describe casts some doubt on the assumption that they can be determined separately and then combined in an attempt to aid decision-making, a point which is taken up in the next section. The complexities of quantitative and qualitative communication of probabilities in genetic counselling are explored in Chapter 2.

## Framing effects

The previous section showed that the interpretation of verbal expressions of probability depends on the salience of the event for the person involved. Such effects run counter to the divide-and-conquer maxim of the decision-aiders. Expected utility theory, the foundation stone of decision-aiding, and of much economics, has been attacked for decades because of similar effects. The expected utility of an action is derived by summing the product of the probability and utility of each possible outcome. The action yielding the highest expected utility should be chosen. The theory has been put forward both as a normative and a descriptive theory of decision-making.

If we are prepared to accept the axioms from which expected utility theory is derived, then the normative status of the theory cannot be questioned. However, its descriptive accuracy can be challenged. Kahneman and Tversky (1979), in their development of Prospect Theory, a descriptive, psychologically based, theory of decision-making, demonstrated a number of ways in which human behaviour departs from the assumptions of expected utility theory. This chapter will not provide a detailed description of Prospect Theory, but will review those findings about framing effects which played a major role in its development, and which have relevance not just to our main concern – how people handle uncertainty – but also to the question of how value is assessed.

Framing effects occur when different ways of presenting (or framing) the same problem result in different decisions: a most undesirable outcome for anyone aspiring to rational decision-making.

Kahneman and Tversky (1979, p. 267) asked participants to choose between:

A: A 50 per cent chance to win a three-week tour of England, France, and Italy.
B: A one-week tour of England, with certainty.

or

C: A 5 per cent chance to win a three-week tour of England, France, and Italy.
D: A 10 per cent chance to win a one-week tour of England.

Of those offered a choice between A and B, 78 per cent chose B. Of those offered the choice between C and D, 67 per cent chose C. The two examples involve identical outcomes, with probabilities in the same ratio. From an expected utility perspective, the problems do not differ. However, the responses show that people do not judge them equivalent. Kahneman and Tversky argue that, in the first example, the 100 per cent chance of the outcome in B is weighted more, relative to the 50 per cent chance of the outcome in A, than is the 10 per cent chance of the outcome in D, relative to the 5 per cent chance of the outcome in C. They describe this as the certainty effect, and go on to show that certain positive and negative outcomes are disproportionately attractive or aversive.

Another finding which conflicts with the expected utility approach is derived from the following problems, in which people were asked to say which of two gambles they would prefer. Kahneman and Tversky (1979, p. 267) asked participants to choose either between:

A: $6000 with probability 0.45 and $0 with probability 0.55.
B: $3000 with probability 0.90 and $0 with probability 0.10.

or

C: $6000 with probability 0.001 and $0 with probability 0.999.
D: $3000 with probability 0.002 and $0 with probability 0.998.

Gamble A says that a participant will win $6000 with probability 0.45, but will win nothing ($0) with probability 0.55. Of those presented with a choice between A and B, 86 per cent chose B. Of those selecting between C and D, 73 per cent chose C. Once again, the outcomes in both versions of the problem have the same utility, and the ratio of the probabilities are equal. According to expected utility theory, then, the same alternative should be more attractive in both versions, but this clearly was not the case. Kahneman and Tversky argue that the difference in the probabilities associated with C and D are so small that participants tend to disregard them, and base their choice on the greater pay-off associated with C. The same ratio of probabilities associated with A and B, in contrast, yields a difference too large to disregard.

Baron (1994) reports the results of a study by Schwalm and Slovic which detected a similar reduced sensitivity to small probabilities. They found that only 10 per cent of their experimental participants said they would wear seatbelts when told that the probability of being killed in an automobile accident was about 0.00000025 per trip, but 39 per cent said they would wear seat belts when informed that the probability of being killed was 0.01 in a lifetime of driving. Here, the probability of death per trip is so small that it can be discounted. Only when the probability is framed in such a way as to make it appear a significant consideration does it affect intended behaviour.

Findings such as these led Kahneman and Tversky to postulate that probabilities do not enter directly into decision processes. Rather, they are subject to an editing process, which might disregard small probabilities, or small differences in probability. The probabilities of events which survive this editing process are then weighted by a function which gives extra importance to certain outcomes, but is badly defined for small probabilities, sometimes giving them a low, and sometimes a high, weighting. Kahneman and Tversky insist that people fully comprehend the figures in the above examples. However, their judgements do not match the predictions of expected utility theory, and require the postulation of an editing process and a weighting function.

Tversky and Kahneman (1981, p. 251) used the following example to demonstrate framing effects for the utilities component of expected utility theory:

> Imagine that the US is preparing for the outbreak of an unusual Asian disease, which is expected to kill 600 people. Two alternative programs to combat the disease have been proposed. Assume that the exact scientific estimates of the consequences of the programs are as follows:

> Version 1
> Program A: (200 saved)
> Program B: (600 saved with probability 0.33)

> Version 2
> Program A: (400 die)
> Program B: (600 die with probability 0.67)

The two versions present the same information, but in positive and negative forms. Participants given Version 1 tended to choose Program A, but those provided with Version 2 favoured Program B. Again, expected utility theory cannot explain the change in preference which is observed for the two versions. Prospect Theory does so by postulating a different value function for gains (Version 1) and losses (Version 2). Li and Adams (1995) reported similar results from Chinese-speaking subjects for one of two scenarios they studied, based around a disaster at a mine.

A final example of a framing effect from Kahneman and Tversky (1979, p. 273) casts doubt on the very distinction between positive and negative outcomes which underlies most definitions of risk. According to expected utility theory, utility is associated with final asset positions. According to Prospect Theory, value is affected by present asset position. By framing a problem in two different ways, the same outcome can appear to involve either a gain or a loss for participants with consequent changes in their behaviour.

*Version 1*
*In addition to whatever you own, you have been given $1000. You are now asked to choose between:*

> *A: $1000 with probability 0.5 and $0 with probability 0.5.*
> *B: $500 with certainty.*

*Version 2*
*In addition to whatever you own, you have been given $2000. You are now asked to choose between:*

> *C: A loss of $1000 with probability 0.5 and $0 with probability 0.5.*
> *D: A loss of $500 with certainty.*

In terms of final positions, alternatives A and C do not differ ($2000 with probability 0.5, or $1000 with probability 0.5). Alternatives B and D also correspond (a certain $1500). However, 84 per cent of participants preferred alternative B to A, while 69 per cent preferred alternative C to D. Kahneman and Tversky argue that, in comparing A and B, people have already incorporated the gift of $1000 into their assets before they are offered a choice between a further $1000 with probability 0.5, or $500 dollars with certainty. They prefer a certain gain of $500 over a 0.5 probability of $1000, and choose alternative B. In comparing C and D, people have incorporated the gift of $2000 dollars into their current assets before they are asked to choose between a loss of $1000 with probability 0.5 or a certain loss of $500 dollars. Certain losses are very aversive, so they choose alternative C, in the hope of avoiding a loss altogether.

The example clearly illustrates the dangers of assuming the equivalence of a given set of gains or losses. Everything depends on how they are expressed. Do the alternatives, in the example above, represent losses or gains? In one version they look like losses, and we get one kind of behaviour. In the other, they look like gains, and we get another kind of behaviour. The question is not which is correct. How can we hope to talk sensibly, in risk analysis, about the risk associated with a negative event if the same event can be evaluated both positively and negatively?

The examples above have used people who shared a common view of value, but were swayed by the framing of the problems. When people value an outcome differently, such as having a child with Down's syndrome, there is obvious room for disagreement and apparent inconsistency (see Chapter 1). Health professionals may inadvertently frame choices in such a way that those who must make the choice, and live with its consequences, do not consider the situation from alternative possible angles. From one perspective, a risk may appear trivial. From another, it may seem unacceptably high.

## Discussion

Where does this overview leave us? Psychologists have found people's dealings with the concepts of probability to be problematic, and their own attempts to study the issue have themselves been beset with difficulties. At an early stage, the attractiveness to some psychologists of the Bayesian position, which treats probability as a subjective quality, seemed to blind them to the possibility that people were acting in a non-Bayesian manner.

The heuristics programme still has an enormous influence, both within psychology, and in many applied areas, including the study of health risk. Humans often employ simple rules of thumb in order to estimate probabilities, and systematic biases may result. However, the results of this research programme have sometimes been taken to imply that human judgements of probability are never accurate: clearly an overstatement. With almost all of Tversky and Kahneman's demonstrations, some participants do not display the expected bias, and biases are more prevalent in some situations than in others. Heuristics will often do their job of providing a simplified short-cut to a reasonable conclusion. Further investigation of these issues is clearly required.

The estimates that people make of their own risk of experiencing a negative event, and those they make of someone else's risk, differ in important respects. The implications for safety campaigns are obvious. It is also well established that attempts to judge the likelihood of occurrence of a negative event will be biased by knowing that the event did subsequently happen. Knowing about this bias does not seem to be sufficient to guard against it. The hindsight effect has important implications for judgements of professional accountability, such as in nursing (Chapters 13–15), child protection (Chapter 16) and care for the seriously mentally ill (Chapter 17).

Expected utility theory is based on the assumption that probabilities and values of outcomes are independent. However, the evidence suggests that judgements of probability are affected by the values of the outcomes to which they apply. Attempts to decompose problems into these two features, then, can be questioned. Even if the probabilities are provided to the decision-maker, their impact is not a simple function of their magnitude. Sometimes small probabilities, or small differences between probabilities, are disregarded. Different ways of framing a problem can lead people to view the same outcome as either a loss or a gain. Given such findings, the definition of risk as the probability of occurrence of a negative event looks precarious.

# PART TWO

# Researching risk rationality in health and social care

# Risk, sex and the very young mother

Joan Aarvold

## Introduction

The construction of labelled groups within society serves political, economic, academic, professional and other purposes. Foucault (Rabinow, 1984) has described a process of social classification and objectification which assigns particular identities to groups, and which may legitimate social exclusion. Labelling, according to Foucault, reflects the power relations within a society. People are grouped as employed or unemployed, deviant or law-abiding, claimants or non-claimants. Culturally derived classification systems become 'larger than life', and are used as a source of expectations about individual behaviour.

School-age mothers are one of the most stereotyped social groups in contemporary British society. They engage in illegal under-age sex according to the Sexual Offences Act of 1956, do not use contraception (Mellanby, Phelps and Tripp, 1993), do not complete their education (Gribben, 1992), or marry (Babb, 1993), and depend on state benefits (Ineichen and Hudson, 1994). Paradoxically, a mother aged 13–16, although deemed to be engaging in risky behaviour (Black, 1986), faces no greater likelihood of serious pregnancy complications than her older sisters, providing that she receives adequate care (Russell, 1988; Konje *et al.*, 1992). Nevertheless, professionals and policy-makers single out this group as a 'problem'.

Many studies have examined the knowledge, attitudes and behaviours of young mothers (Bury, 1985; Coyne, 1986; Phoenix, 1991; Wilson, 1995b). Research in this field has been largely fuelled by the questions, 'Why does it happen?', and 'How can we stop it?' Platt (1995) criticises this literature for its lack of debate about the social construction of the 'problem' itself.

References, in contemporary society, to sexually active young people arouse a variety of emotions. As noted in the Introduction, the tendency of 'primitive' peoples to detest anomalous entities, relative to their own cultural categories (Douglas, 1966), has not disappeared in more complex societies. Few entities are more anomalous, in Western cultures, than 'children' who are also 'sexual'. This cultural difficulty is reflected in the unavailability of a neutral terminology for describing 13–16-year-old pregnant females. Descriptors such as 'schoolgirl mother' and 'pregnant teenager' carry implications of deviance and potential problems (Illsley and Taylor, 1974). However, most very young mothers are aged 15–16, and are marked as a 'problem' by the school-leaving age, not by some natural watershed.

The starting point for much research, that this group is 'at risk' (Griffin, 1993), obscures attempts to understand young people's own rationality. The first part of this chapter locates the 'problem' of young motherhood within its social and political context, and includes a brief discussion on contraceptive choices, with reference to the risks they entail. The second part considers the experiences of eight young mothers and mothers-to-be.

## The social and political context of young motherhood

### CONCEPTION TRENDS

The conception rate for under 16s has gone up and down over the last three decades in response to political and socioeconomic changes. It rose in England and Wales from 6.8 per 1000 in 1969 to 10.1 in 1990 (OPCS, 1993b, p. 74). However, the rate fell between 1974 and 1980 from 8.5 to 7.2 per 1000. The abortion rate during this period also fell from 4.1 to 3.9, after which it has risen to and remained at around 4.8 per 1000 (Brook Advisory Centres, 1994). Since 1990, the conception rate for girls under 16 has gone down, with 8.5 conceptions per 1000 in 1992 compared with the peak of 10.1 in 1990, rates far above *The Health of the Nation* target (DOH, 1992) for the year 2000, of 4.8 per 1000.

A massive rise in relative and absolute family poverty, engineered by British Conservative governments, in power from 1979 to 1997, may have contributed to the overall rise in teenage fertility during the 1980s, since rates are linked to socioeconomic status, as will be shown below. The 'Gillick' factor undoubtedly made a significant contribution (Gillick, 1986). A Health Service Notice (80)46, 1980, emphasised confidentiality between doctor and patient, however young. In consequence, contraceptive advice and treatment could be given to under 16-year-olds without parental consent. Mrs Gillick objected strongly to this principle, with respect to her own daughters. In January 1981, she began proceedings which lasted for five years, and ended up in the House of Lords. New guidelines have been produced for GPs (BMA, 1994) and Family Planning Clinics in response to continuing confusion over young peoples' reproductive rights. The guidelines, based on the current legal position in the UK, state that those aged under 16 are owed the same duty of confidentiality as any other person.

Recent studies (Dillner, 1991; Family Planning Association, 1994; Lo, Kaul and Kaul, 1994; Allaby, 1995; Wellings *et al.*, 1995) of young people's perceptions of contraceptive services demonstrate the continuing impact of the Gillick legacy. Many still believe they cannot seek advice or treatment while under 16 without involving their parents. Some professionals share this view. One survey found that one-third of GPs believed that prescribing contraceptives to under-16s was illegal (Family Planning Association and Contraceptive Education Service, 1995). The fall in under-16 conceptions since 1991 may be associated with a slow increase in the number of under 16-year-olds presenting for contraceptive advice during this period (Brook Press Release, 1995). Other factors possibly contributing to the recent fall include increased pressure on health authorities to provide services to meet *The Health of the Nation* targets (DOH, 1992); more accessible 'out-of-hours' and 'drop-in' provision by family-planning clinics; and young people's gradually increasing trust, post-Gillick, in the confidentiality of contraceptive services.

## SOCIAL CLASS DIFFERENCES

Markedly higher teenage fertility rates are found in areas of low socioeconomic status (Wilson, Brown and Richards, 1992; Babb, 1993; Smith, 1993). Teenage pregnancy is a feature of the 'health divide' in the UK (Whitehead, 1987) and in other countries and cultures (Hudson and Ineichen, 1991; Moore and Rosenthal, 1993; Males, 1995).

The medical risks associated with youthful pregnancy are themselves influenced by social circumstances such as poverty (Whitehead, 1987; Dillner, 1991). According to Platt (1995), no amount of sex education will compensate for social deprivation. However, the relationship between poverty and the incidence of social 'problems' may be overstated. Higher income groups are better able to conceal stigmatised behaviours such as child and sexual abuse, teenage pregnancy and alcoholism. Inevitably, research has homed in on the less powerful social groups, who have more visible 'problems'.

Smith (1993) found a three-times higher pregnancy rate, among girls aged under 16, in the most deprived areas than in the most affluent ones. But a greater proportion of pregnancies ended in abortion in affluent areas (two out of three) than in deprived areas (one out of four). Higher educational and occupational aspirations have been linked to the choice of abortion (Lo, Kaul and Kaul, 1994). This option appears more acceptable to higher income groups (Wilson, Brown and Richards, 1992; Burghes, 1995). However, even under medically controlled 'safe' conditions, the risks associated with abortion are higher for very young women (Russell, 1988). Late abortion brings with it further risks, not only to the immediate physical and emotional health of the woman but also to her future reproductive capability (Edstrom, 1972).

In poorer communities, characterised by high rates of unemployment and limited job prospects, teenage pregnancy occurs normally, across the generations. Where it is less stigmatised, teenage pregnancy will be seen as less of an adversity. Young people, in these circumstances, will be less motivated to take contraceptive measures, and more reluctant to resort to abortion. A purely informational approach to contraception will not reduce pregnancy rates in this cultural context.

## POLICY INFLUENCES

Health-promotional messages are always politically mediated. The prevailing victim-blaming ideology focuses on lifestyles (Bunton, Nettleton and Burrows, 1995). Despite evidence to the contrary, politicians rarely see high adolescent conception rates as a consequence of their own socioeconomic policies (Trussell, 1988; Males, 1995) or inappropriate educational and service strategies (Prendergast and Prout 1990; Gardner, 1991; Platt, 1995).

The thrust behind prevention campaigns has been primarily economic, to reduce the number of young mothers relying on social welfare. Several studies reported by Phoenix (1991) have not supported the belief that young women get pregnant in order to become eligible for state benefits. Indeed, the system encourages young mothers to place themselves in health-demoting environments, such as high-rise flats in run-down areas, as they have to move out of the family home in order to qualify for even the lowest level of benefits (Wilson, 1995b). Material gain, in such cases, often comes at the expense of social support. Under 16s do not qualify for income support or housing benefit. They are only entitled to child benefit with a one-parent supplement, giving them, in 1996, the princely sum of £17.10 per week (Benefits Agency, 1996).

## Contraceptive concerns

Birth control has a very long history (Oakley, 1993). However, with so many methods now available, women have to choose from a large menu. Their decisions are influenced by many factors, including the way in which options are presented. Contraceptive methods can be evaluated in terms of effectiveness against pregnancy and against infection; cost; availability; ease of use; impact on the sexual relationship, for example on negotiation, preparation and pleasure; side effects; reversibility; monitoring and maintenance requirements; consistency with religious principles; and ecological consequences. Individuals' judgements about contraceptive methods will vary considerably, depending on their social position, values, priorities and belief systems.

A study of women aged 16–49 (Walsh, Lythgoe and Peckham, 1996) concluded that pregnancy prevention and the avoidance of side effects were the principal considerations influencing their contraceptive decisions. Women were strongly affected by the negative perceptions of methods they had not chosen, and appeared to select the 'least worst' option (Walsh, Lythgoe and Peckham, 1996, p. 5). Over half had used more than one method, and the most common reason for changing was concern about health side effects. The report also highlighted problems with the quality and quantity of the information available to women, including inconsistencies, inaccuracies, a dearth of written material, and a lack of opportunities to raise personal concerns.

Although the views of women under 16 were not sought in the above study, it has interesting implications for this age group. The report concluded that most women have already chosen a birth-control method before visiting their doctor. Beliefs about the relative risks of different methods may, therefore, have been embedded in the minds of potential users before they took medical advice. However, women's knowledge of side effects can be inaccurate or based on limited data, for example the problems experienced by a family member, as will be shown below. Women cannot make informed choices unless impartial and up-to-date contraceptive information is made more widely available beyond health-care settings (Walshe, Lythgoe and Peckham, 1996, p. 39). More than 30 per cent of girls under 16 have already had sexual intercourse (Wellings et al., 1995), and are unlikely to have visited their doctor for advice (Dillner, 1991). Contraceptive information in libraries, schools, shops and clubs, etc. could help them to make informed choices.

No known contraceptive offers both complete safety and effectiveness. The risks and benefits to health of different methods of contraception have been well debated (Beral, 1979; Bellini, 1986; Oakley, 1993; WHO, 1995). Maternal mortality and morbidity rates have fallen dramatically in the Western world. However, according to Beral (1979), if deaths from contraceptive causes (e.g. thrombo-embolitic and infectious disorders) are included in the 'reproductive' mortality rate, then the apparent downward trend is less marked.

## USING CONTRACEPTION

Health promotional campaigns mainly emphasise avoidance as a means of minimising health risk. However, young people take account of the perceived benefits of prohibited activities, as well as their costs. They are affected by peer pressures, rebelliousness, the need to explore, role modelling, and the desire to attain adult status. Professionals have learned to take the undesirability of various 'risky' behaviours for granted, but these activities have acquired their bad reputation through selective labelling and marketing processes (Cooper, 1985; Beck, 1992; Douglas, 1994).

Women must make decisions about specific contraceptive methods, and their relative effectiveness in preventing pregnancy and infection, while, at the same time, weighing up other risks to their own health. Such complex decision-making requires knowledge, the ability to plan ahead, and autonomy. The sheath seems to provide an ideal contraceptive solution, providing that the user or his partner does not have a rubber allergy. It is safe, easily available, relatively cheap and effective, and reduces the risk of infection. However, as already noted, contraceptive decisions are influenced by more than purely medical considerations. Condom use requires cultural acceptance, partner commitment, access to a steady supply and the ability to plan ahead (Grimley et al., 1995), qualities not generally attributed to adolescents. It can diminish sexual spontaneity and pleasure. Some young women feel that they are just 'too messy' (Moore and Rosenthal, 1993). Wider social attitudes towards teenage sexuality contain a paradox. An adolescent is deemed not to be an adult, and is not supposed to have sex. However, if an adolescent does have sex, then they are expected to behave in an adult way, to seek out the relevant 'health' information, choose a contraceptive in advance, and use it correctly. Many older, more experienced, women find contraceptive-planning difficult (Walsh, Lythgoe and Peckham, 1996).

A woman's choice of contraception is based not only on her beliefs about their costs and benefits, but on their availability. Young people want accessible facilities, and for their views to be listened to in a non-judgemental way (Scott, 1994). They continue to have problems in obtaining sexual health advice. One survey (Family Planning Association, 1994) reported that 20 per cent of 14–17-year-olds did not know where to find a family-planning clinic.

These findings are supported by the author's conversations with pregnant girls and young mothers, to which the chapter now turns.

## Young mothers speak

### INTRODUCTION

This section is based on small group discussions with eight young women, aged 14–17 years, attending a special educational unit. The full-time unit evolved from a weekly session which the author set up to provide social support and antenatal classes for young, pregnant girls excluded from school. Their general education was carried on through the home-tutor system. Once their babies were born, the mothers continued to attend the unit, and to receive postnatal support. After some three years, the local education authority provided a bigger venue, with a head teacher, at which the girls could receive general education, including one session per week devoted to pregnancy, birth and babycare issues. This separate session eventually became subsumed into the main programme. Local politicians came to accept the unit only slowly, but were impressed by the improved outcomes achieved with respect to both educational attainment and the health of mothers and babies.

Girls are referred to the unit from a variety of sources, both formal and informal. Students sometimes bring a friend along, or a teacher, midwife or GP may make direct contact. The age range on referral varies from 13 to 16, with some 17-year-olds continuing to attend beyond their official school-leaving age. Approximately 25 'new' girls join the unit each year. The stage of pregnancy on referral varies, from about 6 weeks to 7 months post-conception. Generally good rates of attendance have been achieved, even though most girls had stopped going to school before coming to the unit, and some girls have attained five or more GCSE passes. As well as meeting their educational needs, the unit allows young mothers to support each other. Their babies thrive in a well-resourced 'nursery' environment, not usually available to older single parents.

Four of the eight research participants already had babies, while the others were at varying stages of pregnancy. Their attendance at the unit must, inevitably, have influenced their views on pregnancy and childbirth, which may not represent those of other very young pregnant women and mothers. The author spent a day at the centre, getting to know the respondents, and explaining the purpose of the research. Three small group interviews (two with three respondents and one with two) were carried out during the following week. Each lasted for approximately one hour. The tapes were fully transcribed, and the data analysed thematically.

The small group discussions had three aims: first, to ascertain participants' knowledge and use of contraceptive methods, and their perceptions of associated risks; second, to explore their more general understanding of health risks; and, third, to examine their own experiences of being a subject of risk assessment by the health-care system. For convenience, the participants are referred to as 'girls'.

## CONTRACEPTIVE RISKS

### Contraceptive knowledge

These girls had some knowledge, at least, about contraception. For example, they could list all currently available methods of contraception without prompting. They had obtained advice within the unit, and most had received information from school, family and friends. Other knowledge sources included television, newspapers, magazines and health-education leaflets.

Several girls (giggling) referred to the relatively new female 'condom', and all knew about 'implants' (mentioned with grimaces). Questionnaire methods do not detect such non-verbal expressions of humour, pain or fear. However, emotional responses to contraceptive methods affect their subsequent acceptance and use.

Prohibitive attitudes towards sex, in some cases, affected contraceptive education at school. One girl, pregnant at 14, felt that sex was a dirty word in her school, and that sex education had come too late for her. Some teachers seemed reluctant to implicitly legitimate sex and contraception for young people.

> They've started doing it [sex education] younger now, which is a good thing. But, I still don't think they [teachers] know that you can, you see, they don't like to say to teenagers, 'You can have sex,' 'You can go on the pill,' sort of thing.

The information given was judged insufficient.

> We had a little bit ... They don't go into proper details about it, just give you brief notes about it, and that's it.

Superficial education generated feelings of uncertainty, and, as in the second example below, serious misunderstanding.

> It's like the needle. I don't even know how that would work. If I have it every three months ... Well, I can't tell you what that would mean.

> I don't know how the pill works. You just take it ... I think it just kills the eggs inside you. I don't think people know enough about it. It may be just me.

In terms of risk analysis, the next quotation, about the 'morning-after' pill, illustrates two important issues.

> *That's just what it is ... It just like gets the ovaries and kills them [eggs] ... before they get there ... I don't like it. I've had it before ... My friend had it and she was sick ... She says she will never have it again.*

First, the above comment shows how induction can be based on a single concrete incident. In this case, the generalisation turns out to have some empirical support (International Medical Advisor Panel, 1994) since approximately half of all women taking emergency oral contraception experience nausea. Second, the quotation illustrates the intimate connection between medical and social analysis. The respondent believes that a fertilised egg is alive, and, therefore, can be killed. Another group participant described the morning-after pill as producing *'an abortion'*. Whether this pill is considered contraceptive or abortive depends on where the line between sperm/eggs and a live being is drawn.

## Contraceptive behaviour

Only one of the eight girls reported using contraception at the time of conception. She had been on the pill, but had had difficulty in remembering to take it. Others admitted that they had been thinking about adopting contraceptive measures, but had not acted in time. All had been sexually active before the current pregnancy, some since the age of 13, as found repeatedly in surveys of young peoples' sexual behaviours (Wellings *et al.*, 1995). Since they would not have received contraceptive advice in school by this age, their sexual activity could not have been encouraged by its receipt.

Some girls' partners had used condoms, but not on a regular basis. One respondent and her boyfriend had used the withdrawal method successfully for one-and-a-half years before she became pregnant. Another girl reported that she had been having sex for two years, and had used a condom twice.

Having escaped pregnancy for so long, these girls may have induced that they were at low risk. Beliefs about the fertilisation process were sometimes used to produce a sense of reduced vulnerability to the risk of unplanned pregnancy. One girl remarked that her friend had only become pregnant after two years of unprotected sex because, *'she's getting older now and her stuff will be fertilising and everything'*. The belief that women are not immediately fertile following the menarche may have a slight empirical basis, in more frequent irregular ovulation at this time (Baldwin, 1983).

The girls drew on a variety of explanations as to why pregnancy sometimes did not result from sexual intercourse. One was male infertility.

> *He might not have been able to produce proper sperm.*

The following explanation illustrates the complexities of risk-reasoning.

> *Mebbe it's just missed. It has to look for it. It has to go through the cervix bit, doesn't it, but it is only about 100–200 get through there.*

Although correct as one explanation of why sexual intercourse frequently does not lead to fertilisation, this way of looking at reproduction could generate a false sense of security. Millions of sperm are produced, and most 'miss', but only one is needed to produce a baby!

The girls' risk-taking behaviour appears to have been based, initially, on a sense of invulnerability stemming from incomplete or incorrect knowledge. The non-occurrence of pregnancy reinforced this sense, and they came to see sexual intercourse without contraception as a low-risk behaviour. As one of the girls put it:

> You know how people do it, and they don't fall pregnant ... So they do it for ages ... And then it happens.

The use of a sense of invulnerability as a 'protective' device has also been found in young people's responses to the threat of HIV (Abrams et al., 1990), as noted in Chapter 2.

The counter case involves girls who became pregnant very quickly, as illustrated by a remark made in response to the last quotation.

> I know. That makes me laugh ... 'cos I only done it a couple of times without using protection, and I fell pregnant straight away ... And this other lass uses nothing.

However, 'first time' pregnancies were dismissed as highly improbable.

> It's very rare, very rare, that that [pregnancy at first intercourse] happens to someone.

Despite this sense of invulnerability, some girls passed judgement on others who, they felt, should somehow have benefited from their own mistakes.

> It shocks us that there is people still coming in here who are pregnant. Sometimes it is a mistake ... There is nothing you can do about it ... But, you know, there are people who are having sex, and not on the pill, nor nothing ... I done it ... but I think, 'Why don't they just go on the pill ... It's not going to do them any harm.'

The notion of a 'mistake' illustrates the use of the idea of residual fatalism in popular risk analysis (Davison, Frankel and Davey Smith, 1992). However, this respondent's comment invited the following riposte which neatly illustrates the way in which a high-risk behaviour, to an external observer, could be seen as safe.

> But them'll just be thinking the same as what you thought ... that you'll not get pregnant.

## Pharmaceuticals and side effects

Group members had strong, but not always shared, feelings about the risks of side effects associated with different contraceptive methods. They had all heard, in 1995, about news reports concerning certain contraceptive pills. All mentioned blood clots and cancer as side effects of the pill. The three girls who were currently taking the pill said that the only side effects they had been told about concerned the possibility of putting on weight. The 'pill-scare' had not troubled one young mother.

> I've never had any problems with it ... makes us feel dead secure with it ... I don't actually want to go to the doctor because they might change us ... I have known people change and fall pregnant ... I'm not worried.

However, she appears to have confused the pregnancy risk associated with coming off the pill with the risk of switching from one brand to another, and so had unnecessarily precluded herself from switching to a safer brand. Some beliefs about the pill's contraceptive effects were seriously mistaken.

> *Say you have stopped taking it after you have been on it for so many years ... The pill can still last for a couple of more years later.*

Since women may not become pregnant for some time after coming off the pill, this incorrect hypothesis could be supported by concrete experience, another example of the trap of induction.

One girl had experienced mood changes which her family had attributed to the pill.

> *I took it again, and me mam says, 'You are getting all angry again ... And you are starting to get dead depressed.'*

This example illustrates the complexity of cost-benefit analysis involving multiple consequences (see Chapter 1). The respondent appears to have accepted a greater risk of pregnancy in order to avoid the adverse social consequences of the emotional side effects which she attributed to the pill.

Another research participant worried about a relative who had been taking the pill.

> *Me nanna's sister ... she died and everyone thinks it was because she took the pill for all them years ... 'cos she took it from being younger ... She didn't smoke or nothing like that.*

Family-planning professionals need to explore clients' personal views during consultations. No matter how obscure a belief may seem to a clinician, it can strongly influence their contraceptive choices.

Other methods of contraception were viewed with some suspicion. One girl, probably influenced by current media horror stories, said of the implant:

> *I wouldn't like things in me arm. In one woman, they lost the rods.*

The following quotations illustrate the concerns expressed about the long-term side effects of injections and implants.

> *It can make you ill, the injections make you infertile.*

> *I was going to get the injections, but I didn't want it. Implants was another, but they leave you for two years and you always put on weight when you go on the implants, and the injections make you infertile ... I don't want to be infertile.*

The second girl quoted had had an intrauterine device fitted. The next quotation shows that she had chosen this method, despite concern about its side effects, because she believed that those associated with the pill were even worse.

> *Well, I had a leaflet on it [intrautrine device]. It said you, most young people, get infections on it, but there's nowt else I can take. I tried the pill, but I don't want to take it no more ... since blood clots, since the stuff that's been on the news. But I always forgot to take it anyway. That's how I got pregnant.*

Far from evading decision-making, this young mother had followed a similar pathway to her older sisters in taking 'the least worst option' (Walsh, Lythgoe and Peckham, 1996). She took account of her own inability to remember to take the pill regularly, and had consciously accepted the risk of infection.

## Risks associated with physical barrier methods of contraception

Contraceptive methods based on relatively simple physical barriers, such as the femidom, condoms and withdrawal, did not arouse the same fears as high-tech interventions which affect the user biochemically. However, the girls associated the former with risks in quite complex ways.

The femidom, referred to by one girl as *'the wife's condom'* was viewed with a kind of music-hall humour.

*I wouldn't dare ... They look funny.*

To use such a contraceptive, a girl must be able to touch herself intimately. Their use raises issues about ownership of one's body, gender and autonomy in sexual relationships (Oakley, 1993). The last quotation illustrates the motivating power of the need to avoid being a target for humour: a need which does not figure in medical cost-benefit analyses, not themselves noted for witticism.

The advantage seen in condoms was their absence of potential, unknown side effects. The following respondent felt that this advantage outweighed any reduction in sexual enjoyment.

*It [condom] feels different, but I wouldn't get needles.*

Others were concerned about the physical security of the condom.

*I always thought the condom would come off and go inside me.*

*You should worry because the condom can split.*

Most research participants believed that withdrawal was risky. But one girl saw it as an acceptably safe contraceptive method providing that her partner was reliable.

*If you trusted your lad, it is a good method.*

Even when told by a midwife that this method was risky, she maintained her belief that it would be safe, because *'not much goes inside you'*. This remark, again, suggests confusion about the redundancy which nature has built into procreational processes. Withdrawal worked for her for more than a year, but she had then become pregnant.

## Risk and sexually transmitted diseases

Unprotected sex exposed girls to a logarithmic risk of infection from partners of partners.

*Even just somebody that's been with one person ... has been with several people ... other people with several people ... It goes on and on.*

The girls could all list the main sexually transmitted diseases, and knew about the risk of HIV and AIDS. However, risk of infection was not continually on their minds and most felt safe with their respective boyfriends.

*He's only been with one [other] and she was a virgin ... She was only 12.*

*He's not been with loads ... like just a few.*

*AIDS. You don't think that your lad's going to have AIDS, do you?*

Abrams *et al.* (1990) found that young people developed a similar sense of security with respect to the risk of AIDS, based on the idea that it was possible to 'trust' your partner not to be HIV positive.

## Access to contraceptive services

Confusion could still be detected, post-Gillick, about confidentiality and the contraceptive rights of under 16-year-olds, as found in a recent survey (Family Planning Association and Contraceptive Education Service, 1995).

*Well, at first, I thought I couldn't go on the pill until I was 16.*

This confusion was, apparently, shared by some professionals.

*I went for the pill, and they sent me home for to go and tell me mam that I needed permission.*

In contrast, some professionals actively sought out contraceptive needs. One girl had seen her doctor about another matter. The doctor had asked her if she was using contraception, and had told her that if a girl came for advice, it would be given, regardless of her age.

Although professionals are required to encourage under 16-year-olds to talk to their parents, they can legally provide contraceptive advice and services in the best interests of the client (BMA, 1994). Ignorant of their legal rights, some girls believed that they had to lie in order to 'work the system'.

*At the Family Planning, you are supposed to be 16, but people just go. Are they going to prove that you are not 16? ... Make your own date of birth up ... It may be deceiving them ... But if that's what it takes to not fall pregnant.*

## PREGNANCY RISKS

### Stigmatisation of young pregnant women

Girls' attitudes towards their pregnancies, and towards professional advice, were coloured by feelings of being unfairly stereotyped as irresponsible because of their age. (Ironically, the 'older' mothers, whose views are discussed in Chapter 7, also felt stigmatised.)

*It's not just young lasses who act stupid.*

*There's more people in their late twenties who take risks.*

Respondents often felt that they had to excel in order to overcome negative stereotyping.

*You try to make yourself a perfect mother ... Young mothers try to make themselves ... try to have everything ... so people can't say nothing about you.*

Several girls encountered negative attitudes on their first visit to the clinic.

*I went there, and they found out I was pregnant, and they said I should get rid of it straight away.*

This respondent did not return to the clinic. The girls clearly grasped the link between supposedly objective risk assessments and moral disapproval.

*I think everyone should get the same treatment ... We should get the same as a 30-year-old ... They don't say, 'There's a big risk there'.*

One girl recounted being told by her doctor that she was *'too young, with her whole life ahead of her, and that she would have risks of losing the baby'*. He changed his attitude when she told him that she was going to keep the baby, stating that risks in pregnancy were usually the same for everyone.

Group participants asserted that they were less at risk of having an abnormal pregnancy than older women, thus rebutting the charge of medical irresponsibility.

*I thought there would have been a lot less risks for younger people than older people ... Down's syndrome, is it? ... They have to have tests and that, when they are older.*

A 14- or 15-year-old girl who presents early in pregnancy can choose to continue with the pregnancy or to have an abortion, and, in the former case, either to keep her baby or to agree to have it adopted. As Illsley and Taylor (1974) remarked, in their study of teenage pregnancy, such choices are highly personal, mediated by social and cultural norms. The girls welcomed being given information, but felt that they should be allowed to make their own decisions. They, thus, recognised an inherent limitation of expertise (see Chapter 1): that it cannot resolve value questions.

*I think they should tell, and let you know everything, but I don't think they should advise you.*

*We should be the ones who have to think it over for ourselves.*

*It's when they start saying you're being silly.*

Konje *et al.* (1992) found, in a retrospective comparison of pregnancy outcomes, that providing girls aged under 16 received adequate antenatal care, their experience and outcomes were no worse than those in a control group of 20–24-year-olds. Anaemia was more of a problem in the younger group, but, contrary to expectations, they had significantly lower Caesarean section and perinatal mortality rates.

Konje *et al.*'s study highlights the social and emotional needs of young mothers, to be accepted, to belong and to identify with others, which are often overlooked within the health-care system. The authors also conclude that improved contraception services and sex education in schools are needed, as does much of the health promotional literature (Macdonald and Smith, 1990). Konje *et al.* found that 92.2 per cent of the under-16s in their study did not use contraception. However, most lived in high-density, low-income council estates where having a baby at 16 was not unusual. Sex education, to be effective, will have to challenge historically established cultural norms.

## HEALTHY INTENTIONS

All of the girls said that they had modified their own behaviours once they knew they were pregnant. Those who smoked had stopped, during pregnancy, and they had shown awareness of the risks of passive smoking. As one pregnant girl put it, *'No one's allowed to smoke in our house now.'* One respondent remarked that some people smoked and had healthy babies, but they all knew about the increased risks of cot death and bad chests for babies living in a household where people smoked.

All the research participants knew about the benefits of certain foodstuffs. Some had modified their habits during pregnancy, eating more fruit, for example. However, a knowledge–behaviour gap was apparent, as two girls said they ate *'mostly crisps and chocolates'*. Respondents also mentioned the risks of eating paté, certain cheeses and other foods, but their knowledge was somewhat vague.

> *Another thing about eggs ... when they're not cooked.*

> *That disease you can get from the fridge ... if it's off.*

The girls wanted to give their babies the 'best' food, although none had breastfed, or intended to breastfeed. They belong to social groups found to be least likely to attempt breastfeeding, where breasts (and exposing them) have different associations (Martin and White, 1985). They did not consider alcohol in moderation, as they defined it, to be risky. One girl said that she only drank *'the odd time ... one or two at Christmas ... We are not alcoholics ... It's only, like, every other weekend.'*

After the births of their babies, all the smokers resumed their habit, and smoked in front of their children. They saw *'getting fat'* as a worse outcome than accepting the risks of smoking, and used cigarettes as a form of hunger control.

> *I tried to stop smoking, but I just eat.*

> *If you go on a diet you smoke more, don't you?*

As previously shown (Graham, 1984; Heyman, 1995b, p. 83), smokers living in poverty see their habit as a necessary evil which enables them to function in harsh conditions.

> *After I had her, I just started again. You go through a phase, and you get sick, and depression, and that's what starts you off ... When they start crying ... you just automatically go for your tabs ... because it's something there.*

All the mothers felt they were unhealthy as a result of being overweight, smoking and not exercising. Heyman (1995b, p. 82) uncovered similarly negative self-assessments of their own health among the poor residents of a socially deprived area. Dissatisfaction with the healthiness of their own lifestyles is not confined to young mothers. Nevertheless, those in the present study attributed their problems to constant childcare. Their replies suggested humorous resignation to the inevitable.

> I'd just love to go on a diet, stop smoking and get myself dead fit and healthy, but I cannot. Even talking about it makes me tired!

As found previously (Davison, Frankel and Davey-Smith, 1992), fatalism was one response to the residual uncertainty inherent in risk analysis.

> Someone who is dead healthy ... could walk out on the road and get run over.

The final quotation illustrates a hedonistic approach to the future, based on discounting the future at a high rate of return (see Chapter 2):

> I would rather have a short life, when you enjoy yourself.

## Discussion

Although the views of these pregnant and young mothers are not necessarily representative, much can be learned from their responses and experiences. A wider debate needs to include the views of young men, but, in the absence of formal provision for schoolboy fathers, they remain less accessible to researchers.

These young people attach as much significance to image as their elders and social betters. Respondents frequently mentioned weight-gain avoidance as a factor in their choice of contraception, and as an important reason for their resumption of smoking. They wanted to be listened to and respected, not castigated. Most attended support sessions regularly, and wished to become good mothers.

Respondents found social attitudes towards young mothers to be negative. They felt that those in authority treated them unfairly, with a systematic lack of respect. The girls saw themselves as subjected to the influence of external agencies which continually attempted to control them. In the discussions, respondents regularly used the term 'they' when referring to doctors, midwives, schools, the government, or newspapers.

The powerlessness of women in lower socioeconomic groups, especially in relation to their health care, has been well documented (Blaxter, 1983; Arber, 1991). Other commentators (Coyne, 1986; Russell, 1988) have represented the futures of teenage mothers as unavoidably impoverished, and have sometimes portrayed them as a drain on the social welfare system.

Contraceptive services seem to be failing young people, as so many do not use them. The experiences of this group match those reported elsewhere (Konje *et al.*, 1992; Scott, 1994). Services designed by professionals at the request of politicians, aimed at young women rather than men, and based on values at odds with those held by the majority of young people, need to be reconsidered. As the Contraceptive Education Service Report (Walsh,

Lythgoe and Peckham, 1996) suggests, services provided outside medical or other official establishments may attract more of the potential client group. But contraceptive services, however user-friendly, cannot mitigate against the pervasive problems of oppression and poverty.

For many young women, motherhood provides a relatively acceptable alternative to menial, poorly paid work or unemployment. Their future prospects are affected not just by becoming mothers at a young age, but by the consequent socioeconomic status, typically of undeserving claimant, awarded to them. This 'grouping', based on the culturally mediated societal response to young motherhood, more or less seals their fate. In such a climate, teenage mothers will always be deemed 'at risk' of poor health and poor mothering.

# Being old and pregnant

## Mette Henriksen and Bob Heyman

| |
|---|
| Introduction |
| Methodology |
| Data analysis |
| Discussion |

*Little girls are born with every egg they're ever going to have, and you wouldn't buy an egg from Sainsbury's if it had been on the shelf for forty years, would you? Why should you expect to make a healthy baby from it? But people do.* (Clinical research fellow in infertility, quoted in Armstrong, 1996, p. 318)

## Introduction

Modern women are plagued by concerns about the wisdom of late childbearing (Mansfield, 1986a). The first part of this chapter examines the origins of the classification of mid-life childbearing as a risk. The second part considers the experiences of some older and younger pregnant women who attended a single hospital in Tyne and Wear.

### THE CULTURAL CLASSIFICATION OF AGE

Cultures divide the human life span into stages linked to age-specific norms (Johnson, 1989). The Nupe of Nigeria, for example, categorise people into three age groups, while the Nandi of Kenya recognise 28 age categories (Eisenstadt, 1956). Western cultures identify six major life stages: infancy; childhood; adolescence; young adulthood; middle age; and old age (Johnson, 1989).

Age groupings provide prescriptive timetables for the ordering of major life events. Most societies define appropriate age ranges at which to marry, raise children, and to retire. Individuals understand these cultural timetables, and readily describe themselves as 'early', 'late', or 'on time' in relation to family and occupational temporal milestones (Neugarten, Moore and Lowe, 1965). Feeling out of step with one's peers in the timing of major life events may contribute to a sense of personal inadequacy and incompetence (Heslon, Mitchell and Moane, 1984). Rook, Catalano and Dooley (1989) found only limited general empirical support for 'social clock theory', but did detect an association between the delayed experience of (presumably) desirable events, including the birth of the first child, and emotional distress.

## AGE NORMS AND PREGNANCY

Western societies, like most others, attach considerable importance to women becoming pregnant at the 'right' age. Those outside this normative age range can experience both social and medical stigmatisation. In Chapter 6, Aarvold discusses the ways in which professionals and policy-makers may categorise teenage pregnancy as a problem despite a lack of evidence that these women face an increased net risk of unpreventable medical complications. Similarly, 'older' pregnant women can be subjected to a barrage of pessimistic views about their reproductive capabilities (Silverton, 1993).

The medical belief that older women, especially first-time mothers, suffer more pregnancy complications dates back hundreds of years. Points (1957, p. 348) cites a French physician, who in 1668 wrote *'Women a little antiquated suffer more in their first labours than other women.'* A medical report from 1932 (cited in Mansfield, 1986a, p. 19) concluded that older women could *'naturally expect longer labour, more toxaemia and a greater likelihood of fetal and maternal morbidity and mortality'*. In 1958, the International Council of Obstetricians and Gynaecologists decided that a woman aged 35 years or older at her first delivery was to be called an 'elderly primigravida', and considered a high-risk patient (Tuck, Yudkin and Turnbull, 1988). Bourne (1995), in a recent medical text, advised that older mothers should be given the 'at risk card', entitling them to increased antenatal surveillance and testing.

Consideration of the cultural context of this medical opinion raises the question of how far it has been unconsciously influenced by wider social attitudes towards the 'proper' age for motherhood. As argued in Chapter 2, with respect to the link between maternal age and Down's syndrome, the treatment of maternal age as a primary risk factor entails a tacit epidemiological decision to elevate this variable to the status of a bedrock cause, not to be investigated further.

## CONCEPTION TRENDS

Despite such gloomy attitudes towards 'older' mothering, the number of women having babies over the age of 35 is increasing in industrialised societies. In England and Wales, the fertility rate for women aged 35–39 years has increased from 18.2 births per 1000 women in 1977 to 31.7 in 1991, and that for women aged over 40 years from 4.4 to 5.3 (OPCS, 1992). By the year 2000, an estimated 40 per cent of all births will occur to women aged 30 and over (Langford, 1992). An increase in births to remarried women and career-related delays in starting a family have contributed to this trend. The profile of the 'older' mother has changed over the past two decades, from the woman who carries on reproducing into her middle years (Milner *et al.*, 1992) to the middle-class postponer of low parity (Hollander and Breen, 1990) and higher socioeconomic status (Jones, 1996).

## THE RISKS ASSOCIATED WITH BEING 'OLD' AND PREGNANT

> *Older women having children is all about beating the odds and turning convention on its head.* (Armstrong, 1996, p. 11.)

Recent critical reviews (Hansen, 1986; Mansfield, 1986b, 1986c; Utian and Kiwi, 1988; Harker and Thorpe, 1992) have pointed out that most studies of relationships between advanced maternal age and pregnancy outcomes have failed to control for important contextual differences between younger and older pregnant women. Recent studies suggest that, except, possibly, in the case of age-related genetic disorders, being older is not associated with additional risk when other factors are taken into account (Ales, Druzin and Santini, 1990; Berkowitz et al., 1990). Duchon and Muise (1993) argue that the excess of adverse outcomes reported in the older group may result from higher rates of pre-existing disease, subfertility, high parity and unplanned pregnancy, rather than the biological effects of ageing, which may provide no more than a proxy variable.

However, being placed in a high-risk category may itself increase a woman's risks of incurring obstetric problems, through processes of reflexive recursion, as argued in Chapter 2. For example, advanced maternal age alone may influence an obstetrician's decision about the method of delivery, thereby placing older women at an unnecessary risk of medical interventions and Caesarean sections (Tuck, Yudkin and Turnbull, 1988; Duchon and Muise, 1993). The stress resulting from being labelled 'high-risk' may also have a negative emotional impact on older women, and, in turn, affect biological outcomes (Blum, 1979; Mansfield, 1988).

## AGE AND GENETIC TESTING

A positive correlation between maternal age and the risk of chromosomal abnormalities has emerged as one of the few consistent findings in the medical literature. Mothers attending antenatal clinics may be quoted the following 'natural' incidence of live born Down's syndrome infants (in the absence of genetic testing and selective abortion): from 1: 1350 at the age of 25 to 1: 30 at 45 (Kennard et al., 1995). However, as already noted, this relationship may not arise from processes unalterably associated with maternal ageing. For example, it might, in theory at least, result partly or wholly from decreased coital frequency at older ages leading to delayed fertilisation in the monthly cycle, increased exposure to X-rays (Rose, 1994), infections and other environmental factors (Takei, et al., 1995), or differences in prior pregnancy history.

Age varies continuously, as does the background incidence of live Down's syndrome births. The associated questions of the age at which pregnant women should be classified as 'older' (DiGuilio, 1957) and, more recently, the age at which they should be offered genetic testing, have aroused controversy. The cut-off age for being offered testing varies considerably, and, in the USA at least, has dropped steadily, from 40 to 38 to 35, and currently to the low thirties (Rapp, 1988a).

Older women are now offered genetic screening as a routine component of antenatal care, shifting attention from the idea of reproduction as an unmitigated right to that of responsibility to produce healthy children (Beck-Gernsheim, 1996). Those older mothers who knowingly beget unhealthy children, or who refuse screening, have to endure mounting social pressure to conform to standards of 'responsible' procreational actions (Blank, 1992). Older women often feel anxious and depressed as they go through tests which themselves carry risks associated with negative emotions, and of miscarriage in the case of amniocentesis (Green, 1994).

## Methodology

The qualitative data discussed in this chapter were collected as part of a larger project undertaken in a single hospital in an urban area of north-east England.

Women's views about age and pregnancy must be understood in their demographic context (Office for National Statistics, 1996). The urban area served by the hospital-research site had relatively high conception rates among younger women, for example 74.1 per thousand women aged 15–19 in 1994, compared with 58.6 in England and Wales. Conversely, conception rates among older women are among the lowest in the UK. In 1994 this area had a conception rate of 24.9 per 1000 among women aged 35–39, compared with 37.8 for England and Wales. Among women aged 40 and over, the conception rate in the research district was 4.0 per 1000, the lowest in England and Wales in 1994, compared with a national average of 7.7 per 1000.

Not surprisingly, given this youthful maternal profile, the area has a low incidence of Down's syndrome births. Only one Down's syndrome birth, out of 4214 live and still births, was notified in 1991 (OPCS, 1993a, p. 7). On the other hand, the relative scarcity of older women may have contributed to the social pressures they experienced, which are discussed below.

Research information has been obtained from interviews with pregnant women, midwives, obstetric consultants and registrars, tape-recordings of genetic counselling sessions, and questionnaires distributed to pregnant women. Since the samples were all associated with a single hospital, the research must be treated as a case study. Its findings cannot be generalised beyond the site investigated. Some additional data from the project have been presented in Chapters 1 and 2.

The material considered in this chapter derives mainly from intensive, open-ended interviews with a convenience sample of 40 women (36 pregnant and 4 post-partum), 21 of whom were aged 35 or over. A further 6 women declined to be interviewed, giving an 87 per cent participation rate. All interviewees considered their pregnancy normal, and as requiring only routine antenatal care. Respondents chose their own interview location, with 35 opting to be interviewed in their own homes, and 5 in the antenatal clinic. All interviews were tape-recorded, transcribed, and at least partially analysed before the next interview, thus facilitating theoretical sampling, the use of emerging themes to guide subsequent data collection (Strauss, 1987). Interviews ranged in length from 45 minutes to two-and-a-half hours, with most taking approximately one hour. Nine women chose to invite friends, partners, parents or grandparents to participate, while the other 31 were interviewed individually.

Each interview began with a general question, asking the respondent how she had found her pregnancy so far. Follow-up questions were open-ended, designed to encourage the woman to expand on her comments, and to speak at length about her experiences of pregnancy, responses to pregnancy advice, attitudes and plans. Although the interviewer deliberately avoided initiating discussion of risk, or age, data collection focused on the women's accounts of risks in their pregnancy, and the impact of risk appraisal on their decision-making.

A grounded theory approach (Strauss and Corbin, 1990) was adopted in order to explore the experienced worlds of the pregnant women. This approach uses defined analytic procedures to categorise and connect social phenomena in ways that are grounded in the empirical world, rather than superimposed on it by the researchers' preconceptions. Analysis began with the first interview, and was carried out concurrently with the collection of new material (Glaser and Strauss, 1967). As it became possible to discern the functions that might be served by the women's ways of perceiving risk information, the content categories were developed into analytic categories (e.g. being on the right side of risk, induced expectations about risk, acquiring risk knowledge). These interpretive categories were used to describe and analyse what the women were saying about themselves and their concerns.

The picture of pregnant women's perceptions of risks during normal pregnancy that emerged from the interviews was based on the integration of many comments made by different women about a variety of situations. Excerpts from the interviews are presented to illustrate emergent themes. All names have been changed in order to preserve the anonymity of the participants.

## Data analysis

### AGE AND PREGNANCY

#### Being 'old' and pregnant

Most respondents, young and old, reflected on their age in relation to being pregnant. Some older women felt that the category of being 'old' had been imposed on them by clinicians or peers.

> I gets booked in, you know, and she went, 'And how old are you?' And I went, 'I'm 40.' So she writes 40, and then she underlines it in red three times. (Alison, aged 40)

The next quotation illustrates the way in which the possibility of testing generated a sense of being 'old', even where it was rejected.

> No, they didn't mention it last time [prenatal screening], but this time they did. To be quite honest I came out feeling more like 58 rather than 38, and after a lot of soul-searching, I just decided not to bother with anything. (Jane, aged 38)

Respondents resented the professional choice of language which demeaned them because of their age.

> Yeah, so the doctor said to me with the second one, 'Well, if you want any more, you're getting on a bit, perhaps you'd better bang it out quick'. That was his exact words. 'Bang it out quick.' (Carol, aged 38)

A woman's status as 'old' was also linked to her appearance in a wider family and social context.

> *I feel people are looking at us all the time ... I've never been one of these that looks young, so sometimes people think I look older than what I am. And people's looking at me, and he [husband] says, 'You're imagining it,' and I'd say, 'I'm not.'* (Linda, aged 36)

A number of respondents mentioned the importance, to them, of experiencing pregnancy at the same time as their peers. The following quotation comes from an obstetric registrar who was discussing her own personal views about becoming pregnant while in her mid-thirties.

> *Most of the circle of friends and professional friends that I have are around the same age anyway, so it is not as if I would feel like I was an old mum among lots of 25-year-olds', because I'm sure that, within my circle of friends, we would all be within five years of each other. And so that wouldn't be a problem.* (Obstetric registrar)

Complicating the apparently simple matter of chronicity still further, the age at which a pregnant woman was judged to be 'old' could depend on parity.

> *I must say, I had a worse reaction to my age with my first baby. And that was really, you know, 'How old are you, how old? And this is your first, your first?' And I was thinking, 'I'm not old' ... I was only 33.* (Carol, aged 38)

## Age as a binary category

In classifying themselves and others as 'old' and 'young', women had to decide where the boundary lay. Judgements varied, but were bound up with the perceived need to have genetic tests. The location of the boundary between being 'young', and not being routinely required to consider testing, and being 'old', and expected to make decisions about testing, depended both on the information women received, and how they interpreted it.

> *They said with my age, I wasn't over 40, so really it [testing] wasn't necessary.* (Helen, aged 36)

> *I suppose, maybe, if I was like older, maybe 35 or something, I would think a lot more about it [testing].* (Joan, aged 31)

> *I think once you're over 30 ... I wouldn't have tests like that, so I wouldn't put myself in that position.* (Lisa, aged 28)

Each of these women (Tversky and Kahneman, 1973) anchored the cut-off point for being old a few years above her own age. Possibly, women may move the testing boundary upwards as they get older. As the quotes illustrate, some women excluded themselves from the 'older' category because they wished to avoid being eligible for testing. However, one woman felt the dividing line was an arbitrary one, created by service-providers in order to balance costs and benefits.

> *The only thing that makes me think is, why is amnio[centesis] only offered to 35-year-olds and over ... I suppose they've got to draw the line somewhere.* (Glenda, aged 37)

Some women discovered that registrars and consultants within the hospital had different individual policies with respect to the age at which genetic screening should be routinely discussed (see Chapter 2).

> I was asking them [other mothers] about the blood test, and they were just saying that some of them were offered them when they were 33. So, just different cases, different doctors. (Anna, aged 35)

Since being 'old' and pregnant was constituted, within the hospital, by the requirement to consider testing, a doctor's testing policy determined whether a borderline woman was 'old' or not.

## Age and moral responsibility

'Older' women and their partners sometimes felt they were deemed morally irresponsible because they had chosen to take risks by deciding to have a baby while 'old'.

> WIFE: I thought, I am 46 and having my first baby, people will think I ought to know better.
> HUSBAND: We both thought that when we started telling everyone people would say you are too old ...
> WIFE: And ought to know better, and should be using something ... I did, as I said before, I wanted one [a baby], as I am coming up to 45. And I am going to get the same thing, 'You should have known better at your age. You shouldn't be having kids.' (Sophie and Toby, both aged 46)

However, health professionals could also judge a woman to be morally irresponsible for having a baby whilst 'too young.'

> INTERVIEWER: How did you cope with having a miscarriage at 22 weeks at such an early age [18]?
> INTERVIEWEE: I think I coped because I was still with my mum. I didn't think the hospital was good ... I didn't get any support, and the nurse treated us as if it was my fault. (Lisa, aged 28)

While 'older' women resisted the idea that they were being irresponsible, 'younger' women were more likely to see problems in having a baby later in life. They were as much concerned with their own health and functioning as with the risk to the baby.

> I want to be young enough to think that I'm fit enough to enjoy them while I'm young. But I don't think the fact of being older, as a risk to the baby, entered my head. (Sam, aged 25)

## COST-BENEFIT ANALYSIS

Women used age, reduced to a binary category with a variable boundary, to determine their eligibility for genetic testing. However, those who felt medically eligible, through being 'old', were not necessarily willing to be tested. The women employed a form of cost-benefit analysis in which they first decided whether they might be willing to have a termination. Women who had rejected termination in any circumstances mostly, but not invariably, concluded that, therefore, testing served no purpose. In contrast, those women who had tests did so usually because they had already decided to consider termination if a genetic abnormality was detected.

Thus, in both cases, women reasoned rationally, but from different value positions. However, four important asymmetries, discussed below, were found in their reasoning. First, those willing to consider termination invoked wider family considerations, while women who rejected testing focused on the loss of the baby. Second, the decision to be tested affected women's attitudes towards the baby in the period before the results were known. Third, women who contemplated termination encountered uncertainty about their future intentions should the test result prove positive which, in turn, affected the rationality of the initial decision. Fourth, the decision to be tested often stimulated intense anxiety, not experienced by those who had rejected it.

## Rejection of termination

The women who chose not to be tested mostly reasoned that, since they did not want a termination under any circumstances, being tested served no purpose and, in the case of amniocentesis, would lead to an increased risk of miscarriage.

> If there is a problem, would I want to put the baby at risk with amniocentesis or an abortion? Could I do that? I don't think, personally, I could. And that way, I probably wouldn't have screening done. The consequences, I'm going to be left with, fair enough. But, there again, I could have a nice healthy normal baby. I don't need it. I could have had a Down's syndrome baby at 26. (Faye, aged 34)

A few women rejected testing because they did not want to risk knowing that they would give birth to a Down's syndrome child.

> I didn't want to be placed in a position of having to decide about a termination, because I knew I wouldn't want one. But I thought, 'Once you know for a fact that you have a Down's syndrome child, would that change you?' (Joanne, aged 36)

This woman was also concerned to avoid moral censure which she felt might arise from knowingly deciding to have a child with Down's syndrome.

> Would I feel pressure from people out there [if tested with a positive result], who would say, 'You knew you were having a Down's syndrome child, and you brought it into the world,' you know? So I didn't even want to run the risk of going down that road. (Joanne, aged 36)

This reasoning illustrates one of the main points made in Chapter 2: that individuals have some choice over the probabilities entered into the cost-benefit equation, since they can opt to seek or avoid further information which would either increase or decrease a more global estimate. By deciding not to be tested, the above respondent accepted an intermediate probability of having a baby with a genetic abnormality, lower than that which she would have had to face if she had tested positive, but higher than the one she would have gained from a negative test result. As argued in Chapter 2, people managing risks can accomplish the apparently impossible feat of controlling the probability of an event through their decisions about its investigation because probability statements entail the externalisation of uncertainty on to the world.

Having made their decision, the women had to negotiate their relationships with health professionals. Their experiences, and the problems they gave rise to, varied. Some considered they had been given a genuine choice, but others felt under pressure to be tested. One woman accepted serum-screening, even though she was not prepared to have amniocentesis or a termination, out of a sense of obligation.

> They looked at me history, and then they said, 'Well you are 35, so I think we'll give you the, would you like the blood test?' They says, 'You don't have to have it.' But, I think, when you are offered something I think you feel, well, I feel guilty, so I took it. (Anna, aged 35)

Exceptionally, overt conflict arose between a woman who had rejected testing and a health professional.

> I had to wait for ages, and I saw a lady doctor who said she wanted to talk to me about Down's. And I said, 'Well, actually I have no questions. We've done our own research, and we're quite happy about it and that, we will get on with it.' And she said, 'Well, you should have a test'. And I said, 'Well, no. I know that the test carries a risk of a miscarriage' ... And then I had to wait there, and wait there, and wait there, while she tried to persuade me to have this test ... A just plain headache was turning into a migraine. And she said, 'Well, I can't just let you go with that. You'll have to talk to the consultant.' Then the consultant came by He said, 'What's it all about?' ... And I said, 'Look, I've talked it over with my husband, and this is what we've decided, and I don't see the point in doing it.' [The consultant said] 'Aha, very sensible,' and left. (Carol, aged 38)

The account of the first exchange, between the respondent and the lady doctor, illustrates the way in which a professional's undelimited claim to expertise (a claim to be able to resolve value questions through expert knowledge) will be refuted by clients on the grounds that only they can decide such matters. The consultant whose response is discussed in the second part of the quotation appears to have adopted a liberal position, rejecting this undelimited claim out of hand. The very brevity of his response, as communicated by the client, conveys an attitude of taking for granted her right and ability to make her own 'sensible' decision.

## Consideration of termination of pregnancy

As already noted, women who accepted testing were mostly willing to contemplate the possibility of termination, which they justified in terms both of life quality for the child and the impact on other family members, particularly siblings. They did not mention the consequences for the mother herself, perhaps because they regarded a rationale for termination based on the welfare of others as more morally acceptable.

> I just felt that with the children, I mean his five and my two, that being as old, that if anything was wrong with the child, that it wouldn't be fair on the child or the kids to bring up, you know, another one, that we would all have to look after. (Sue, aged 41)

The decision to be tested had three important consequences. First, as reported elsewhere (McGeary, 1994) these women often avoided identifying with the baby, in case the test result turned out to be positive.

> I must admit I was trying not to think about it, and not to think of it as a baby. I thought I wouldn't ... buy anything ... The kids were talking about it. I would say, 'We will wait and see if everything's alright.' And I don't know, I just felt as if I didn't want to get too attached to it. (Judith, aged 40)

Second, the rationality of most women's decisions to be tested depended on their willingness to terminate the pregnancy following a positive result. But some respondents felt they could not know what they would do in this eventuality.

> So I went in for the amniocentesis. And, well, even then, we thought that by the time we get that done, and then the results back, it's going to be too late in any case ... And I thought it would be a terrible ordeal to go through an abortion then, like. And we just said, we'll decide if it came up that there was something wrong then. (Sue, aged 41)

Third, many women experienced intense anxiety during the period of waiting for the test results.

> Oh it [waiting] was awful ... I was just crying and everything again like I did when I found out I was pregnant. Cos I was saying, 'This baby will come out a miserable little thing!' 'Cos I was just so worried, you know. And, like I say, you think, ee, it was going to be another decision after that, you know. But it's a long time to wait, you know. I mean, when you read the books and that, you think, 'Oh well,' you know, 'Three, four weeks,' but, like, you're wishing your life away, and it's awful. (Alison, aged 40)

The above quotation brings out three important features of the risk context for those who had chosen testing. First, anxiety was, itself, experienced as a significant adverse event. Second, the women could not fully anticipate how worried they would feel when they opted for testing, even though doctors did sometimes warn them, in genetic counselling sessions, about what to expect. Third, this respondent feared that her anxiety might affect the development of the fetus, through the process described in Chapter 2 as reflexive recursion.

Other women expressed concern about the impact on other family members of having to live through such an anxious period.

> I remember feeling guilty, that I thought about the baby more than the kids around us ... I felt guilty that I was em, not as actively involved with them two for a short period of time ... because I was bogged down with worry. (Wendy, aged 36)

## RISK KNOWLEDGE

### Induction from concrete experience

In making decisions about testing, the women tried to appraise the risks involved in the various choices open to them. Despite the problems involved in inducing probabilities from very small numbers, they most commonly made inferences from positive and negative exemplars.

*I think you always worry to a certain extent, whether everything is going to be alright. I have got a couple of friends where the babies haven't been alright, so it crosses your mind.* (Sheila, aged 34)

*My friend is 40, and has just had a baby, and is fine ... I don't think it is a bleak picture that I am going to have a Downs syndrome baby. But, yes, it does cause some reassurance, especially of someone who is 40, and has had a very healthy baby, and had a very healthy pregnancy as well. She had no problems.* (Kim, aged 36)

On occasion, women would reason in a way which avoided generalisation from concrete experiences, in order to counter potentially negative predictions.

*There aren't anything in the family, really. Nobody's had ... apart from my grandparents, which is years ago, my grandmother had two hydrocephalus babies ... and my sister ... she [baby] died when she was 11 weeks old, at [other hospital]. She was born with a liver disorder, but [sister] has had a perfectly normal healthy girl after ... I mean, it's not something that was in the family. That was just something that unfortunately happened.* (Sarah, aged 37)

The implicit reasoning in the above quotation contains a number of steps. First, the respondent lumped together a variety of clinician conditions which might or might not be genetic, and reasoned from this supposed general category to the risk for her own baby. Second, she temporally distanced her own case from that of her grandmother, thus reducing its apparent relevance to herself. Third, she judged that since her sister had a second healthy baby, the problem with the first baby could be put into the residual category of luck or chance (Davison, Frankel and Davey Smith, 1992), and dismissed as 'unfortunate'.

Concrete experiences could override the general knowledge of probability.

*I think at the time it was 1 in 200 or something like that. I mean the odds are still great and my husband knows someone who was only in his early forties now, and he's got a Down's syndrome boy ... and both him and his wife were in their early twenties when they had him. And I think, 'Well, if it can happen at that age, it can happen any time.'* (Jane, aged 38)

## Risk knowledge and professional expertise

Respondents made little use of professional knowledge. One woman actively resisted statistical reasoning on the grounds of its impersonality. She had perhaps implicitly understood that probability statements involve attributing characteristics of populations to individuals, and so entail the ecological fallacy, as discussed in Chapter 2.

*But, then, when he [consultant] was saying, like, I think there's one in 200, and one in 100 miscarriages, or whatever it was. I felt that was a little bit, em, daunting really ... To me, it had nothing to do with, like, what was happening, you know ... You want to be told that there's a risk, but you don't want to be quoted numbers. I felt that was, like, a bit impersonal, you know, to be told about statistics ... I didn't want to hear that. I just wanted to know what, what could be done and what couldn't be done.* (Alison, aged 40)

The women may have felt that the professionals were biased, and that, there-fore, their codified knowledge could not be trusted. Where women did draw on health professional expertise, they sometimes used information about the latter's personal trustworthiness for quality-assurance purposes.

> We had a good bit chat, and she [midwife], well, she was more down to earth and matter of fact, and she helped a lot. And the fact that she was 35, and she had no children, and she wasn't unduly worried, and she did want a family, you know. I think they can relate to you, and they must have come across virtually every problem there is to come across. (Jane, aged 38)

This midwife's credibility arose from her status as a person who intended to become an older mother.

One of the few women whose thinking had been clearly affected by prob-abilistic information was an ex-midwife researcher married to a university lecturer. She cited a probability of 1 in 311 of having a baby with Down's syn-drome, while the other women gave rounded figures such as 1 in 200. Rapp (1988b) found that, in the USA, genetic counsellors were more likely to give exact probabilities if they felt the woman was 'intelligent'. Most of the women using the hospital in the present study came from working-class backgrounds, and professionals, particularly registrars and consultants, may have been influenced by stereotypes about their capabilities, as suggested by the following two quotations from medical staff who undertook genetic counselling.

> I think sometimes, if you've got simple folk whose only, who don't do any reading, whose basic level of education is watching the television set and reading the Sun newspaper, then, obviously, it is going to be difficult to communicate. It may be impossible.

> I think they are probably more educated [in Midlands town]. They want to know every-thing in more detail than the [north-east town] people who accept everything you say and are happy with it.

The second quotation suggests that less-educated women place more trust in experts, a conclusion which our interviews with pregnant women did not support. This doctor may have incorrectly inferred patient compliance from an absence of communication across the social class divide.

Data from our questionnaire survey of 1000 consecutive maternity admis-sions suggest that the probability of a woman aged 35 and over being offered genetic testing was influenced by her socioeconomic status. A highly statisti-callly significant relationship, independent of maternal age, was found (using the statistical technique of logistic regression) between a socioeco-nomic indicator (household owns residence plus use of car) and reporting having been offered genetic testing. This relationship is shown in Table 7.1 on page 183 for respondents aged 35 and over.

Consultants and registrars might have unconsciously avoided offering genetic testing to women of lower socioeconomic status because they believed these women would find probabilistic reasoning too difficult, as suggested by the first quotation, above. The likelihood of women reporting having been asked about cervical screening, and about the number of scans

**Table 7.1**   The relationship between socioeconomic status and reporting having been offered genetic testing among women aged 35 and over (n=64)

|  | Home owner and car user | Not home owner and/or not car user |
|---|---|---|
| Reports being offered testing | 84.4% (38) | 52.6% (10) |
| Reports not being offered testing | 15.6% (7) | 47.4% (9) |

Chi-square with Yates correction = 5.61 with 1 d.f., p = .018.

they stated they had received, were both unrelated to socioeconomic status. The inequality identified in Table 7.1 was confined to the specific, complex issue of genetic testing.

## Intuition

Some women had strong prior convictions about their baby's health which affected their attitudes towards testing. One respondent had decided to have serum-screening (AFP), even though she had ruled out both amniocentesis and termination. She felt the result would be reassuring, and, by implication, negative.

> And if I had the AFP test, that would let me know when it was a high risk or a low risk. And if it were a low risk, well, I could practically rule out having a Down's baby anyway. So that was brilliant anyway because that give me peace of mind. (Glenda, aged 37)

However, drawing inferences from screening tests such as AFP entails grappling with complex statistical issues (Guidotti, 1986, p. 110). Information provided regionally for health-care professionals (Northern Region Genetics Service, 1995, p. 27) advises them to inform women that those whose test result places them in the high-risk group face a probability of 1: 35 of carrying a fetus with Down's syndrome. This means that most positive results will be false. However, as with all inductive probability estimates, the figures obtained depend on how the data is grouped. If both age and AFP result are taken into account, the proportion of false results among those who tested positive varies between 1: 200 and 1: 2, according to the above source.

As Dracup notes in Chapter 5, the probability of A, given B (a positive test result, given genetic problems) differs from the probability of B, given A (genetic problems, given a positive test result). Most of the small number of women who test positive with AFP, and who may risk miscarriage through amniocentesis, or suffer emotional harm, will be carrying babies without genetic defects. Women may not appreciate that tests which give accurate predictions for a population can generate a high proportion of errors for the relatively rare events they are designed to predict, such as Down's syndrome.

Probability tables, like that produced by Cuckle, Wald and Thompson (1987, p. 391) rely on the tacit assumption, justified or not, that sensitivity and specificity remain constant over the entire age range. Moreover, the above authors point out that AFP yields a continuous, quantitative marker for the probability of Down's syndrome. The balance of sensitivity and specificity depends on the test-designer's decision about where to draw the line delimiting 'positive' and 'negative' results.

Some women who rejected testing used epidemiologically unreliable signs such as family history, the baby's movements and scans to reassure themselves that testing was unnecessary.

> *I come from a disgustingly healthy family, where if you don't make it to 90, well, you're not trying, you know, so that aspect of it doesn't worry me.* (Sheila, aged 34)

> *I never felt that things were wrong. Well, I suppose in the beginning, but I think the baby's movements are very reassuring.* (Carol, aged 38)

## Fatalism

The above women managed an uncertain future by anticipating a positive outcome. Others fatalistically rejected testing, concluding from the random element in genetic disorders that they could not control the future.

> *And you think, well, you can test for this, and test for that, and, at the end of the day, it could be something totally different. And, as I say, I've just got my fingers crossed. I've put it to the back of my mind, and hope that everything is alright.* (Jane, aged 38)

The quotation below is based on the notion that each person is 'given' so much luck. However, statistically, an absence of family history, would, if anything, indicate a reduced risk of Downs's syndrome.

> *It was like, ee, I've got three, I shouldn't go in for any more, because it's pushing fate, you know.* (Wendy, aged 36)

## Discussion

At first sight, the probabilistic reasoning of the pregnant, mainly working-class, women whose views were explored in this chapter might be dismissed as falling well short of the standards of scientific rationality. Respondents mostly eschewed statistical quantification, generalised from single cases, and constructed *ad hoc* risk categories. However, closer inspection shows up the logic underlying their reasoning about uncertain costs and benefits. At the same time, as some women recognised, arbitrary and variable age cut-offs for routinely offering genetic tests cannot be scientifically justified. Some felt stigmatised for being too 'old', and others for being too 'young'. Epidemiological analysis of risks cannot be easily divorced from wider cultural notions about age-appropriate behaviour.

The survey finding, admittedly tentative because of the crudity of the socioeconomic status indicator, that better-off older women were significantly more likely to report having been offered genetic testing, suggests that clinical decisions in individual cases were heavily influenced by cultural stereotypes. This conclusion fits with Fielding and Evered's (1980) finding, discussed in Chapter 1, that middle-class patients were more likely than working-class patients to be given a psychological explanation of ambiguous symptoms, because medical personnel (or trainee doctors at least) assume that the former will find such a diagnosis more acceptable.

Current genetic testing technology, itself rapidly changing, offers women only awkward choices. Serum-screening has limited accuracy, and the results take some time to process, facing women with the possibility of amniocentesis and late termination. Amniocentesis is associated with a risk of miscarriage and the prospect of losing a healthy baby. Respondents approached their decision, which most felt that they had to make alone, by reasoning backwards from their willingness to terminate. However, some women who ruled out termination accepted serum-screening because they thought it was expected of them, or because they anticipated a negative result.

Consultants, registrars and midwives mostly expressed respect for women's right to make their own choices. The incident, quoted at length, in which a registrar tried unsuccessfully to compel a woman to accept testing stands out as exceptional. In relation to the conceptual framework developed in Chapter 1, the professionals adopted a 'liberal' rather than an 'undelimited' approach to expertise. However, they may not have always appreciated the logic of the link between rejection of termination and declining genetic tests. A midwife, quoted in Chapter 1, had learnt from her own pregnancy that *'If you are against terminating the baby, then there is no point in having the bloods [AFP] done in the first place.'* Professionals who have not fully internalised this logic may give women 'choice' while covertly regarding the rejection of testing as irrational.

Although based on a small, qualitative sample drawn from a single site, this picture corresponds to that obtained from a recent large National Childbirth Trust survey (Dodds, 1997) which concluded that about two-thirds of women felt they had made the decisions about genetic testing, but that 10 per cent had felt pressurised, while nearly one-fifth said that the hospital had made assumptions about what they should want.

Many women who opted for genetic testing experienced intense and unanticipated anxiety while waiting for the results. Some feared that their anxiety might damage the baby, or harm their other children, and these concerns added to the vortex of negative emotions. Some delayed identifying with the baby until the testing process had been completed. Recordings of genetic counselling sessions suggest that consultants and registrars did mention the emotional ramifications of testing, but the women may have found it difficult to imagine how distressed they would feel during the waiting period.

The limited accuracy of AFP serum-screening raises ethical and risk-management dilemmas, because of the large percentage of false positive results it produces. This shortcoming may explain why, as noted in Chapter 1, only 3 out of 19 (15 per cent) of consultants registrars and midwives interviewed for the research would accept AFP for their own offspring. In contrast, our survey showed that 49 per cent of 107 women who were offered genetic screening accepted AFP. New techniques may spare women who wish to be tested from having to choose between the inaccuracy of serum-screening and the risk of miscarriage associated with amniocentesis. Nevertheless, an investigation of current dilemmas can provide valuable insights into the ways in which organisations and their clients adapt to imperfectly predictive technologies.

# Risk and coping with diabetes

Bill Watson and Bob Heyman

| |
|---|
| Introduction |
| Methodology |
| Data analysis |
| Discussion |

## Introduction

This chapter explores the ways in which people with diabetes manage the risks associated with this condition. It concentrates on their experiences and attempts to portray their perspectives.

Diabetes is a chronic condition with a prevalence of around 4 per cent (MacKinnon, 1993). Onset can occur at any age and, in the absence of a cure, medical treatment focuses on control. Short-term problems, such as fluctuations in blood sugar and metabolic abnormalities, can lead to ill-health, but long-term complications are potentially more serious. Damage to blood vessels can lead to heart attacks, strokes and problems with kidneys or eyes. Diabetes can take two forms Type 1, which usually develops during childhood or early adulthood, and Type 2, which tends to develop later in life. Those with Type 1 diabetes require daily insulin injections, whereas Type 2 patients may be treated with either tablets or insulin, or a combination. Restriction of carbohydrate intake is recommended for people with both forms.

As well as causing physical problems, diabetes can have serious social consequences. The changes in behaviour and cognition that result from hypoglycaemia (low blood sugar), including confusion, slurred speech and aggression, can be highly embarrassing and demoralising. Many people are advised to adjust their diet, omitting sweet foods, or eating at times determined by their treatment rather than by hunger or social routines. Injections may have to be carried out in public, at work, in a restaurant or on public transport.

Self-care is a large and important part of life with diabetes, as with many other chronic illnesses. Regardless of the amount of clinical support available, patients must take daily decisions about their health, and undertake many aspects of treatment for themselves (Coates and Boore, 1995). Reif (1973), in a study of people living with ulcerative colitis, showed that self-management involved much more than following advice from health professionals. She found that people learnt complex strategies for coping with symptoms and the effects of treatment. They would restrict their diet, restructure their time management, and modify their social interaction. Personal strategies would often conflict with medical regimens. For example, patients would alter the dosage and timing of their medication to make them compatible with other aspects of their lives.

A considerable literature explores the psychosocial effects of diabetes and its associated self-management activities. Living with the risks arising from diabetes can place great psychological stress on the individual (Armstrong, 1987b), leading to feelings of fear and uncertainty (Charmaz, 1983). However, research gives a less clear picture of how individuals respond to these stresses. Ternulf-Nyhlin (1990), for example, found that diabetics developed adaptive cognitive and behavioural strategies to 'make sense' of their situation and 'keep going' with their lives. Robinson (1993) reported that people with diabetes try to limit the impact of living with risk through attempted normalisation. The work described in this chapter focuses on individuals' experience of life with diabetes, with particular reference to their strategies for managing the risks which the condition entails.

## Methodology

### THE SAMPLE

Participants had recently taken part in a cross-sectional survey investigating a sample of 200 patients' views of hospital-clinic services and their reasons for not keeping clinic appointments. A small purposive subsample was invited to take part in the second study. Questionnaires were used to select people with divergent views of hospital services.

Fifteen people were invited to participate in the study, and seven agreed. Of the eight who declined, four did not respond to written invitations, or did not return telephone calls, two were too busy, one was not at home at the arranged time, and one withdrew after becoming upset during the interview. The sample contained four men and three women, aged 32–61 years. Four members of the sample had Type 1 diabetes, and three had Type 2.

### METHODS

Semi-structured interviews, organised around the 'diabetes life history', were used. This method allows a personalised and longitudinal account of an individual's health to be obtained (Leininger, 1985). In the present study, interviewees were asked to describe their experiences of diabetes in chronological order, from the time before diagnosis up to the present day, and to discuss their expectations for the future. Respondents were asked to explore events associated with diagnosis, its immediate impact, how they had adjusted to having diabetes, the support needed and received from professionals, family and friends, and their future prospects. Discussion of these topics focused on perceptions of risks and personal coping strategies.

Interviews, which lasted about 45 minutes, were taped, with respondent permission, and transcribed verbatim. Interviewees were offered the chance to read the transcript prior to analysis. Data was analysed using the open and axial coding methods of Grounded Theory (Strauss and Corbin, 1990). Emergent themes related to risk and coping strategies were grouped into categories, and their properties and relationships explored.

## Data analysis

The results are presented in two sections. The first focuses on individuals' views about diabetes, its associated risks, and their future prospects with the condition. The second section explores the ways people cope with diabetes at a day-to-day level. The life-history format of the interviews made it possible to generate retrospective personal biographies, beginning with the initial diagnosis, and working through to the emergence of personal management strategies and future trajectories.

### PERCEPTIONS OF DIABETES AND ASSOCIATED RISKS

#### Causal explanations

Several medical explanations of diabetes aetiology have been proposed, involving, for example, viral illness, genetics and diet. Medicine does not provide a clear or simple explanatory story. In Western, science-based societies, lay beliefs are both derived from, and distinct from, medical theories. Herzlich (1979) argues that people in such societies actively seek out explanations for their illnesses to a greater extent than those in many other cultures. Furnham (1994) found that personal explanations of health and illness were closely related to individuals' political, religious and health beliefs, as well as their attitudes to medicine.

The lay accounts given below illustrate the ways in which respondents selected causal explanations from the menu of current medical theories.

> I just put it down to being overweight. I mean, I always eat loads of sugary stuff, or at least I used to, and I just thought it was because I had eaten all this sugary stuff. (Woman aged 32)

> Just that with it running in the family, you know. My mam had it, me dad had it, me oldest brother he had it and I thought to myself, 'Well, if they've had it,' you know, 'It's gonna come out again.' (Man aged 55).

Individuals who have regular contact with health professionals can be expected to share some of their views. However, a study of individuals without diabetes (Rankin, 1996) found that they also offer explanations of diabetes which are closely related to medical thought. The two explanations quoted above are both monocausal, but differ in emphasising lifestyle and genetic factors respectively. While this difference can be put down to the presence of a visible family history in the second example, the two quotations illustrate the way in which lay explanations can simplify the often complex, multifactoral, interactive epidemiology of modern diseases by latching on to single causes.

## Perceptions of risk

The medical view of risk tends to be dominated by the physical complications of diabetes. Since a clinical trial (The Diabetes Control and Complications Trial Research Group, 1993) showed that diligent management can yield benefits, in terms of fewer complications, up to nine years in the future, health professionals have tended to adopt long-term views of risk. If patients share the professional view of risk, they should also adopt a similarly extended time frame. However, many of their concerns raised related to immediate problems.

> It's me eyes I'm most bothered about. I've had that laser treatment on them. (Man aged 61)

> Well, I get this tingling in my feet sometimes. It even keeps me awake in the night. I think that's what most worries me. (Woman aged 39)

Other concerns show how the risk of adverse social consequences could override medical considerations. Neither of the respondents quoted below mentioned physical problems when asked what concerned them most.

> The worst thing for me would be to lose my driving licence [as a taxi driver]. (Man aged 42)

> Well, with being an insulin dependent diabetic, I can't get my PPL [private pilot's licence], and I think that's probably the hardest thing about it. (Man aged 49)

Although non-medical, these concerns do not necessarily reflect a shorter time frame than that adopted by professionals concerned with preventing future physical complications. For example, losing one's livelihood can have a long-term impact on the quality of daily life, both for patients and their families.

## Views of the future

Attitudes to the future provide a telling insight into individuals' priorities. Some respondents displayed considerable concern, while others, quoted below, appeared indifferent to what the future might hold.

> I mean, I'm not particularly worried about the future. It doesn't prey on my mind. (Woman aged 32)

> I just try to take things as they come. I think if you worry about things sometimes it just makes it more of a problem. Worrying about it won't help anyway. I think if you are aware of the problems, you've just got to take it as it comes. (Woman aged 47)

From a medical perspective such attitudes could be viewed as a frustrating barrier to treatment. Lack of clear recognition of a future threat has been linked to poor compliance with diabetes treatment (Rosenstock, 1985). The first quotation illustrates an approach to the future, based on heavy time discounting, which was labelled as hedonism in Chapter 2. Individuals, faced with a doubtful future trajectory, may decide to live for the present. The second quotation seems to entail an implicitly fatalistic attitude to the future. Furnham (1994) argues that certain non-Western cultures are characterised by a widespread social attitude of fatalism. However, closer inspection of cultures uncovers pluralism in health beliefs (Unschuld, 1986). Fatalism is an important ingredient in the lay management of the future in Western cultures (Davison, Frankel and Davey Smith, 1992). The second quotation illustrates the respondent's belief in the process described in Chapter 2 as 'reflexive recursion'. The respondent suggests that worrying about a problem makes it worse.

Whether valid or not, this way of thinking implicitly rejects a purely mechanical, physical approach to diabetes management. Health professionals who view diabetes from a biomedical perspective could easily construe both patients' attitudes as demonstrating culpable negligence towards the future. Reading such responses in this way may prevent professionals from finessing the conflict between the need for arduous physical treatment on the one hand, and the need to sustain as normal a life as possible, both mentally and physically, on the other.

Others appeared to think in ways which matched the current medical position, demonstrating their concern about the physical complications of diabetes.

*I feel that if you keep tighter control there should be fewer problems in the future.* (Man aged 49)

*I'm really concerned about [my eyes] for the future, because I know that it can cause blindness. I have my eyes checked regularly at my local opticians, because I don't want to go blind.* (Woman aged 39)

According to the health-belief model (Rosenstock, 1985), the acceptance of personal vulnerability is an essential prerequisite to behavioural compliance with medical advice. Health professionals may feel more comfortable with patients who think in this way than with those who do not worry about the future, or who emphasise recursive processes.

## PERSONAL COPING STRATEGIES

Several models have been developed to explain strategies for coping with health problems. Early models (Gleser and Ihilevich, 1969) assumed that people progressed through predictable and easily measurable sequences, for example denial, anger and acceptance. Later models (Lazarus and Folkman, 1984) treat coping with illness, and its associated risks, as a more complex and variable activity. These researchers see coping as a constantly changing behavioural and cognitive effort to manage specific external and/or internal demands.

The data from the present study support the latter definition of coping. Those interviewed displayed a number of coping strategies, which they employed concurrently. The use of a life-history methodology made it possible to see how these strategies developed and changed over time, although these shifts can only be viewed, in the present research, through patients' retrospective accounts.

The results are presented in terms of two subcategories of behavioural and cognitive coping, corresponding to the two main elements identified by Lazarus and Folkman (1984).

## BEHAVIOURAL COPING STRATEGIES

Coping actively with an illness through behavioural strategies requires a foundation of faith that the causes and consequences of the underlying disease are understood, and that its course can be at least partially controlled. As will be seen, patients who adopted such strategies mostly adapted expert medical knowledge to their own personal ends. A typology is presented below.

### Self-care

The St Vincent Declaration – the mission statement for diabetes management – emphasises the importance of promoting self-care. Patients and significant others need to be more actively and directly involved in their treatment than would be the case for many other conditions. Professionals are enjoined, in the Declaration, to 'organise training and teaching in diabetes management and care for people of all ages with diabetes, for their families, friends and working associates and for the health care team' (DOH/British Diabetes Association, 1995, p. 2). The data presented here describe the steps that interviewees took in their daily life to keep themselves well, and to minimise the effects of diabetes. By taking such steps, patients implicitly accepted the validity of medical knowledge about diabetes, while trying to modify its effects on their quality of life.

All interviewees described some degree of active self-care. The responses can be grouped into three distinct but overlapping subcategories. One strategy involved **planful problem-solving** (Lazarus, 1992).

> With modern day food labelling, you can tell straight away what the carbohydrate content of the food is. And this is something that I'm quite aware of. (Man aged 49)

This patient accepted the medical view that the amount and type of carbohydrate in the diet should be regulated, and used food-labelling in planning his diet.

A second example of planful problem-solving involves the maintenance of stable blood sugar. Health professionals recommend that diabetics should keep their blood sugar as stable as possible, in order to reduce the risk of physical complications. In practice, full stability is almost unattainable, and the achievement of even a degree of control requires great motivation and effort. The interviewee quoted below had been talking about his struggle to stabilise his blood sugar.

*With blood monitoring, you can adjust your insulin. So, if you're going out for the night, you can alter your insulin to accommodate for what you might eat, and you have a lot more flexibility.* (Man aged 42)

Blood-monitoring allowed this patient to determine his blood-sugar value, and alter his insulin dose as required. Actively managing one's own blood-sugar levels in this way requires considerable understanding of their desirable range, appropriate insulin doses, and the relative effects of different activities and foods.

A second behavioural strategy involved the **establishment of a safety net**. The interviewees quoted below accepted that lapses in glucose control were unavoidable, but had developed contingency plans to deal with them.

*I carry sweets with me all the time just in case I go hypo.* (Woman aged 47)

*I had a bad hypo last week. My blood sugar was down to 1. I was taken into — hospital, and that gave me a fright. Now I always carry Lucozade, and I make sure my blood's over 7 before I go out shopping.* (Woman aged 39)

Patients will usually get warning signs of falling blood sugar. If these signs go unheeded, confusion and, ultimately, coma will ensue. However, taking sugar in the form of sweets or drinks can quickly reverse the process. The risk of going 'hypo' can be reduced by artificially elevating the blood sugar before starting an activity such as shopping.

The coping strategies discussed above were based on an acceptance of medical principles. However, over time, the patient may develop personal expertise in the self-management of diabetes, and assume control of their condition, building up detailed experiential knowledge of their individual responses to different circumstances (Paterson, 1994). Patients may use this personal knowledge to modify the rigours of the medical regime, safely as they see it, thus **synthesising medical perspectives with personal experience**. The patient quoted below had only had diabetes for one year, but had build up an elaborate belief system about the dietary lapses which her body could tolerate.

*I don't really feel that bad because I know how much to eat. I've learnt myself how much [chocolate] I can have. Like, I'll only eat one piece. I've learnt to cut the piece in half of what I used to have. And whereas, before, I'd have two sausages, now I'll only have one.* (Woman aged 32)

The respondent had learnt to adapt medical prescriptions by working out, through practical experimentation, how much of her favourite foods she could eat without feeling ill. This example can be used to illustrate three important issues concerning risk analysis for diabetic patients.

First, medical knowledge about conditions such as diabetes is more or less nomothetic, allowing prediction only about average persons. But individuals respond differently, and the effect of one person's treatment regimen on their blood-sugar level is subject, potentially, to the mediating influence of many interacting factors, such as age, gender, disease duration, social support and stress level. Medical knowledge cannot hope to track the effects of so many factors and their interactions. To the extent to which these complexities affect clinical condition, patients have an advantage over professionals in applying general medical principles to their own cases.

Second, the example illustrates the way in which patients use informal cost-benefit analysis in deciding how far to comply with medical advice. The woman quoted above balanced medical risk against her desire to continue to eat certain foods, and had tried to develop an optimum balance through experimentation.

Third, the experiential side of the personal–medical synthesis could only take into account immediate, apparent effects. Possible long-term risks would only be controlled in so far as they correlated with immediate symptomatic indicators. The patient just quoted may have been mortgaging her longer-term future.

## Support and advice from others

The coping strategies discussed so far involved the take-up of medical advice, or its synthesis, with personal experience. Respondents also drew on advice and support from various lay sources. Helman (1989) argues that some people are used as a source of health advice more often than others, for example those with personal experience of a particular disease, women who have acquired extensive life experience through childrearing. The use of lay sources is illustrated in the next two examples.

*J — two doors down, was the one who told me to go to the doctors with this, because her son's got the diabetes. So if I get a problem, I always go to her. She's a bit like a mother figure to me, really. I tend to go to Joan first even if I needed practical advice. She's one of these people, she'll know how bad you are, and she's one of these that she knows exactly what to do for every thing.* (Woman aged 32)

*If I had a problem with the diabetes, well, the wife's always with me. She would take it from there.* (Man aged 61)

In both cases, the credibility of the source derived from their personal relationship with the patient, not their technical expertise. Interactions with the medical world were mediated through personal ties. However, lay influences often reinforced the medical order.

*INTERVIEWER: Do the people around you help you look after the diabetes?*
*RESPONDENT: Well I get told not to eat this and that now. If I'm going for bags of crisps, I'll hear, 'You only get one bag, you can't have two,' and they'll put the rest away. And he's [husband] always saying, 'Have you pricked your finger yet?' Then, when the kids come in from school, they'll say, 'Have you done your [blood test]?'* (Woman aged 32)

The three quotations illustrate the multidimensional nature of social support (Woods, Yates and Primomo, 1989). The first involves support from someone outside the family. According to Helman's framework (1989), J—'s importance as a source of support arose from her life experience, including personal involvement with diabetes. She also provided an opening for illness-related social exchanges outside the family setting (Bloom, 1982). The other two extracts show how support was given and received within the family. Role reversal, with children adopting a parental, carer role, and checking that the medical regime is being followed, as seen in the last quotation, has also been observed by Stetz, Lewis and Primomo (1986). However, in our example, the reversal contains a joking element, and illustrates the role of humour in social support and risk management.

## COGNITIVE COPING STRATEGIES

The strategies discussed below involve cognitive and emotional processes which appear to help patients come to terms with having diabetes, rather than directly health-related behavioural responses. By developing these strategies, respondents could make sense of their symptoms, and locate themselves in relation to other people with diabetes.

### Reframing symptoms as normal

Robinson (1993) found that people with a long-term condition were able to create a 'life as normal' by **reframing** its negotiated meaning. The following examples show how respondents, in their first reactions to being told they had diabetes, normalised their symptoms by linking them to non-pathological reactions.

> I was thinking to myself that I'd been eating loads of sweet stuff, and I'd been doing that the day before they brought me to the hospital. I just thought that the more sweet stuff I eat, the higher my blood sugar would go. (Woman aged 32)

> I couldn't believe I was diabetic when the doctor told me. I mean, I had been drinking a lot, and he said that that was often how it started. But it had been hot, you know, and I just put it down to that. (Man aged 61)

It is not surprising that newly diagnosed patients saw 'symptoms' as a normal response to life events (e.g. feeling thirsty because it was hot) since a disease framework would not have been readily available to them when the symptoms first occurred. They may have found it disorienting to reframe, after the diagnosis, responses which they had previously normalised, and, therefore, clung on to previously developed explanations. Such retention of the familiar may have helped them to cope with the first stage of their transition to being diabetic.

The main early medical manifestation of diabetes, for many patients, is the need to self-administer regular injections. The respondent quoted below isolated this procedure from the rest of her life, thus preserving its non-medical normality as far as possible.

> I really don't think I'm bad. You have your injection, and you think, 'Oh well, I must have it.' But, afterwards, I totally forget I've got it. It's just something that you do, and that you know you've got to do. (Woman aged 39)

### Down-scaling severity

Type 2 diabetes has an insidious onset, often involving no tangible symptoms other than thirst or feeling tired. New patients can find it difficult to appreciate that they have just been diagnosed with a serious illness.

*It was a shock seeing all these people around you, and you think, 'Oh no, there's nothing the matter with me.' And they've got all these drips hanging from them, and I was thinking, 'What am I doing here?'* (Man aged 55)

*It didn't feel like an illness. I'd been ill, and in hospital, before. It wasn't like I'd been ill before.* (Man aged 61)

**Down-scaling**, a process of minimising the seriousness of their condition can, as with normalising, be understood simply in terms of patients' cognitive frameworks, rather than as a behavioural strategy. People exposed to popular medical culture, through the mass media, may naturally confound serious disease with serious symptoms. However, down-scaling may, again, help new patients to cope with the early impact of seeing themselves as having a long-term health concern.

The first respondent quoted above interpreted his predicament in relation to the much worse condition, as he saw it, of others. The second patient used his own previous experience of 'real' illness as a source of favourable comparison. Such comparisons, which made the respondent's condition appear relatively unserious, can perhaps be understood in terms of the more general cognitive phenomenon of 'unrealistic optimism' (Weinstein, 1980), discussed by Dracup in Chapter 5. Unrealistic optimism is inferred when people, on average, believe themselves significantly better off than the average, for example in terms of their risk of developing a serious disease, a logical impossibility. Although it was not possible to decide how 'realistic' optimistic individuals were, favourable comparisons with others may have helped them come to terms with becoming diabetic.

## Embracing specialism

Finally, the cognitive coping strategy of **embracing specialism** involved placing faith in the ability of hospital-based experts to protect the individual from the complications of diabetes.

*I feel happier with their [hospital] expertise than with my own doctor.* (Woman aged 39)

*I like to go somewhere technical to find out what is it actually wrong.* (Man aged 42)

*They know all the up-to-date things.* (Man aged 61)

These accounts did not acknowledge the limitations of medical expertise, in the absence of a cure or fully effective treatment. The above examples describe a type of attitude which Thorne and Robinson (1989) have termed 'hero worship'. In their study, 'hero worship' relationships with professionals were characterised by a strong element of naïve trust, and discounting, by patients, of possible flaws in the system.

Embracing specialism may have given patients faith, realistic or misplaced, that *'As long as you stick by the rules, stick to your diet and take your insulin you'll be OK'* (man aged 42).

# Discussion

This study used a qualitative, inductive approach to explore the ways in which adults with Type 1 and Type 2 diabetes perceived current and future risk, and the coping strategies they adopted. The results suggest several areas in which lay and medical perspectives differ. For the person living with diabetes, social or economic risks may outweigh physical ones. Some may concentrate on current concerns, and actively avoid dwelling on their uncertain future. Patients adopt complex, varied cognitive and behavioural coping strategies, which can go far beyond complying to prescribed medical treatments. For example, daily activities may be planned with diabetes-related considerations in mind. Patients may synthesise medical advice with their personal experience, or subsume their initial symptoms in non-pathological explanations.

These findings match those of other research. Burckhardt (1987), in a study exploring coping with long-term conditions, concluded that individuals employ both direct actions and intrapyschic processes. This study also found social support to be an important coping element. Respondents often talked about turning to others for advice and support, having their medical treatments verified and policed by their family, or having contact with health professionals mediated through significant others. The importance of significant others has been reported by other authors (Butcher, 1994; Newby, 1996). Edelstein and Linn (1985) linked survey with clinical data, and concluded that family support correlated positively with glycaemic control. This study also found that individuals may, at particular times, cope with diabetes by adopting the 'patient role' and relying heavily on professional expertise. The need to become a patient should not be overlooked in the drive towards participative care.

The Royal Society (1992, p. 2) defined risk as the probability of 'an adverse event'. However, the nature of the adverse event involved in diabetes is somewhat ambiguous. Its probability of occurrence is affected by a variety of factors such as family history, diet and body weight which are more or less under individual control. But the potential impact of the disease on new patients arises as much from the risks it opens up, such as blindness and heart disease, as from immediate symptoms such as tiredness and hypoglycaemia. Diabetes can be seen, Janus-like, both as an adverse event and as a major risk factor requiring preventive strategies. Respondents in the present study had varying views about their illness status, if any. Description of diabetes as a 'chronic illness', however justified on medical grounds, may not match up with patients' own approach to the condition, and so may act as a barrier to communication between individual patients and professionals.

In this respect, diabetes can be compared with other long-term conditions the onset of which is marked by relatively mild symptoms, such as HIV (Chapter 4) and high blood pressure (Chapter 14). Diabetes has had, until very recently, a medical risk status somewhat intermediate between these two conditions. HIV has a trajectory of almost certain decline and death, while, as O'Brien and Davison point out in Chapter 12, the outcome for individuals with high blood pressure is uncertain. The long-term consequences of diabetes cannot be easily avoided, but they may be delayed and mitigated through arduous effort, mostly required of the patient.

Although diabetic patients and their families bear the main burden of care, the knowledge base on which prevention is founded is highly medicalised. Tight glycaemic control confers long-term benefits, which are only loosely correlated with immediate health, and which only show up in random control experiments such as The Diabetes Control and Complications Trial (1993). Hence, proper medical care requires patients to make major changes to their lifestyles in order to conform to the requirements of a system of expertise which they cannot evaluate directly, and which has often been found wanting. However well-founded diabetes treatment recommendations may be, patients will approach them with various degrees of scepticism.

From a medical perspective, compliance becomes the critical issue. From this point of view, diabetic patients face high risk, and both the quantity and quality of their futures could be dramatically improved if they would only obey doctors' instructions. However, qualitative research suggests that the attitudes of diabetic patients are too complex to be simply dismissed as 'non-compliant' (Trostle, 1988). They may normalise or minimise their condition, worry more about social than medical consequences, or adopt a short time frame. Patients who do comply can have unrealistically 'heroic' expectations about what medicine can do for them, and be doomed to disillusion.

Professionals and diabetic patients face the dilemma of balancing the latter's sense of wellbeing against the demanding physical requirements of managing the disease. Over the last 5–10 years, diabetes has been placed at the forefront of participatory care and patient-centred research. However, it is becoming increasingly apparent that the individual with diabetes is the true expert on how to live with the disease. For this reason, practitioners and researchers must continue to listen carefully to patients' voices. Only by trying to understand what our patients already know can we hope to be able to offer accurate and useful advice. For example, worry avoidance should not be dismissed as just a 'defence mechanism'. It should be seen as an element in personal functioning which, ironically, may contribute to health maintenance, through the therapeutic processes of reflexive recursion.

# Freedom of the locality for people with learning difficulties

Bob Heyman, Sarah Huckle and Elizabeth C. Handyside

| Introduction |
| --- |
| Methodology |
| Data analysis |
| Discussion |

## Introduction

This chapter explores the negotiation of local autonomy for adults with learning difficulties (referred to in the following text as adults) living with parents or other family carers. The chapter links their spatial freedom to the quality of life for adults with learning difficulties, on the one hand, and to family approaches to risk management on the other. The chapter draws on qualitative data obtained from adults themselves, and from their family and professional carers.

The direction of this risk concern can, itself, be historically located. In the first part of the twentieth century, policy-makers were influenced by eugenic notions, and driven by fears of being genetically overwhelmed. They worried more about the dangers which people with learning difficulties purportedly posed to the social order than about their needs and aspirations (Ryan and Thomas, 1987, p. 107). The same social group has shifted from being regarded as a source of danger to being seen as a target for protection.

Cultures develop norms about the age-appropriateness of socially significant accomplishments such as working, developing sexual relationships, having children and living independently. Individuals do not agree perfectly, even at the subcultural and family levels, but most members of modern Western societies would object, for example, to a 10-year-old getting married, working full-time, or being 'home alone' for more than a short time. Although seemingly natural, such perceptions vary culturally (Neugarten, Moore and Lowe, 1965; Neugarten, 1979), as pointed out in Chapter 7.

In the wealthy Western societies of the late twentieth century, adult–child relationships are generally understood through an ideology of beneficence (see Chapter 15). Children are not expected to pay their way, or to care for their families, only to enjoy themselves, and acquire the skills which will enable them to cope with adult life. However, parents who attempt to manage the lives of their children according to the principle of beneficence are faced with a risk-management dilemma. If children's autonomy is restricted for the sake of their safety, their learning opportunities will be limited, and their development may be retarded. On the other hand, allowing children more autonomy than they can handle puts them at risk in a dangerous world.

Spatial autonomy for adults with learning difficulties, the focus of this chapter, can be graded in terms of the degree of autonomy/risk involved. Our familiarity with suburban life enables us to immediately recognise the approximately ordinal structure of the series of steps shown in Table 9.1.

The sequence below should not be thought of as a series of developmental stages, but as a set of unreflexive, although socially shared, tactical balances which have evolved as a means of managing the safety/autonomy dilemma in a modern urban ecology. Two of the present researchers agreed perfectly in 'blind' rankings of the amount of freedom of locality attained by 14 adults with learning difficulties, suggesting that this dimension is well understood. The double line below *'locally constrained'* reflects the researchers' judgement that this level represents a watershed in terms of wider autonomy. Adults whose spatial passports took them beyond local constraint could undertake activities, outside the home or day centre,

**Table 9.1**  Levels of spatial autonomy

| | |
|---|---|
| Closed, fully monitored | Moving in a closed environment in the visual presence of an adult carer (e.g. playing in a room with a carer present) |
| Closed, partly monitored | Moving in a closed environment in the near non-visual presence of an adult carer (e.g. carer in the next room) |
| Confined within potential monitoring range | Staying within monitoring/recall distance within an open environment (e.g. playing in the street) |
| Locally constrained | Making specific local journeys, spatially and temporally authorised by carers (e.g. an errand to a local shop) |
| Freedom of the locality, temporally constrained | Making non-specific local journeys, temporally authorised by carers (e.g. going round the town centre) |
| Freedom of the locality | Making non-specific, unauthorised local journeys, without temporal constraint |
| Globally constrained | Making specific non-local journeys, spatially and temporally authorised by carers (e.g. a train journey to visit relatives) |
| Globally autonomous | Making non-specific, unauthorised journeys outside the locality (e.g. roaming the world) |

which they chose and initiated. However, as will be shown below, such autonomy was usually achieved at the price of considerable anxiety, particularly for family carers. We therefore describe those who had gone beyond local constraint as *'limited risk-taking'*, and those who had not as *'danger avoiding'* (Heyman and Huckle, 1993b).

The details of the spatial licences which parents and children negotiate will vary, depending on culture, subculture and individual circumstances. For example, as noted in the Introduction to this book, German children go to school unaccompanied at an earlier age than do those living in England (Hillman, Adams and Whitelegg, 1990). The norms about spatial autonomy which children are subjected to may be affected by their social class background, their gender, and the kind of urban/rural environment in which they live.

Family microcultural variations can be expected both in risk tolerance, and in views about the ages at which the various stages of letting go become acceptable. The acquisition of spatial autonomy involves processes of negotiation between family members who will draw on local exemplars in order to legitimate claims to age-specific competencies or incompetencies. Parents may find it difficult to refuse their own child permission to go into town if their child says that Johnny down the street has been doing so since time immemorial.

A step-by-step expansion of the spatial and temporal boundaries of their worlds enables children to learn through the beneficial processes of reflexive recursion, as discussed in Chapter 2. Thus, a child who ventures into the town centre on specific spatially and temporally monitored errands acquires skills which can be utilised on more complex, unregulated local journeys. The development of spatial autonomy normally involves travelling on a downward risk escalator (see Chapter 2), since carers progressively reduce the intensity of their control of a child's spatial movements as their ability to manage potential danger improves through experience.

This spatial and temporal expansion cannot be separated from the broader development of personal autonomy. For example, young adults who can move freely around the locality whenever they wish have a greater choice of potential personal activities than children who can leave their local street only on specified errands. Their wider autonomy also gives young people opportunities to undertake activities of which the wider society or their parents might disapprove, such as joy-riding, the development of sexual relationships, or the consumption of prohibited substances. Hence, spatial autonomy involves more than the acquisition of geographical skills. Again, a normal form of beneficial reflexive recursion can be identified, in which a demonstration of the ability to handle limited freedom responsibly, according to prevailing cultural definitions, is rewarded by new visas in a child's metaphorical passport.

Family carers and adults with learning difficulties may feel unable to draw unproblematically and unreflexively on age-specific norms about spatial autonomy. Family carers may not credit adults with 'grown up' developmental status and, as will be shown below, may believe them incapable

of learning through reflexive recursion. The dilemma of balancing autonomy and safety must appear much more acute if the fledgling's first risky
wing-flappings are judged (rightly or wrongly) to take it to the limits of its
capability.

One American survey (Thorin, Yovanoff and Irvin, 1996, p. 118) asked parents of young adults with learning difficulties to assess 14 dilemmas, and
found that they were most concerned about the dilemma of wanting *'to create
opportunities for independence for the young adults and wanting to assure that
health and safety needs are met'*.

Family traditions and local exemplars do not provide a guide to age-
appropriate levels of spatial autonomy, which must be decided on in individual cases, depending on an assessment of the riskiness of the environment,
the perceived competence of the adult and, more nebulously, their potential
for improvement. The classical principle of normalisation (Wolfensberger,
1983) helps little, because of the difficulty of defining normality. Adults normally take for granted their right to full global autonomy, but they also normally avoid excessive risk. In the absence of clear cultural indicators
(Cicourel, 1973), for adults with learning difficulties families invent their own
varying solutions to the risk/autonomy dilemma.

For most of the families whose views we have considered in the research
discussed below, the debatable boundary for spatial mobility involved freedom of the locality. The majority of family carers believed that it was too
dangerous for the adult whom they cared for to undertake more than locally
constrained journeys, such as errands to local shops, trips to and from the
day centre. Adults, mostly aged 25–40, generally concurred with this view, at
least in interview, although many regretted the consequential loss of personal autonomy, for example being unable to visit friends who lived locally.
However, about one-third of our sample of family carers did give adults
some freedom of the locality, usually with considerable anxiety. This freedom, as will be seen from the quotations below, was, in all but a few cases,
hedged with spatial and temporal restrictions.

Acceptance of perceived risks was socially patterned. Middle-class families
which contained two parental carers were much less likely to give adults
with learning difficulties freedom of the locality (Heyman and Huckle, 1993a,
1993b). It has not been possible to separate out these two factors, since poorer
families were also much more likely to be headed by a single parent.
(However, we have one case study of an elderly, middle-class widow who
prevented her son from making other than highly restricted local journeys.)
Two non-exclusive possible explanations of the association between social
background and attitude to risk in this context can be suggested. First, the
middle classes may be culturally more risk-averse. Second, lack of material
resources makes risk intolerance more costly. For example, family carers can
more easily provide substitutes for personal mobility and leisure activities if
they possess cars and can afford to pay for entertainment. This cost-benefit
analysis may explain why poorer people tend to be more risk-tolerant (Beck,
1992).

The data analysis presented below will be concerned with the ways in which families attempted to manage the risks they associated with freedom of the locality for people with learning difficulties. After briefly setting the scene by illustrating different attitudes, we focus on aspects of risk management considered in Chapter 2, including reflexive recursion, differentiation/generalisation, the tactical use of risk communication and cost-benefit analysis.

## Methodology

The data discussed below is derived from a series of studies of the views of family carers (Heyman and Huckle, 1993a, 1993b, 1995a, 1995b, 1995c; Gillman, Heyman and Swain, 1997; Heyman et al., 1997; Swain, Heyman and Gilman, 1997). Their methodology has been discussed in the above papers, and will only be outlined here. In brief, extensive, qualitative interviews were carried out with adults with learning difficulties, and with family and professional carers. Interview topics included developmental history and present life, with reference to mobility, friendships, sexual relationships, work, leisure, and home and future aspirations. Risk management emerged as an important theme in the first interviews, and became an important focus for subsequent work. The quotations given below are derived from transcripts of taped, confidential interviews, with authors' emphases in bold. All names have been changed.

The sample for the first study (Heyman and Huckle, 1993a, 1993b, 1995a, 1995b, 1995c) included 20 adults who lived at home with family carers and attended one of two adult-training centres (ATCs) situated in a single town within Tyne and Wear, at least one family carer looking after each adult, and a sample of staff from the two ATCs. Subsequently, further data has been collected from 32 adults and associated carers living in two other towns within Tyne and Wear (Heyman et al., 1997). The total sample includes 52 adults, 29 men and 23 women, most of whom were aged 25–40. Thirteen of the adults involved in the second-stage studies lived independently, or with paid carers (Heyman et al., 1997). However, this chapter focuses on adults living at home with family carers. All names have been changed.

Total interview times have varied, depending on respondents' willingness to participate and the quality of information obtained. Key informants have been interviewed for 8–10 hours, over several sessions, with all interviews taped and transcribed. Research participants needed to have some verbal communication ability, however limited. The sample, therefore, does not fully represent the highly varied population of those labelled as having a learning difficulty. A number of techniques were used, in the second-stage studies (Heyman et al., 1997) to enhance communication with adults with learning difficulties. The more successful techniques included talking about adults' own photo albums; asking them to discuss photographs which they took with a disposable camera supplied by the researchers; use of the *Just About Me* game which invites the adult and the interviewer to talk in response to open-ended cards, with messages such as 'I feel sad when ... '; and use of the *People I Know* diagram, a series of concentric circles, with a heart at the centre, to map how close the adult felt to significant others. Such techniques facilitated exploration of the lives of adults with very limited speech, but required considerable time inputs over a series of sessions.

## Data analysis

### FREEDOM OF THE LOCALITY AS A POTENTIAL HAZARD

Freedom of the locality was viewed, variously, as not a hazard, as unacceptably dangerous, and as a risk worth taking. Individual family carers and adults mostly agreed about its dangerousness for the adult, and about risk-taking in general, although a few overt conflicts were found. In the first study (Heyman and Huckle, 1993b), we found a statistically significant correlation of 0.75 (N=20) between the number of mentions by the adult and by their family carer, in separate interviews, of themes involving danger avoidance. This finding suggests a powerful family influence on attitudes to risk. It seems likely, in view of the power differences between adults and family carers, that, in most cases, adults acquired their attitudes towards freedom of the locality from family carers.

Families in our sample only rarely saw freedom of the locality as non-hazardous, and so unproblematic.

> INTERVIEWER: *How well do you manage when you go out on your own?*
> JANE: *I manage well. I have no problems.*
> INTERVIEWER: *How do your parents feel about you going out on your own?*
> JANE: *They don't worry.*

And:

> INTERVIEWER: *Can Jane use public transport on her own?*
> JANE'S MOTHER: *Yes, she manages well.*

Although unusual, this example demonstrates the need for a two-stage analysis of risk involving, first, hazard identification and, second, risk management. Unless a situation is seen as hazardous, questions about its safety will not arise.

Other family carers expressed anxieties about giving adults with learning difficulties freedom of the locality, while adults' views depended on whether they were able to move around relatively freely, as will be shown below. Family carers and/or adults were concerned that the adult might get ridiculed, lost, run over, mugged, kidnapped or physically attacked. These sources of hazard can be classified as originating from various combinations of adults' lack of normal competencies (e.g. inability to navigate) and the dangerousness of the environment (e.g. stigmatisation of people with learning difficulties, physical threats towards those who could not defend themselves). Hence, the ecological context for anxiety about the risks associated with spatial autonomy was a 'community' which was often seen as a dangerous locality (Heyman and Huckle, 1995a).

Because of concern about such hazards, about two-thirds of the families whom we interviewed rejected freedom of the locality for the adult as unacceptably dangerous.

INTERVIEWER: *Would you like to be able to go out on your own?*
DONALD: *No.*
INTERVIEWER: *Why?*
DONALD: **It's very dangerous.**

And:

INTERVIEWER: *Can Donald use public transport on his own?*
DONALD'S MOTHER: *No. I've never allowed him to travel on a bus on his own.* **I would worry too much.** *It is a difficult situation.*

The following quotation vividly illustrates both the sense which many adults who could not move around freely had of the locality as a highly dangerous place, and the way in which this perception legitimated family carer authority.

INTERVIEWER: *Do you go out on your own?*
BRENDA: *No. I go out with my parents. I can't go out on my own. Say if my mum wants me to do the shopping I can in the daytime, not in the dark.*
INTERVIEWER: *Why not in the dark?*
BRENDA: *Because people in cars might take you away.*
INTERVIEWER: *So are you afraid on a night time because of these people?*
BRENDA: **You don't know what they are like. They might hurt you. They might kidnap me.**
INTERVIEWER: *Would you like to be able to go out on your own?*
BRENDA: *No.*
INTERVIEWER: *Why?*
BRENDA: *Because of what I've just told you.*
INTERVIEWER: *What if it was the daytime?*
BRENDA: **With my parents, yes.**

About one-third of the families had a different approach to freedom of the locality, which we have described as limited risk-taking (Heyman and Huckle, 1993b). The adult felt that they coped well with going out independently, but agreed to temporal and spatial constraints insisted on by family carers. The family carer worried about the adult, but accepted the risk because of the perceived benefits. We return to this divergence of views when we consider communication tactics in risk management.

INTERVIEWER: *When you go out on your own, where do you go?*
PERRY: *To the pub, grandma's, my sisters, and my aunties ...*
INTERVIEWER: *How well do you manage when you go out on your own?*
PERRY: **I manage well.**
INTERVIEWER: *Do you have any difficulties?*
PERRY: *No. Only if I get drunk.*
INTERVIEWER: *Why do you get drunk?*
PERRY: *Because people always buy me drinks.*
INTERVIEWER: *When you go out do you have to be back by a certain time?*
PERRY: *Ten o'clock. If I am not back my mother comes and looks for me.*
INTERVIEWER: *Do you ever stay out after ten o'clock.*
PERRY: *Always home by ten.*

And:

*INTERVIEWER: How do you feel about him going out on his own?*
*PERRY'S MOTHER: Well. **He seems to enjoy it, but I worry about him** until he comes in.*
*INTERVIEWER: What type of things do you worry about?*
*PERRY'S MOTHER: Is he still in the place, and is he wandering all over?*

As the above quotations show, adults who had freedom of the locality could achieve some limited degree of social integration with the wider community. Family carers recognised its value to the adult, and were prepared to tolerate the resulting anxiety.

## REFLEXIVE RECURSION AND RISK ESCALATORS

We have argued above that, in circumstances defined as culturally normal, children acquire spatial autonomy through a series of small stages. Each step requires the acceptance of a relatively small risk which opens up learning opportunities, leading to increased competency, and reduced risk at the next stage. The counterfactual belief that individuals can develop skills which they do not presently possess entails the assumption that they are capable of learning from experience at progressively more advanced levels.

The significance of this issue can be seen in the sharply contrasting views of professional and family carers. In general, professional carers believed strongly that adults could learn recursively, while family carers in our sample, including those who were prepared to give the adult freedom of the locality, considered that their relatives had reached the limits of their potential capabilities. These contrasting views of 'reality' are illustrated by the following quotations.

*ATC STAFF MEMBER: **If you don't give them experience, they aren't going to learn.** We try to push them as far as we can with their potential. I only offer as much help as they need to do each task they are given. Then, the next time they do it, they don't need as much help, because they have remembered from the last time ... **Most parents have got the wrong idea of reality**, and they tend to look on the black side of things, not to the benefits for their son or daughter.*

And:

*MAUD'S BROTHER: There are too many dangers for them to lead a normal life, and let's face it, she is not normal, and will never be normal. There are only so many things that she is capable of doing. If she could do more we would let her. **We have tried to show her how to do things, but she cannot do them properly no matter how much time you spend training her.** We have tried for years. It is because of their handicap that they can never achieve a standard that is OK. If she could do more we would let her.*

The above family carer had given his sister considerable spatial freedom, but worried about her safety. The two quotations illustrate the sharply conflicting 'realities' generated by professional and family carers. Different assumptions about the highly conjectural issue of how much an adult with learning difficulties could potentially learn lay underneath this difference of opinion.

The impact of such differences on relationships between professional and family carers is illustrated in the following quotations.

*ATC STAFF MEMBER: Parents are overprotective. Like road safety, to use independent travel. We ask them if they want to do it, and they say no, because their mum won't let them.*

And:

*ANDREA'S MOTHER: It is alright the authority saying do this and that, but who is more qualified to say what should be done than the parent who has lived with them for 40 years? I know what they can do. An awful lot of them can't even cross the road properly. They can't judge gaps.*

Family carers who rejected freedom of the locality for their relative also feared that increased personal mobility would lead the adult into new areas of risk. If they experienced a first taste of free travel, they might demand more. The respondent quoted below was worried about her son's poor eyesight, and because *'he hasn't got any sense'*.

*JOHN'S MOTHER: I don't like him doing too much, you know. If he can [travel to work independently], maybe the next thing, he can start and go up [elsewhere] by himself.*

Freedom of the locality could also be feared because of dangers associated with other areas of personal autonomy which it could lead adults into.

*INTERVIEWER: Has Cliff ever visited Veronica's [girlfriend's house]?*
*CLIFF'S MOTHER: No. I wouldn't let him. I would be worried that something might develop.*

In contrast, one young man, Peter, unusually, had almost total freedom of the locality. He could use public transport, and successfully navigated long journeys on foot, returning home at times of his own choosing. His mother was not concerned about him getting lost or run over, but was worried that he might be attacked by *'nasty people'*, be led astray by law-breaking acquaintances, or get into trouble with the police. He had an obsession with cars, and had once been driven home in a police vehicle, having been picked up looking at cars, while carrying a bunch of keys. Peter's mother accepted the risks which his spatial autonomy generated because she felt that it provided his only source of quality of life.

One family carer, exceptionally, as she herself recognised, believed that her son could improve his navigational skills through experience. He had an unusually high degree of spatial autonomy, and travelled to local towns by bus.

*KEITH'S MOTHER: I had to trust him to travel himself, you know. A lot of people have said that they would not let my daughter [sic] go out by himself – he would get lost. I said that I had to let Keith, **because he is not going to have me here some day, and I have just had to let him do things himself**. He goes anywhere now. I used to say, 'What happens if you get lost, Keith?' And he would say, 'Well, I've got a tongue in my mouth. I can ask a policeman.'*

The next quotation, also exceptional, reveals the negotiated character of family risk-management strategies.

*JIM'S MOTHER: Well, I think he has achieved a lot more, **despite my efforts to stop him**. He's achieved a lot more then I thought he would. I never ever visualised him travel-*

*ling on his own, going on the Metro on his own, even having a job. It's just been sheer*
*determination and will-power on his part.*

The above respondent concluded, in retrospect, that she had underestimated her son's learning potential. This reappraisal had only become possible because her son had insisted on taking risks, supported by a local authority 'base' which provided more encouragement for independence than traditional day centres. However, if he had not learnt to cope with greater spatial mobility, irreversible damage might have resulted, either through a seriously adverse event, or through him becoming more discontented, after sampling the world beyond, with the narrow confines he could not safely leave.

## DIFFERENTIATION AND GENERALISATION

The use of differentiation and generalisation in the management of risk acceptability was discussed in Chapter 2. It was argued that a person who wishes to maximise the acceptability of an activity, the safety of which is questioned, may differentiate risk situations as much as possible, disaggregating situations involving a higher or lower probability of an adverse event. In effect, a single event class is divided into multiple event subclasses, only some of which need to be avoided. Family carers who gave adults local autonomy nearly always hedged this freedom with spatial and temporal restrictions designed to avoid the most dangerous situations, as illustrated by the next two quotations.

PERRY'S MOTHER: *I wouldn't ever want him to go night-clubbing.*
INTERVIEWER: *Why is that?*
PERRY'S MOTHER: *I don't know, but I just prefer him to be at the pub.* **I'd rather him be among the people that he knows.**

MAUD: *I get the bus to George's [daytime].* **He gets the bus back with me on a night to make sure I'm alright**, *and then he will get the bus back to his house again. In the summer I walk or go out on my bike myself.*

In contrast, generalisation from a relatively narrow class of events of doubtful safety can be used as a means of maximising the unacceptability of a wider category of events. The family carer quoted below generalised from a single event involving a child to danger for adults with learning difficulties.

BRENDA'S MOTHER: *It is this element of being protective really* **because once upon a time** *there was a case in Hebburn where this little girl had got on the bus, and she did not know that she had not got off the bus until she reached Hartlepool. She had gone to sleep on the back seat.* **It's that type of thing.** *As much as you would like her to use it, I don't know if it's worth the hassle.*

The impact of 'horror stories' such as the above depended on how far, and in what ways, they were seen as illustrating the dangers faced by adults with learning difficulties who went out on their own. One family carer, whose sister did have some freedom of the locality, described an incident in which a man had attempted to sexually molest her in a local pub. She had been banned from visiting this particular pub, but was otherwise allowed to go where she liked in the local area. Generalisation of danger, and restriction on this woman's spatial autonomy, were thus minimised. The family carer could easily have ruled out visiting any pub, or travel in general, on the basis of induction from this single adverse experience.

## COMMUNICATION OF ANXIETY AS A RISK-MANAGEMENT TACTIC

Spatial autonomy, within the boundaries of the culturally acceptable, is negotiated within families. In contemporary Britain, for example, locking a relative permanently in a room, or allowing a very young child to undertake a long solo journey, would provoke almost universal censure. Adults with learning difficulties and family carers undoubtedly negotiated the former's freedom of movement, although the notion of a two-way process of mutual influence does not imply that each party necessarily has equal power.

Family carers who did not wish to accept the risks they associated with adults having freedom of the locality used their own anxiety as a way of legitimating constraints on adults' spatial autonomy.

> INTERVIEWER: *Do you tell Audrey you are worried?*
> AUDREY'S MOTHER: *Yes **I tell her I worry** ... I always wait for her getting of the bus, and I have told her not to talk to strangers.*

In contrast, those family carers who had accepted the risks associated with adult freedom of the locality tended to suppress expressions of anxiety because of their potentially inhibiting effect.

> INTERVIEWER: *Do you tell Mandy you are worried [about her going out alone]?*
> MANDY'S MOTHER: *No.*
> INTERVIEWER: *Why is that?*
> MANDY'S MOTHER: ***I think that it would only worry her more.***

Through the use of follow-up telephone interviews, it was possible to establish, for 16 of the 20 families who participated in the first study, whether the main family carer would communicate worry about the adult going out alone. We determined whether the adult felt that the family carer was worried about them going out alone from the original interviews. The results of this analysis are summarised in Table 9.2.

The above table shows up a strong communication effect. In all 12 cases where family carers said that they would communicate worry about the adult going out independently, the adult felt that the carer was worried about this happening. In all four cases where family carers said they would not communicate worry, the adults believed that they were not worried. Family carer communication of worry was significantly associated with the absence of adult freedom of the locality ($P < .01$, Fisher's exact test, 2-tailed).

## COST-BENEFIT ANALYSIS

The above data provide numerous examples of the ways in which adults and carers based their attitudes to adults' freedom of the locality on an informal

Table 9.2   Communication of carer worry about a family member with learning difficulties going out alone (N=16)[1]

| | Families in which the adult had freedom of the locality 'limited risk-taking' | | Families in which the adult did not have freedom of the locality 'danger-avoiding' | |
|---|---|---|---|---|
| | Adult sees family carer as worried | Adult sees family carer as NOT worried | Adult sees family carer as worried | Adult sees family carer as NOT worried |
| Family carer would communicate worry[2] | 2 | 0 | 10 | 0 |
| Family carer would NOT communicate worry | 0 | 4 | 0 | 0 |

[1] Four of the 20 families in the sample (1 'limited risk-taking' and 3 'danger-avoiding') were excluded from this analysis because the family carer could not be contacted for the follow-up interview.
[2] Based on follow-up telephone interviews with family carers.

cost-benefit analysis. This analysis took into account family carer worry, the benefits to adults of being able to go out independently, and the risks entailed. For example, one family carer, quoted above, felt that allowing her daughter to use the bus was not *'worth the hassle'*. In contrast, the mother of Peter, who had maximal temporal and spatial freedom of the locality, said that she *'couldn't stop him, no. I mean, he would have no life at all, you know'* even though she couldn't *'relax until he's actually come in through the door'*.

Family carers rarely mentioned benefits to themselves, in terms of a reduced workload, of enabling adults to develop social outlets outside the family. They, perhaps, discounted their own needs within a research interview concerned with caring roles. Few family carers mentioned the potential benefits for adults of practising and improving mobility skills. As noted above, most believed, rightly or wrongly, that their relatives had developed to the limit of their potential, a view which professional carers strongly contested.

As discussed above, families who gave adults some spatial autonomy, despite the hazards they felt that it entailed, nearly always adopted a strategy of risk minimisation based on differentiating times and places where freedom of movement involved more or less risk. Temporal delimitation of freedom of the locality allowed them to recognise quickly if anything had gone wrong, and to minimise their own anxiety, since the adults had to return by a certain time. They were, like Cinderella, given spatial autonomy on a temporary licence.

Spatial autonomy was not valued, primarily, for its own sake, but as a means of gaining independent access to extra-familial social activities. Families who rejected freedom of the locality as too dangerous adopted one of two methods of coming to terms with the resulting preclusion of such activities, facilitation and minimisation (Heyman and Huckle, 1995a). Facilitation involved family carers taking responsibility for the adult's personal life, attempting to compensate for the loss of personal autonomy which they saw as a consequence of disability.

> DONALD'S MOTHER: *All my money goes on him. He doesn't get no rubbish gear, and they wouldn't pay £100 odd for a leather jacket. You can't get in his wardrobe for clothes. My sister has taken him to Florida and I am always taking him on holidays, so he gets all over.* **He's OK. He does alright by me.**

Facilitation, as a means of compensating for the consequences of danger avoidance, had three potential disadvantages. First, as the last quotation makes clear, it placed considerable financial and personal demands on family carers. However, some had integrated their own social lives with those of the person they were looking after, for example enjoying visits to segregated social clubs where they could meet other parents. Second, adults' autonomy was inevitably curtailed since they could not make independent choices about how to spend their time. Third, because their time was managed for them, incentives and opportunities for adults to develop daily living skills were limited.

Perhaps because of the personal and financial costs involved in facilitation, some danger-avoiding family carers adopted a strategy of need minimisation. They reasoned that the person they were caring for did not need social outlets beyond those obtained at a day centre, and through family activities. If this premise was accepted, then a cautious strategy which precluded freedom of the locality became cost-free. However, adults could not so easily dismiss their own need to experience a less limited social environment. Hence, need minimisation depended on achieving non-communication, as illustrated below.

> MICHAEL'S MOTHER: *No. He [friend] has not visited.*
> INTERVIEWER: *Would you ever let him?*
> MICHAEL'S MOTHER: *I think he sees him enough at work. But if Michael asked me, I would say yes.* **But he has never said, so I don't think he is bothered either way.**

And:

> INTERVIEWER: *Do your friends visit?*
> MICHAEL: *I would like them to, if my mum would let us.*
> INTERVIEWER: *Would you ever ask your mum?*
> MICHAEL: *No.* **I would wait for her to ask me.**

## Discussion

The academic literature on the lives of people with learning difficulties strongly favours risk. Perske (1972) refers to *'the dignity of risk'* for the mentally retarded. The notion of parental *'overprotection'* (Block, 1980) incorporates a covert value judgement that parents **ought** to encourage people with learning difficulties to take more risks. The concept of *'letting go'* (Richardson and Richie, 1989) implies that parents avoid risk for adults with learning difficulties for selfish reasons, because they do not want to give up the parental role. The unspoken assumption that it is **not rational** for parents to put the safety of their offspring above their autonomy is embedded in these analyses. In taking such a stance, academic writers side with the professional carers whose views have been quoted above.

The research discussed in this chapter has attempted to understand risk management from the perspectives of adults with learning difficulties and family carers. An *a priori* assumption of the irrationality of a safety first strategy precludes this kind of enquiry. Much can be learnt from the study of freedom of the locality, for two reasons. First, the extent of a person's spatial licence strongly affects the range of other life choices open to them. The achievement of freedom of the locality does not in itself guarantee a rich quality of life. People with learning difficulties who do attain such freedom may wander aimlessly, as did Peter, discussed above. However, a spatial licence is a necessary, although not sufficient, condition for opening up wider areas of autonomy in a modern urban ecology. Some adults who have been granted a restricted licence do achieve some degree of integration into the wider community. For example, among the adults discussed in this chapter, Perry socialised in his local pub, and Maud went to social clubs with her boyfriend, who also had learning difficulties.

Second, within the samples studied, freedom of the locality had a marginal status, more or less just within or just outside adults' perceived capabilities, and so proved to be a rich source of variation in family risk-management strategy. In contrast, families mostly agreed, rightly or wrongly, that living independently, having a sexual relationship, getting married or holding down a job involved unacceptable risks for their relative. Practice guides for professionals (Michaels, 1994; Stone, 1995) mainly emphasise these larger areas of autonomy. However, they cannot be achieved unless more basic freedoms can be established as routine. One adult participant in our first study rebelled for a time against his mother's risk-avoidance strategy, and sought to marry, live independently and obtain full employment. But he also believed himself incapable of going out safely on his own, and his girlfriend, who had been given a little more spatial autonomy, had to visit him. Because of its marginal acceptability, freedom of the locality may provide the most promising area for professionals to begin to attempt to synthesise their own risk perspectives with those of adults with learning difficulties and family carers.

Although family attitudes towards freedom of the locality differed, they arose from a similar starting point, based on two related assumptions: first, that the wider urban world, sometimes fancifully described as 'the community' was packed with dangers; and, second, that their relative had reached the limit of their potential, and so could not learn through experience, thus reducing the level of risk. Not all family carers saw freedom of the locality as hazardous, or regarded their relative as incapable of learning to cope with its dangers, but most did. The promotion of spatial autonomy for this client group involves more than acquisition of the transportation skills discussed by Bosch (1994, pp. 217–18), and requires professionals to engage both with family politics and risk-management dilemmas. As the data presented above has shown, professional interventions designed to expand adult zones of autonomy, and so of risk-taking, will fail unless they are supported by family carers. Such support will not be achieved unless professionals treat risk-management policy as an area of genuine uncertainty, requiring dialogue rather than the imposition of their own line, legitimated by claims to expertise which provoke sceptical responses.

Perceptions of the locality as a dangerous place cannot be divorced from wider cultural attitudes towards urban life in the UK, as evinced, for example, by the media attention given to assaults on children by strangers. Although rare in Western European countries, such incidents touch a raw cultural nerve, and family carer attitudes have to be understood in the context of this wider concern. In consequence, most family carers hedged adult freedom of the locality with temporal and spatial constraints, and experienced considerable anxiety when the person they were looking after went on an unsupervised journey.

The second common component of family carers' approach to freedom of the locality for adults with learning difficulties was a pessimistic view of the potential recursive benefits of practice. Professional carers tended to believe that if adults took risks, they would learn from experience, thus reducing future risks, while most family carers considered that adults had reached the limits of their capabilities. We have adopted a studiously neutral position on this issue, since we have aimed to illuminate the rationality behind conflicting lay and professional approaches to risk, not to judge their relative merits. It is worth speculating analytically about why family carers minimised, but professional carers maximised, the potential for positive recursion.

Learning potential has a nebulous quality, as any struggling teacher can testify. It can be demonstrated through success, but can never be totally ruled out. Theoretically, at least, if suitable methods could be found, anyone could learn anything. The editor of this volume might even fulfil his ambition to become a passable violin-player. Professionals had a stronger, counterfactual sense than family carers of what adults with learning difficulties might become in appropriate circumstances. Their legitimacy as experts depended on such possibilities, and their experience with particular individuals was limited. Family carers, in contrast, had had a lifetime of experience of what the adult could *not* do. They may have found it harder to visualise alternatives. And, as several family carers pointed out, if anything went wrong, they, not day centre staff, would be left to pick up the pieces.

Some family carers accused professionals of being biased by organisational interests, pushing adults beyond safe limits so as to justify moving them out of the day centre, in order to free-up places for individuals with worse disabilities. Others felt that professionals who encouraged their children to take risks were exploiting them as guineapigs:

> I think to a certain extent they [adults] are being used, aren't they. Maybe I am being nasty, but I suppose they are used in an experimental way.

Ferrara (1979) found that parents favoured normalisation for people with learning difficulties in general more than for their own child. A parallel may be drawn between this situation and so-called *'courage to fail'* at the frontiers of medicine. Typically, radical new procedures, for example in transplant surgery, yield a low initial success rate, and a poor cost-benefit ratio when balanced against the pain and distress they cause. However, unless doctors are given opportunities to improve their skills, such innovations will never succeed. Levels of risk may be reduced through early failures, and potentially beneficial procedures cannot be identified in advance. Doctors' courage to fail may be bolstered by the realisation that the consequences fall primarily on their patients. Similarly, professionals ask a great deal of family carers when they seek to persuade them to modify patterns of behaviour which have protected close relatives from the terrors of the modern world.

# The resettlement of people with severe learning difficulties

## Chris Corkish and Bob Heyman

## Introduction

> *The world in which we live is not always safe, secure and predictable. It does not always say 'please' or 'excuse me'. Every day there is a possibility of being thrown up against a situation where we may have to risk everything, even our lives. This is the real world.*
> (Perske, 1972, p. 24)

This chapter is based on a research project which is examining quality of life issues for people with severe and profound learning difficulties who are currently resettling from a long-stay institution. The chapter begins with a discussion of the influence of learning difficulty on the development of styles of personal risk management. The history of institutional care is then briefly reviewed with respect to its influence on family and staff views of resettlement and risk-taking for long-stay residents. Finally, the risk-management strategies employed by service-providers, and their impact on users, are considered.

### Learning difficulties and the development of personal risk management

Human development depends on exploration and experimentation (Piaget and Inhelder, 1958). Children naturally discover, through trial and error, pleasure and pain. The frequent minor accidents experienced by infants seem almost to be a rite of passage. Young children explore common hazards but, through lack of experience, may not be able to predict the possible adverse consequences of their actions. Parents invest considerable effort in ensuring children's safety, giving them time to learn to progressively manage more demanding risks. As children mature, their autonomy, and exposure to risks, increases. Although cultural attitudes vary, older children and adolescents in many societies explore the cultural boundaries of risk. Joyriding, for example, may be confined to a minority of mainly young men in specific subcultures, but comparable behaviour can be observed elsewhere among adults who enjoy risky sports or gang conflict.

For individuals who have learning difficulties, this developmental path may be delayed or diverted. Children and adults with severe disabilities often experience sensory difficulties (Woodhouse *et al.*, 1996; Mazzoni, Ackley and Nash, 1994) as well as difficulties in processing and organising sensory information. More able individuals may have memory problems, an inability to predict events on the basis of previous experience, or attention deficits. Accompanying physical disabilities may restrict their capacity to explore the environment. Many people with learning difficulties also suffer from epilepsy (Brandford and Collacott, 1994). Seizures cannot be predicted, and can have a significant impact on individuals' ability to manage risky situations. Sufferers may experience disorientation, poor attention and tiredness, all of which affect judgement. Modern antiepileptic drugs can impair attention and perception, both essential to risk judgement, either through provoking drowsiness or through long-term iatrogenic effects.

The effects of impairment cannot be readily separated from those resulting from societal responses. Low expectations, stigmatisation, strategies which attempt to make the environment totally safe, and institutionalisation may deprive individuals of essential risk-management learning experiences. In a reductionist culture, which implicitly regards biological explanations as more 'real' than social ones, the resulting lack of confidence can be all too easily attributed in total to the initial impairment.

Cultural and domestic factors mediate the ways in which people with learning difficulties encounter risks (Perske 1972; Edgerton 1975; Edgerton, Bollinger and Herr, 1984; Edgerton, 1988; Heyman and Huckle 1993a, 1993b). This research, in general, portrays adults as restricted by their care environment, and family carers have been represented as trying to maintain their offspring in a childlike state (Richardson, 1989; Richardson and Ritchie, 1989). However, this view of the family carer role discounts as irrational parents' fears about the dangers which they see people with learning difficulties as facing, and overlooks cultural variations. Heyman and Huckle (1993a, 1993b) found that adults with relatively mild learning difficulties who came from better-off, two-parent families, generally had less autonomy and were more protected than those from poorer, single carer, families. Ironically, the children from more prosperous families appeared to be achieving less of their potential with respect to everyday living skills.

Cultural beliefs, material wealth, ethnic origin, parental marital status, the gender of the main carer, and of the person with learning difficulties, the health status of both, and the local environment may influence family attitudes towards risks. People with learning difficulties cannot learn how to manage risk for themselves unless they are given the opportunity to practise. Incompetence resulting from lack of practice reinforces the impression that they can never learn. Conversely, as argued in Chapter 9, the view held by many parents that their offspring have reached the limit of their potential, and therefore should not be exposed to additional risks, should not be dismissed *a priori*.

## An historical context for institutional care

### THE ORIGINS OF INSTITUTIONAL CARE FOR PEOPLE WITH LEARNING DIFFICULTIES

The history of long-stay hospitals may explain, in part, why, as will be shown below, many relatives see them as safe havens. Such hospitals, now being largely phased out, have often been condemned as incapable of providing a good quality of life for people with learning difficulties (Townsend, 1962; Goffman, 1968; Morris, 1969; HMS0, 1979). However, at their inception, in the early nineteenth century, long-stay institutions were widely seen as a positive step. Baldwin, Craddock and Joy, in their 1815 report to the Committee of the House of Commons on Madhouses in England, maintained that institutional care was needed:

> *in order to prevent the intolerable evil of these unhappy persons being imprisoned in gaols or in parish workhouses, or permitted to wander about the country in a state of total helplessness and neglect.* (Cited in Alaszewski, 1986, p. 10)

These reformers felt optimistic that the new institutions would provide places of refuge, offering specialist care, in small, purpose-built environments, for people who could not cope with the outside world. Later in the century, however, the reformers' original idealism was replaced by pessimism as the size of the institutions grew, and they became increasingly impersonal. Scull (1979, p. 198) records a steady increase in the number of asylums in England, from nine in 1827, to 66 in 1890, and in their average inmate population from 116 to 802 over the same period. He suggests that they simply became warehouses of the insane.

Although categories of inmate were differentiated to some extent, in section 17 of the Idiots Act of 1886, separate provision for the 'mentally defective' was not proposed until the early twentieth century (HMSO, 1908). The 'colonies' were eventually introduced after the First World War. These reproduced many of the geographical, architectural and care-practice features of the nineteenth-century traditional asylum. They grew in popularity and, between 1924 and 1954, the population of people with learning difficulties in the colonies rose from 17 104 to 55 984 (Rooff, 1957). Sixteen per cent of the individuals participating in the present research project were admitted during this period. Many are now returning to their home town after a considerable period in hospital (see Table 10.1, on page 221), and first went into institutional care when its value was largely unquestioned.

For their parents and grandparents, the then new models of care would have seemed to offer a significant improvement over care at home, the workhouse or the madhouse. Many of the relatives contacted for the present study, usually surviving parents or siblings, reported that professionals and family members had put significant pressure on them to have the disabled person 'committed' in that person's own best interests. At the same time, the segregation of intellectually impaired individuals was justified in terms of the protection of society. The 1913 Mental Deficiency Act, influenced by prevailing eugenic beliefs, forbad sexual intercourse between an intellectually impaired female and any man.

The geographical isolation of the institutions ensured minimal contact with the outside world, including family members. With food produced on site through residents' cheap labour, the colonies soon became detached from the rest of society. This physical separation protected the institutionalised from the world outside, and vice versa. However, institutions, isolated from the wider society, become communities in their own rights and generate their own risks. For example, an apocryphal story, known to insiders at the hospital site for the present research, advises walkers to a certain spot in the grounds to carry a Mars bar with them, allegedly the normal currency within that community for sexual favours. The authors cannot judge the truth of such stories, but they do illustrate the dangers which, undoubtedly, are found in such isolated environments, for example that a more able person will take sexual advantage of a resident who cannot give fully informed consent or understand the risks associated with casual sex.

## THE ORIGINS OF COMMUNITY CARE

Criticisms of institutions (Lomax, 1921) generated little response from governments until the 1950s, when anti-institutional ideology began to gain momentum. Examination of long-stay hospital care (Ministry of Health, 1965) generated a depressing picture of personal, environmental, occupational and social deprivation among residents. Morris (1969), in her study of institutional life for people with learning difficulties, found that 61 per cent of hospitals had 1000 or more beds, with only 1 per cent of patients in single rooms. The majority slept in dormitories, many with less than 2 feet between beds. Only 21 per cent possessed their own toiletries, and most wore communal clothing. Life for a person who had a learning difficulty, and lived in an institution, offered little.

Much has changed within hospitals for people with learning difficulties. Between 1969 and 1983, the government paid considerable attention to their condition (HMSO, 1969, 1978, 1979; DHSS, 1971, 1976, 1980). Staff training improved, and wards became smaller, as the more able residents moved back into the community. Greater emphasis was placed on the quality of the physical condition of the wards, and on individual autonomy.

Data collected in 1994, for the present research, showed that considerable emphasis was being placed, within the large residential hospital studied, on living conditions, personal choice and individualised care. Considerable effort had been put into making living areas homely, and improving their material quality. However, the legacy of the colony still remained, with mass living, institutional architecture, limited resident choice, and a power inequality between staff and service-users. Many staff recognised difficulties, but felt powerless to change the institutional structure. As one staff member wrote:

> Staff work towards ensuring dignity, respect, equality and privacy is given. However, this would be greatly improved if the home was of a smaller scale.

The disadvantages of hospital life may be concealed because institutionalised residents do not wish to challenge the prevailing order. A staff member said of one long-standing resident:

> One gentleman states he is wary of speaking up about any odd problem in case he causes trouble, despite constant reassurance he won't.

In a mass living environment, with a low ratio of staff to residents, practical safety strategies are geared to the needs of the least able. Typically, institutions will limit residents' access to potentially hazardous situations through the design of buildings and the organisation of care. Within the hospital studied, stairs to private areas like dormitories were often closed to residents, and outer doors were frequently locked for their safety, to prevent residents from getting out, as well as to stop unauthorised individuals from getting in. Most kitchen areas on the wards visited were not accessible to residents, because a minority were judged incapable of appreciating the dangers to be found there. Hazards were minimised even for less-dependent individuals who could travel freely within the grounds without support. For instance, visitors to the hospital who arrive by car are reminded by a sign on the approach road to drive with care, and to be aware of 'Handicapped Residents', who enjoy the enviable situation of having right of way on the road.

The minimisation of environmental hazards would, at first sight, appear to benefit those who cannot manage personal risks competently, but it does not encourage the development of self-protection skills. Such hazards cannot be so easily controlled when institutionalised individuals are discharged into the community. The inexperience of the newly discharged hospital patient in dealing with everyday hazards increases their dangerousness. For example, a person who has spent most of his life in an environment where traffic is controlled for his benefit has a greater chance of suffering a road-traffic accident once resettled, unless appropriate learning opportunities are provided.

Professionals who avoid potential accidents minimise the risk of expensive and time-consuming incident enquiries, litigation and career damage. However, a totally safe environment may restrict an individual's life experiences and potential for growth. Perske (1972, p.24) wrote that:

> such overprotection endangers the retarded person's human dignity and tends to keep him from experiencing the normal taking of risks in life which is necessary for normal human growth and development.

Large-scale, long-term, residential care produces an environment which tends to override the needs of the individual in favour of organisational requirements. Managerially, it is easier to maintain a relationship of authority over residents, and to discourage them from achieving self-determination in the name of safety. One staff member described the hospital as *'very safety conscious. Regular health and safety checks.'* However, another felt that her colleagues were *'very overprotective to all people'*. She went on to say that residents *'were not allowed to think for themselves. Staff tend to be in charge.'*

## A study of a resettlement scheme

Central government policy (HMSO, 1989, 1990) requires all long-stay hospitals to close, and their residents to be returned to the community. The hospital in question provides a large regional facility, and the present project concerns individuals returning to one town, over 20 miles away from the hospital.

For individuals who originally came from this town, and have lived for longer than 10 years in long-stay voluntary hospitals, the resettlement process has progressed in two stages. Selection criteria for those moving out in Stage I were based on residents' abilities in terms of self-care, mobility, continence, communication and independence. The abilities of those selected and those left in the hospital differed considerably, although a small proportion of more independent residents chose not to leave in Stage I.

Similar selection processes operated nationally, and quality of life studies at the time (Jones and Bassell, 1987; Cattermole, Jahoda and Markova, 1990) used samples of more able individuals who resettled early, and had the ability to express their views in research interviews. The present study involves 98 residents who were not selected for Stage I resettlement, and who began to move back to their town of origin during Stage II, early in 1994. As noted, these residents tend to have the most severe learning difficulties. Some also have other difficulties, including mobility disabilities, communication problems, challenging behaviours, incontinence or health problems relating to the ageing process.

The present research project, an evaluation of the Stage II resettlement programme, is examining changes which occur in quality of life for residents before, during and after the process of moving out of hospital. Qualitative and quantitative data are being collected from a variety of sources, including observation, interviews where possible, skills' assessment and the measurement of adaptive behaviour. Longitudinal comparisons are being performed, with individuals acting as their own controls.

Some background information on Stage II residents is given in Table 10.1. All hospital residents will have returned to their town of origin by March 1998, when the hospital's long-term residential facilities should close. Some individuals will move directly into existing provision, while most will spend a period of up to a year in a 15-place residential facility in their town of origin, before moving to their final homes.

Community-care providers are faced with the difficult task of balancing the promotion of service-user autonomy against the maintenance of their safety. For example, independent travelling is fraught with potential dangers

**Table 10.1**   The backgrounds of discharged hospital residents (N=98)

|  | Men | Women |
|---|---|---|
| Number of residents | 61 | 37 |
| Average age | 50.6 | 57.9 |
| Age range | 29–90 | 30–84 |
| Average length of hospital stay (years) | 32.6 | 40.8 |
| Range of length of hospital stay (years) | 10–65 | 20–65 |

for residents, including getting lost, road accidents and abuse from a small minority of the population. Community nurses have received frequent requests to assist with independence training for returning residents.

Few, if any, of the individuals being resettled in Stage II will ever gain sufficient daily living skills to become independent in the local community. Most will need to be accompanied by paid workers when they access local amenities. Many will need assistance or total help with feeding, hygiene and clothing. Others may develop some cooking skills, but are currently unable to assess the hazards involved, and need help to avoid injury. Service-providers planning risk management for this group need to employ different criteria to those used for more independent individuals. For instance, it can not be assumed that residents have developed basic life-preserving skills, such as predicting the consequences of touching very hot objects, or eating the indigestible. One practical risk-management method used widely in hospital and community provision involves locking external doors in order to prevent severely disabled residents from unaccompanied exposure to external dangers. Such restrictions can, arguably, be justified for the most severely disabled on the grounds of safety, but raise questions about the meaningfulness of 'community' care.

## Formal and informal carer perspectives on risk management

### FORMAL CARERS PERSPECTIVES ON RISK MANAGEMENT

Life in any environment, inescapably, entails risk. However, paid carers who take decisions on behalf of people currently undergoing resettlement are faced with a risk-management dilemma. At one extreme, environments which maximise safety may severely limit individuals' life experiences. At the other, environments designed to enrich life experience may generate demands on a person which they cannot, currently, manage safely. Professional care staff need to develop environments which optimise the balance of autonomy and safety, and to identify ways in which service users' existing skills can be improved upon, so that the zone of acceptable risk-taking can be expanded.

In theory, more personalised care can be provided in smaller community homes. However, paid carers who wish to enhance service-user autonomy have to continually appraise and manage situations involving potential risk to individuals with severe disabilities. If, for example, a client wished to visit the local public house, the carer would need to assess the risks entailed on the basis of previous knowledge of the individual's capabilities and anticipation of possible negative outcomes. The carer would then need to attempt to plan to me*et all* anticipated contingencies. In practice, restrained by staffing and other resource limitations, formal carers may be tempted to access local facilities by taking all the residents out collectively. Although service-users may value such activities, they do little to promote personal autonomy or competence.

When adversity does strike, judgements about the actions of responsible staff may be subject to hindsight effects (see Chapter 5). Fear of punitive action by employers and professional bodies, and of litigation, can dissuade formal carers from exposing service-users to avoidable risks. Anecdotal evidence from colleagues, and press reports of staff negligence, can serve to reinforce an atmosphere of uncertainty, while formal carers have very little personal incentive to allow service-users to take risks. Not surprisingly, they often adopt a risk-minimisation strategy.

Staff balance resident safety and autonomy in different ways. A few of those responsible for the different residences within the hospital studied took service-users on regular weekend trips to a large shopping centre, 11 miles away, or to a more local swimming-pool and pubs. Staff who adopted this line saw access to the local community as relatively easy to obtain. One staff member wrote that the hospital was *'rather central, walking distance to local shops, on a regular bus route. Hospital has contract with a local taxi firm,'* and that *'Residents are accepted in local community.'*

Most hospital formal carers, however, rated accessibility as a major problem which limited external activities, and highlighted the disabilities of the residents. As one staff member wrote:

> Most residents are disabled and use wheelchairs [for] most trips out, visits to shops even local are made by taxi or bus. Distance for wheelchair users too far.

This staff member also took a much more pessimistic view of community integration, stating that there was *'very little contact with local people'*.

Variations in staff attitudes may have arisen because of differences in the disabilities of service-users living in particular residences, since similar clients tended to be grouped together. One ward, for example, catered for the more elderly population. However, each residential area housed at least a few individuals, dissimilar from the rest, who needed extra support when engaged in potentially hazardous activities. Given the need to manage groups of residents *en masse*, the balance of personal development versus safety tended to be struck at the level of safety which was deemed appropriate for the most vulnerable members of the group. One staff member responded to the questionnaire items on risk management and community access as follows:

*Normality can only be taken so far, depending upon the type of resident living within the home. Abilities differ dramatically.*

This carer had had to cope with an increased number of people who had challenging behaviours moving on to the ward as the hospital rationalised its resources. These individuals, although a minority, needed a greater level of support, taking staff away from the rest. This 'lowest common denominator effect' may intensify when residents move out into community facilities, and are exposed to new internal and external hazards.

How should professional carers differentiate between acceptable risks and dangers to be avoided? The rational individualistic model of care, which many hospital and community establishments purport to employ, would utilise information from a wide variety of sources. Details of individuals' skills, physical and mental state, history and personality would all contribute to an assessment of their present abilities. Risks could then be considered in relation to environmental hazards. For the fictitious character, mentioned earlier in the chapter, who wanted to visit a local pub, the relevant information might include his knowledge of geography, purchasing skills, drug/alcohol contraindications, ability to manage alcohol consumption, mental state, previous experience of the pub and general demeanour. Knowledge of the fictitious public house, especially its safety for the individual concerned, would figure largely in the equation. As a result of this calculation, the level of necessary support could be determined, or an alternative provided if necessary. In this way, probabilistic reasoning could be used to shift the balance from dangerousness to risk for the individual.

Unfortunately, such individualised risk appraisal cannot be achieved in current conditions. Care staff do not enjoy the luxury of making decisions solely on the basis of information about individual service-users and their environment. They have to consider issues such as professional accountability, staffing ratios, previous experiences, political pressure, the needs of other service-users and relatives' demands. However, as people who have learning difficulties resettle from institutional into community facilities, the opportunities for experiencing healthy risk should increase. Long-stay hospitals, by their design and organisation, have achieved the objective of the early reformers, to provide safe segregated care, but have generated dehumanising, overprotective living conditions.

Formal carers working in the new community-based environment have the opportunity to break away from the old institutional culture. They should be able to find the appropriate means to restore the balance between risk and safety for each individual, provided that the institutional mentality does not merely relocate as the hospitals close. The processes through which a new community home developed risk-management practice are illustrated below with respect to two critical incidents, involving access to the outside world and to the kitchen. In both cases, staff, coping with novel circumstances, developed more restrictive risk-management rules in response to adverse events.

## The gateway to the outside

Few people with learning difficulties living in long-term residential care have their freedom legally restricted under the terms of the Mental Health Act 1983, on the grounds that they are judged to be a danger to themselves or others. But, despite being full citizens, their liberty is limited by others. A locked door policy was operated on most wards within the hospital studied. Staff at the community home, to which residents were initially sent, at first kept the door to the outside world open as a matter of principle. They were obliged to modify this line when a known 'absconder' escaped and only just avoided being run over on a nearby busy road. Staff compromised their integrationist principles by introducing an electronic locking system which they felt would, somehow, be less oppressive than a traditional lock and key.

In this instance, risk management had to be based on the lowest common denominator. Service-providers ensured the safety of some residents, but limited the freedom of others who could have been safely allowed out. However, the electronic lock, fortuitously, provided a way of protecting the safety of the majority, while giving access to the outside world to those residents judged capable of coping safely. The minority who had some self-preservation skills were also those few who could operate the lock without help. One individual in this small group had a manipulation disability which would have precluded the operation of a mechanical lock. The installation of the electronic device enabled him to open the external door independently.

Even if physical barriers between residents and the outside world had not been set up, restrictions to their freedom would still have been needed for safety reasons. The two most capable individuals (out of 15 at this residence), whom hospital staff judged to need only minimal help in road-crossing, were thought by community residential carers to need full support. Their extra caution probably arose from the presence of a nearby busy road. The level of spatial autonomy (see Chapter 9) judged acceptably safe for service-users, thus, depended on features of the wider environment.

## In the kitchen

In the hospital setting, as mentioned earlier, only a few relatively skilled residents, and those receiving instruction, were ever allowed access to ward-cooking areas. Within the community facility all residents had the opportunity to participate in, or at least observe, food preparation. Minor accidents were accepted as normal.

However, even in this more open environment, some limitations had to be imposed because of potential dangers to one individual. This person, unaware of the potential consequences, had found an unopened loaf of bread in one of the kitchens and proceeded to eat it too quickly. He suffered a serious choking episode which would probably have killed him if staff had not quickly intervened. Subsequently all food was placed out of reach, and the main kitchen, where the majority of meals were prepared, was locked when staff were unable to supervise.

This example, as with the locked door discussed above, suggests that community residents may gradually find their autonomy eroded as staff respond to adverse events, and adopt a lowest common denominator approach to risk management. However, individual occurrences do not provide a good inductive guide to underlying probabilities. Theoretically, such choking episodes might happen very infrequently where residents have open access to food. But once an activity has been ruled out as too dangerous, further inductive evidence about its safety cannot be obtained. Since unlikely events will happen, an atmosphere in which the occurrence of adversity leads to the withdrawal of an activity will generate a continually shrinking zone of autonomy. Over the longer term, as will be argued in the Discussion, organisations caring for vulnerable groups may oscillate between prioritising safety and autonomy for service-users.

## FAMILY CARER PERSPECTIVES ON RISK

Professional and family carers differ considerably in their attitude to risks. Family carers, most commonly parents, looking after a relative at home may worry continually about their relative's personal safety, and fear for their future after they have died (see Chapter 9). The close relatives of people who have lived most of their lives in hospital face different issues. Direct responsibility for day-to-day care has been transferred to formal carers, who make judgements about the persons' risk-taking capabilities from a different viewpoint. Although concerned for residents' welfare, they are unlikely to have the same degree of emotional involvement as family members. They can appraise risks in a more detached way, but have to take into account the requirement to manage groups of vulnerable people, and the risks associated with professional accountability, as discussed above.

Some residents within the hospital were originally admitted through necessity, for example following the death of the main carer. However, the majority moved to the hospital as a result of decisions made by their next of kin. Of the 98 residents being resettled, 68 per cent were under 18 when they were admitted to hospital. Accounts given by the 51 next of kin who visited residents regularly suggest that their original decision to have a relative admitted was influenced by the concern expressed by health professionals and other family members about the safety and wellbeing of the person with learning difficulties. Having made the decision to admit their relative, family carers had to rely on the expertise and trustworthiness of hospital staff.

The impending closure of the hospitals will dramatically affect those moving out. On average, the hospital residents included in the present study have spent 36.7 years (range 10–65 years) in the same environment. During this time, friendships between residents, and between residents and staff, have developed. Routines necessary to the smooth running of the organisation have become well-established. Residents may find resettlement difficult to cope with, and service-providers have given some consideration to overcoming 'transition shock' (Booth, Simmons and Booth, 1989). The emotional consequence for their next of kin is, perhaps, given less attention. Many family members participating in the present research discussed their feelings and actions at the time their relative was admitted to hospital, and spoke of admission as a recent event despite the long time period which had since elapsed: a testimony to its significance for them. Of the 51 people visited, all but one expressed confidence in the hospital staff and in the quality of care provided.

Relatives' feelings about the impending resettlement were, however, more mixed. Eighty-one per cent (41) of those contacted expressed concern about the safety of their kin in the new environment, and about the ability of care staff to recognise potentially dangerous situations. Relatives cited well-publicised cases, in which individuals moving out of long-stay mental illness hospitals had encountered problems, as evidence of poor community-care practice.

A minority of family members opposed resettlement completely, and had formed protest groups which sought to maintain hospital-based care. However, none of those whose relatives had already been resettled expressed anxiety about the risks associated with the new environment. Those next of kin who had been visited by members of staff from the community home before their relative moved there were, also, generally less anxious than those who had not. Direct or indirect experience of the new environment appeared to rapidly assuage family carer apprehension. Relatives may have been reassured by the rapid erosion of risk-taking in the new community homes which was discussed above.

## Discussion

Few of the service-users participating in the present study will ever be able to fully understand the issues involved in risk management. Decisions affecting their health and safety will always be made by others. However, people who have severe and profound learning difficulties are capable, to varying degrees, of learning how to manage some hazardous situations successfully. For example, many residents excluded from hospital kitchens could, with support, learn how to negotiate this dangerous environment safely. Some risks must be accepted if residents' quality of life is to improve in the new community setting.

Formal carers need to find an appropriate balance between risk-taking and danger avoidance. Staff are, inevitably, influenced by factors other than the needs of individual service-users. They have to manage groups of residents, and must seek to protect their own professional status by avoiding disasters for which they would be held accountable. There is a risk that any adverse events which do occur will be subject to media amplification and overreaction, leading to the reinstitution of the hospital environment in a community setting.

Alternatively, as suggested in Chapter 15, with respect to services for the elderly, care systems for vulnerable people may respond to the dilemma of autonomy promotion versus hazard avoidance by oscillating between the two over the longer term. A trend towards prioritising safety may be eventually corrected, perhaps in response to outside criticism, because life for residents has become too stultifying. When disasters occur, they are then blamed on the risk-accepting line, and the regime becomes more restrictive.

Closely regulated systems may be criticised for failing to promote as normal a life as possible for residents of institutions, while more risk-tolerant systems can be accused of recklessness if accidents occur.

Service-user risk-taking ability is, at present, assessed informally in the community. Safety rules commonly evolve in response to specific incidents, as in the examples, discussed above, of the gateway to the outside world and kitchen access. This reactive approach to accidents needs to be replaced with proactive planning based on detailed knowledge of individuals. It should be possible to predict how much autonomy each resident can be given in different zones of everyday living, and to plan accordingly. The establishment of formal risk-assessment procedures in community settings would help carers to design systematic risk-management programmes which balance costs and benefits, and do not depend on responses to the vagaries of chance. Documented risk assessment would also protect professional carers from litigation by enabling them to demonstrate that they had employed reasonable care in taking risks. Professionals who feel confident that they have only accepted appropriate risks, in line with organisational policies, may not need to adopt protective strategies which will defeat the purpose of the community-care reforms, and provoke an eventual counterreaction.

MERTHYR TYDFIL COLLEGE
LIBRARY

# 11 Risk management for people with dementia

Charlotte L. Clarke and Bob Heyman

| |
|---|
| Introduction |
| Risk knowledge and risk-reasoning |
| The process of interfacing |
| Discussion |

## Introduction

Mrs G cares for her mother, Mrs S, who has had dementia for many years, and now depends totally on her daughter for her care. They live happily together, but are faced with the same problem each morning: how to get downstairs. For Mrs G, sleeping upstairs is an important aspect of her mother's life. For their district nurse, the journey downstairs entails avoidable danger to staff, Mrs G and Mrs S. The professional response is to require Mrs S to sleep downstairs. Mrs G, however, does not lack ingenuity. Each morning she helps Mrs S downstairs herself, having first opened the front door so that she can call on a passer-by for help if she gets stuck on the way down.

The district nurse judges that both Mrs G and Mrs S risk injuring themselves on their perilous daily journey, and is concerned about her own professional accountability in the event of an accident. Mrs G considers this risk worth taking, as its acceptance enables her mother to sleep upstairs, an important anchor in normality. But she feels that health and social services have been unhelpful and unwilling to respond to her wishes.

Ms Y's father is determined to wander from their house at any time of the day or night, and to approach strangers. She is faced with two choices: either to sedate her father with medication, or to allow him to wander despite the risk of physical harm from traffic, and of him being reported to the police for accosting people. She chose the latter option to preserve his right to self-determination. As in the case of Mrs G, a risk-management strategy which might be dismissed, at first glance, as rash, makes sense when put in the context of attempts to preserve life quality, and to lead as normal a life as possible, in the face of serious health problems.

This chapter compares the risk perspectives of family and professional carers, drawing on relevant risk theories, and on theory developed during a study which explored caregiving for people with dementia (Clarke, 1995b). The two examples just outlined derived from this study. Data was collected in three phases. In Phase 1, 14 family carers of people with dementia completed diaries and semi-structured interviews (Clarke and Watson, 1991). In Phase 2, questionnaire data was collected from a multidisciplinary sample of 60 professional carers (Clarke *et al.*, 1993). In Phase 3, case studies of an additional nine families were undertaken. family carers kept a diary, and were interviewed, as were all 25 of their professional carers, including staff from health, social and voluntary care organisations.

Analysis of the research data led to the development of a theory of normalisation. This theory proposes that family carers work to give meaning to their caregiving relationship by defining and redefining that which is perceived to be normal in their own lives, that of the person with dementia, and in their relationship. Three processes are identified: normalising, in which family carers employ the strategies of pacing, confiding and rationalising in attempting to preserve a self-defined 'normality'; interfacing, in which family carers negotiate the involvement of professional carers; and interacting, in which family carers work with professionals in order to support their normalising strategies.

Professional predictions about health, ill-health and the effects of health-care interventions depend on beliefs about established evidence (Sackett and Haynes, 1995). However, those who base their advice on this evidence often fail to acknowledge the complexity of its relationship with social environments, discounting the cultural and political dimension of risk knowledge (Douglas, 1994). The research discussed in this chapter sought to articulate non-professional evidence in a context, that of families caring for people with dementia, in which they draw on rich individual and culturally specific knowledge.

The Alzheimer's Disease Society (1993) has estimated that around 650 000 people in Britain have dementia. Much is known about the pathophysiology of dementia, but the experiences of individuals who have the disorder, and the social and psychological factors which affect them, are less well understood (Kitwood and Bredin, 1992).

The knowledge base of family carers has remained largely unarticulated in the face of the dominant, medically driven, approach to dementia care. Professional and family carers utilise quite different sources of knowledge, however. Whereas professionals draw on research evidence, and on generalised beliefs derived from their training, socialisation and clinical experience, family carers have detailed experience of the person with dementia as an individual, and of their particular circumstances. Professionals are primarily concerned with pathology, and its prognosis; family carers with the wider social meaning of disease. Family carers, therefore, need to negotiate professional involvement so that it fits with their own concerns. This 'interfacing' process with respect to risk management is the main focus of the rest of the chapter.

## Risk knowledge and risk-reasoning

Dementia care, by either family- or professional carers, is guided by the identification, assessment and management of need. Where care involves risk concerns, decisions about the likelihood of possible future events must utilise a stock of knowledge which is founded on past events and assumptively extrapolated into the future. Family and professional carers, however, have very different histories, and so draw on different knowledge bases. A schema which elaborates these differences is presented in Table 11.1.

The polarity between family and professional perspectives suggested in Table 11.1 has been overstated for presentational purposes. Both parties share a common culture. Family carers will have been exposed to the culture of health-care through the mass media, and previous interactions with the health-care system. Most professionals will have encountered ill-health personally, for example through involvement with the problems of other family members. Given the prevalence of dementia, professionals and their families are, like everybody else, personally at risk of being affected by the disorder in the future. A considerable crossover between family carer and professional perspectives can, therefore, be identified.

### FAMILY CARER RISK PERSPECTIVES

The family carer of a person with dementia can access knowledge about that person's particular situation and individual character which is largely denied to professional carers. Mrs G, for example, felt that professional carers would not be able to care for her mother in the way that she could, because of her personal knowledge of her mother's needs.

> One day I'll say I'm not giving her this [food] because of this, I'll give her the other. You feed her according to how her bowels are, etc. (Mrs G, caring for her mother, interview)

In order to protect this individual knowledge base, and to find the evidence to support it, family carers seek out exceptions to the professionally defined, pathological, view of dementia. They do not necessarily deny the inevitabil-

**Table 11.1**   A comparison of family and professional carers' risk knowledge

| Family carer perspectives | Professional carer perspectives |
| --- | --- |
| Specific knowledge of person | General knowledge of disorder |
| Knowledge of individual need | Knowledge of aggregate need |
| Seek to normalise situation | Seek to pathologise situation |
| Seek to disconfirm expected trajectory of decline | Seek to confirm expected trajectory of decline |
| Personal/political knowledge claims | Evidence based knowledge claims |
| Values/meaning discourse | Facts discourse |

ity of deterioration, but use any signs of intact personhood in their relative as evidence that they are still the human being known in the past. For example, Mrs G cited her mother's response to the presence of her great-grandchildren, and her alertness to protect their safety, as an indication that she retained her previous character.

> You see there must be something there, because, when the babies come in, she'll [mother] do 'ah ah ah'. Now, on a Sunday, when they're in the highchairs and one of them stands up, there'll be 'aaah', and you look and one of them's standing up. (Mrs G, caring for her mother, interview)

Another family carer normalised deterioration as part of a natural ageing process.

> I just accepted it [confusion]. I thought it's just a piece of getting older. (Mrs U, caring for her husband, interview)

Management of the trajectory of decline by family carers can also be seen in the control family carers maintain over information, which they selectively acknowledge and dismiss according to its congruence with the trajectory of normalisation.

> All the time, along the line, we kept saying, we tried to tell [family carer] the next possible step, and what we could do about that. And he kept saying, 'I don't want to know.' So we said, 'Well, fair enough, but just we'll tell you about it anyway.' (Community psychiatric nurse, interview)

In terms of the framework presented in Chapter 2, the above family carer resisted getting on to a risk escalator. Going up the escalator would bring more intensive support designed to reduce risk to both carer and the person with dementia, but at the price of increased dependency and disruption of the current state of self-defined normality.

Ironically, however, family carers would sometimes embrace a pathological framework in order to normalise the relationship with the person with dementia.

> If he says horrible things to me I get really upset ... I've got to take into consideration that he doesn't know what he's saying, but it still hurts when he says nasty things to me. (Mrs D, caring for her husband, interview)

In this example, the family carer used her husband's pathology to explain away his personal attacks on her. Distinguishing between the person and the illness provided family carers with one means of actively maintaining sight of the person despite their illness. They, thus, used the dementia label strategically in order to protect a close relationship.

As well as 'hearing' information provided by professionals selectively, family carers released information to them in ways which supported their own approaches to normalisation. As also found by Keady and Nolan (1994), family carers 'covered' for the person with dementia in the period before the official diagnosis. One family carer withheld information about the severity of her husband's illness for several years in case he was 'taken away' from her into permanent residential care.

*Nobody can take him from us, I was frightened of that.* (Mrs P, caring for her husband, interview)

Whether or not there was a real risk of professionals institutionalising this woman's husband against her will, her fear meant that professionals who depended on her for information did not find out promptly about the severity of his condition. Fear that a loved one could be 'taken away' has historical roots. Older people would be used to a pre-community care society which institutionalised its members much more readily. A similar point is made in Chapter 10 about the attitude of older parents to the institutionalisation of people with severe learning difficulties.

family carer perceptions of institutionalisation were affected by their exposure to the mass media (Gabe, 1995). The following quotation shows how family carers could acquire a generalised, highly negative, picture of institutional care, as an adversity to be avoided at all costs, for the sake of their relative.

*I know the hospitals can't do any other, but when you see them on TV, I mean I've only seen them on the news or in plays, but from what I can gather, to me, they're all sitting there like zombies waiting to die. They just give them tablets to sedate them, as obviously there's not enough staff to look after them.* (Mrs G, caring for her mother, interview)

At times, risk-reasoning may lie outside mainstream, science-based modes of analysis altogether, and be based on notions of fatalism, divine justice and punishment (Gellner, 1992).

*I keep thinking to myself, when I see couples out and about together, and you're stuck in the house all the time, 'Where have I gone wrong?' It is hard sometimes.* (Mrs D, caring for her husband, interview)

## PROFESSIONAL CARER RISK PERSPECTIVES

Professional carers drew on a system of beliefs about the 'normal' pathology of dementia. This knowledge base provides information about the average expected future of persons with the disease, not the fate of individuals, and about biomedical disability rather than social functioning. It generates an unremittingly gloomy view of the 'natural' course of the disease, and about the current inability of medicine to modify the inevitable downward trajectory. Clashes of perspective between professional and family carers could arise when professionals, uncritically, tried to force family carers to accept management strategies which focused on aggregate pathology rather than on individual social functioning.

*There was one doctor from the surgery, a woman doctor who said, 'You want to have him put away.' You know, when she said that, I didn't like her after that.* (Mrs P, caring for her husband, interview)

family carers have to make value judgements about the relative merits of a range of negative and undesirable options (Wilson, 1989). Even if the consequences of different management strategies for the parties involved could be fully specified, cost-benefit analysis could not generate a single, rationally based, 'best' decision about how to manage the care of someone with dementia because qualitatively different negativities cannot be compared directly (Rescher, 1983, p. 20), as pointed out in Chapter 1. For example, weighing the negative consequences for a person with dementia of being institutionalised against the negative effects on their carer of looking after that person at home requires judgements, implicit or explicit, about the value of these two forms of adversity. Specific advice given by professional carers, for example to institutionalise a close relative with dementia, contained embedded value judgements. Such advice could threaten family carers intensely, as in the last example, because the professionals' implicit values were legitimated by their claim to expertise.

However, professionals also came to know people with dementia more or less well individually, depending on their role and their personal relationships with particular families.

> *Listening? Well, how else are you going to learn about that person?* (Domiciliary care worker, interview)

Hence, professional carers, potentially, could draw on two sources of knowledge: one 'scientific' and general, the other personal and individual. Professional carers actively sought to learn about the person with dementia as an individual.

> *If you know someone well, and know them like your own mother or father, then I think you have a better understanding of that person as a person, which is different with someone you don't really know.* (Staff nurse, interview)

## The process of interfacing

Grinyer (1995, p. 31) argues that policy-makers tend to see risk in *'a one-dimensional context, rather than being part of a multidimensional, complex and socially embedded process'*. Although science offers certain forms of 'fact', for example about average disease trajectories, family carers' risk knowledge is underpinned by their own personal and political values. Since family carers understood that professionals did not necessarily share their values, they managed their relationships with the latter through processes of interfacing (Clarke, 1995b).

In normalising a continued relationship with their relative, family carers deconstruct the pathology both of the person with dementia and of their relationship together, and may reject the dominant professional trajectory of inevitable decline (Gubrium, 1987; Clarke, 1995b). From this position, family carers may adopt a utilitarian approach to their relationships with health professionals, pragmatically balancing the costs and benefits of engagement with systems whose underlying values they do not necessarily share. Becker and Nachtigall (1992, p. 469) have highlighted the perils of entangling with a system which approaches chronic ill-health problems biomedically.

> *For those who turn to the health-care system for a condition that has been redefined as a disease yet fail to meet medical criteria for successful cure or management, the consequences of medicalisation may be severe.*

The course of negotiations between family- and professional carers will depend on the degree of congruence between the professional carer's plan of care and the wishes of family members. Unless needs, for example for greater social contact, are identified, they cannot be entered into the cost-benefit calculation.

## MEETING NEEDS

When considering possible service interventions, family carers appraised their own needs, those of the person with dementia, and the availability of services. For example, the family carer quoted below rejected respite care for her father because she felt it would not meet her needs at that time, a concern also identified by Smith, Cantley and Ritman (1983).

> Everybody said after my Mum died, 'Well why not have a break, have a week or something.' But, I really feel that that, to me, would probably do more harm than good. (Ms Y, caring for her father, interview)

family carers, and people with dementia, often had clear ideas about what assistance they required, but found the services available too inflexible to meet their needs.

> What I wanted a home help for was just to chat to her, and they wouldn't do it. They would only provide a home help to do housework which she wouldn't stand for. (Mr 0, caring for his mother, interview)

family carers often refused a service intervention, if it would have resulted in the replacement of an activity which was important to the family carer, or which reinforced the family carer's sense of continuing with normal activities.

> I don't bother with the home help. If I didn't have any work to do, I'd go crackers. (Mrs D, caring for her husband, interview)

Even when care was wanted, it was not always available. Service-providers themselves recognised that they had to spread their resources thinly, and so could not respond fully to the wishes of individual carers.

> You can't always give them what they want, because they may well want five days' care, and you can't do that. (Enrolled nurse, psychiatric day centre, interview)

In the next example, the social worker appears to have attempted to break up the family carer's time frame in order to encourage him to continue in this role.

> [A few years ago] I had said I would like her in permanent care and the social worker had preyed on me, the better side of my nature if you like, and said, 'Oh, we'll put you on a decent package. Could you not try to cope with her for a few months at home?' (Mr O, caring for his mother, interview)

## FAMILY CARER PERCEPTIONS OF PROFESSIONAL CARER INTERVENTIONS

family carers considered professional carer interventions in relation to the needs of the person with dementia. However, professionals often felt that service-users had unrealistic expectations about services, or were unclear about their aims. Thorne and Robinson (1988) have suggested that the professional/user relationship has its own typical dynamic, with naïve trust gradually replaced by disenchantment and eventual guarded alliance.

> *People assume you can move mountains for them but you can't.* (Community care manager, interview)

family carers developed metaperspectives about professional interventions, varying in the extent to which they believed they had control over the actions of statutory and voluntary service-providers. As in most health-care relationships (Brooking, 1989), family carers were inclined to be diffident. For example, they frequently used a mediator before approaching medical staff if they felt unsure of their position.

> *I think in a lot of cases they tend to use us as an intermediary between them and the GP. They like to bounce a lot of things off us which they would feel embarrassed about calling the GP about.* (District nurse G, interview)

Making decisions about accepting support from voluntary or statutory services poses many dilemmas for family carers. They may, at some point, have to decide between continuing to attempt to normalise their relative's situation and accepting a trajectory of decline. For example, a son and his wife had the following dialogue about the possibility of his mother going into permanent residential accommodation.

> MRS Z: *I mean, you've really kept her until the last, sort of thing. I mean ... if we weren't moving, she'd still be with us maybe.*
> MR Z: *Sometimes I think it would be better if she just died. I know it's not a nice thing to say that.*
> MRS Z: *But I think it's, it must be awful, to think she's your mother.* (Mr and Mrs Z, caring for his mother, interview)

## BENEFITS OF PROFESSIONAL CARER INTERVENTION

Family carers valued services which supported their normalisation strategies. Clarke (1995b) identified three types of strategy. Pacing enabled family carers to limit their physical and emotional exposure to the person with dementia. Confiding allowed them to 'off-load' feelings about caregiving without necessarily expecting tangible help or advice. Rationalising involved family carers in cognitively managing their relationship with the person with dementia through a process of selectively seeking and acknowledging information, and selectively attributing this information to either the individual or the illness.

Benefits were also obtained if the professional carer provided instrumental care, meeting the functional needs of the person with dementia. However, as pointed out above, family carers' attitudes towards offers of tangible services have to be understood in the context of their normalising strategies. Similarly family carers negotiated their contact with other family members, for example, rejecting offers of physical help while accepting opportunities to confide in other family members.

## Supporting normalising strategies

Professional carers had a potential contribution to make to each of the three normalising strategies. Physical pacing sometimes required professional carer support. It gave family carers some space in which to maintain their own self-identities.

> *Only when I go out on a Saturday do I get a break from him. The carers' support woman [who sits with person with dementia], they've got a rota once a fortnight. If it wasn't for that, I wouldn't get out at all.* (Mrs D, caring for her husband, interview)

Professional carer interventions also supported the normalising strategies of confiding and, to a lesser extent, rationalising. At times, professionals sought to gently push the family carer into discussing the personal impact of what was happening. In this way a mutual understanding of need and therefore risk knowledge could be sought.

> *I had a feeling he was trying to talk to me about sex and love. And I said to him, 'How do you feel about warmth with [wife], how do the two of you get on?' because she was so restless and agitated you know. 'How do you cope with, you know, if you're sitting of a night time, [wife's] sitting beside you.' And his eyes filled straight away. 'Well, I can't even hold her hand now, she just won't let us.'* (Community psychiatric nurse, interview)

## Instrumental intervention

family carers saw an instrumental intervention as beneficial if it fulfilled a need which they, themselves, had identified, and if the intervention supported their normalisation strategy. In the following example, the son's sense that his mother was still a person with rights was protected by the human quality of the paid carer's interventions.

> *The home help came this morning, she is a wonderful, helpful, and caring person who I rely on to do things for my mother that I obviously couldn't do, such as changing her underwear, etc. A girl comes every Friday to give my mother a bath who is also very nice and caring.* (Mr K, caring for his mother, diary)

## COSTS OF PROFESSIONAL CARER INTERVENTION

The main potential costs of involvement with professionals for family carers and people with dementia arose from threats which it could pose to their normalising strategies, particularly where the professional approach to care focused on the person with dementia's trajectory of decline. The three principal areas of risk were that the person with dementia might be pathologised and devalued; that interactions between the family carer and the person with dementia might become restricted; and that conflicts of interest between the family carer and the person with dementia might be opened up.

### Devaluing the person with dementia

Acceptance of any professional carer intervention entailed the implicit or explicit admission that there was 'something wrong' with the person with dementia, and could increase the interpersonal distance between the 'normal' family carer and the 'not quite normal' person with dementia. family carers stepped on to this potentially dangerous ground cautiously, testing the impact of professional interventions by monitoring the response of the person with dementia. If this response was positive, the service on offer could be accepted in relative safety.

> He went to the Alzheimer's group today, he seems to enjoy this day out. (Mrs U, caring for her husband, diary)

However, family carers were likely to reject a service if the person with dementia received it negatively. The person with dementia, thus, played an active role in this part of the process of interfacing, and, ultimately, normalisation.

> He was only there [residential home] three days, but when he came back he hated the place and wouldn't go back. (Mrs D, caring for her husband, interview)

## Restricting personal care

The use of services such as daycentres and respite care had the effect of taking people with dementia out of their customary environment for segments of time. This removal could disrupt the pattern of family life, and the maintenance of wider relationships, and so threaten family carers' efforts to emphasise the person rather than the illness.

> He went [to daycentre] last Friday. So that's three days they're going to let him in, which I feel terrible about, because you see I take him out on a Friday to meet some of his friends. But, maybe, in the summer, I'll let him go two days, and I'll take him down the coast. (Mrs N, caring for her husband, interview)

family carers also worried that the person with dementia might not be cared for as well as they would have been at home, that their individual preferences might not be respected, and that their dignity might not be protected by others. They feared that professional carers, who did not know their relative personally, would treat them as just somebody with dementia. Other studies (Bowers, 1987; Pratt, Schmall and Wright, 1987) have also found evidence of family carers' wish to protect the character of a vulnerable family member. family carers know the person with dementia as an individual, but may fear that professionals will see them as no more than a member of an aggregated category. An important part of personhood for relatives is a shared history, which the person with dementia may have forgotten in whole or in part, and which professionals cannot readily access or value.

## Conflicting needs

It was pointed out, in Chapter 1, that, since events generate potentially infinite consequences, cost-benefit analysis involving risk requires a prior selection of which consequences to include in the calculation. Dementia affects both the person with dementia and members of their family. Management strategies which minimise risk for the person with dementia may increase the risk for the family carer, or vice versa.

*He's [person with dementia] managed by keeping him flat [with medication] if he's vio-lent. If that's the way she [wife] can manage him, then that's OK.* (Enrolled nurse, interview, day unit)

Separating the needs of the family carer and their dependant, and minimising the meaning of their relationship, undermines family-normalising strategies. However, in many situations, family carers rationalised this potential conflict into a redefined normality by working out a compromise between their own needs and the rights of the person with dementia. This process of rationalising service intervention could be done in two ways. First, family carers could emphasise the person with dementia's enjoyment of participation in activities organised by service-providers, as in the case of Mr U's involvement with an Alzheimer's group, discussed above. Second, family carers could justify falling back on services by depersonalising their relative to some extent, on the grounds of their mental state. However, in so doing, they accepted the trajectory of unmodifiable decline. The following quotation closes off the risk that placing the person with dementia in residential care could, recursively, lead to further deterioration.

*I don't think she'll really know where she is [in residential home].* (Mr Z, caring for his mother, interview)

## Discussion

### SYNTHESISING RISK KNOWLEDGE

At first sight, the study of dementia looks like unpromising territory for risk analysis, since the disease carries a trajectory of inevitable, irreversible decline, rather than of conditional probability. Dementia is, medically, an adversity which has already happened. Its trajectory can be contrasted sharply with those for conditions such as diabetes (Chapter 8): a disease which has relatively mild consequences in its early stages, but which puts patients at heightened risk of avoidable medical complications, and so requires arduous preventive endeavour.

However, dementia looks quite different from the viewpoint of family carers, for whom the person with dementia counts as a major figure in their own personal biographies. family carers attempt to normalise their relationship with the person with dementia as much as possible, focusing on functioning rather than disability, on individual personhood rather than pathology. Professionals may inadvertently threaten the normalising process simply by offering services, or by emphasising the physical and psychological risks faced by family carers, and so implicitly writing-off the humanity of the person with dementia. Because events have potentially infinite consequences, selective attention to risk factors cannot be avoided. If professional carers, sometimes blinded by an overmedicalised training, only see the person with dementia as a source of risk to family carers, they will fail to consider the risks their professional response to the condition creates for family carers.

The multiple consequences of any event or action often provide mixed blessings. As a result, minimising one risk frequently exacerbates another (Firth, 1991). Diagnosis of dementia can allow access to professional support, but can also medicalise the person with dementia, and pathologise family relationships (Clarke and Keady, 1996), placing clients on an upward escalator of care and societal reaction (see Chapter 2). Such dilemmas are inherent in most forms of health-risk management, for instance with respect to the iatrogenic effects of child-protection orders (Chapter 16) or labelling an individual as having a learning difficulty (Chapter 9).

Bradbury (1989) argues that science-based approaches to risk presume the superiority of expert over lay knowledge. Professionals who uncritically take for granted their epistemological superiority may seek to educate family carers, through a one-way communication process, about the risks they face, and to promote compliance with their advice. However, the effective management of health problems requires mutual client and professional understanding of each other's risk knowledge. Otherwise, professionals will not value family carers' knowledge, and family carers will dismiss professionals' advice as inappropriate.

Because they approach risk from different perspectives, each party can have difficulty understanding the other's perspective. Synthesis of their risk-reasoning, a prerequisite for mutually acceptable collaboration, depends on a shared understanding of difference, but also requires partnership and willingness to accommodate. How can professional carers work with individuals to manage future risks when their knowledge is inductively derived from the average behaviour of aggregated groups? Similarly, how can family carers predict the likelihood of future events when their knowledge is based on the past and present behaviour of one particular individual whose biography has been fractured?

Misunderstandings and tensions between families and professionals arise not so much from absolute differences in the interpretation of 'evidence', or from value conflicts, but from limits in the forms of knowledge on which the actions of each are grounded. There are inherent difficulties in moving between the specific and the aggregate. Professional carers' risk judgements are based, primarily, on extrapolation from past frequencies, and depend on the assumption that aggregate rates are a good guide to what happens individually (Gigerenzer, et al., 1990, p. 45). family carers extrapolate the future from past experience of a specific individual. For them, knowledge of other individuals, and of aggregates, provides, at most, a background.

McKee (1991) sees movement between the individual and the aggregate as a defining characteristic of humanistic nursing. However, there are both cultural and organisational barriers to the attainment of such fluency. The requirement, in modern health systems, for professionals to manage large caseloads, frequently en masse, works against making allowances for individuals. Corkish and Heyman, in Chapter 10, discuss a similar problem with respect to care for people with severe and profound learning difficulties, where the lowest common safety denominator, such as locked doors, often rules. Even where resources can be found to personalise care, concern about accountability, and fear of litigation, make it difficult for professionals to tolerate exceptions which involve the acceptance of risk.

## FAMILY CARER RISK MANAGEMENT

family carers often manage the risks which concern them without any professional intervention at all. For example, Mrs G placed a sensor pad under a bedside rug which activated the house-security alarms so that she knew if her mother got out of bed. family carers' personal expertise and commitment was counterbalanced by their lack of medical knowledge. Mrs N fed her husband liver 'to give him blood', because he looked so cold and pale, several months before he was diagnosed as anaemic. She also gave him aspirin because she had read that it could help to prevent further mental confusion. Unfortunately, the anaemia may have been exacerbated by the aspirin, through its irritant effect on the gastric-intestinal system.

Having admitted professionals into their lives, family carers purposefully modify and adapt professional carer interventions, as observed by Hasselkus (1988). Their acceptance of information and advice provided by professionals depends on its congruence with the particular normalising strategies they have adopted. They treat professionals as a resource enabling them to get on with their lives, as Kitson (1987) has also pointed out. They make decisions about any potential professional involvement on the basis of its anticipated costs and benefits. For example, Mr C discontinued the district nursing service because it came too early in the evening. Mr K liked his mother to receive daycare because she enjoyed it, and it enabled him to get out of the house. Mr O refused a home help because he really wanted someone who would just talk to his mother.

This notion of health and social care as a resource, to be drawn on according to the perceived needs of the person with dementia and their family carers, fits with a consumer-orientated philosophy of health care. But it stands in contrast to the idea, commonly expressed in the sociological and professional literature, that professional/client interactions are dominated by professional ideology, at the expense of the patient (Rundle, 1992). The results of the present study, however, suggest that health and social care is often 'let in' to peoples' lives through the interactive process of interfacing, rather than being imposed by professionals on passive recipients.

Professionals often see client non-compliance with their risk-management recommendations as irrational: as rash or overprotective. family carers, such as Mrs G, discussed in the opening example, who insisted that her mother should sleep upstairs despite the risks involved in getting her downstairs, and Mrs Y, who allowed her father to wander rather than have him put on medication, are very much 'risk experts', with their own distinct forms of contextualised risk knowledge and reasoning. They actively manage risks, on the basis of this knowledge, through the process of interfacing.

# Care and protection for older people

## Jan Reed

I should like to acknowledge the work of Dr Valerie Roskell Payton, who worked on the research project and data analysis on which this chapter is based. Responsibility for its contents rests solely with the author.

**BUDGET FOR A BETTER BRITAIN**

> *'Shut old people's homes down,'*
> *A minister declares.*
> *Well, that's a ringing clarion call,*
> *Which shows he really cares.*
> *Zimmer frames in doorways,*
> *Wheelchairs in the street.*
> *It's crowded on the pavement, but*
> *They'll soon learn to compete.*

(From a poem by Simon Rae, published in the *Guardian*, 20 April 1996)

## Introduction

Newspaper stories about an older person whose body has been found in their home days or weeks after their death evoke a range of responses. The story is tragic because it points to a life which was not valued, a person who was not cared for, and a 'system' that has failed. It becomes emblematic of a society which neglects its elders, of a community subject to the jungle law of survival of the fittest. We feel guilty about what our society has become, and about our failure to remedy this state of affairs.

Our feeling of responsibility for events like these, or our sense, at least, that someone else should take responsibility, perhaps indicates something about the way in which we think about the risks faced by older people. It differs from the way in which we appraise risks for other adult age groups.

While we might still find the lonely death of a younger adult shocking, we would generally expect them to take responsibility for themselves. However, our response to risks faced by older people cannot be simply described as parental, and therefore demeaning. Assumptions about the inability of older people to look after themselves, or to make rational decisions, are mixed-up with valid concerns about their welfare.

The cultural context for such concerns is, one of stereotyping and ageism. The latter can be defined as an attitude leading to negative expectations of the category of older people regardless of their individual characteristics. Ageism is communicated, in our culture, through mass-media images of sweet old grannies who fail to understand the modern world, of senile, socially embarrassing, old men, and of cantankerous curmudgeons who disapprove of anything new or different. These stereotypes impinge on other debates about the care and welfare of older people, who are often portrayed as both dependent and incapable of making rational decisions.

A broad historical sweep suggests that our conceptions of older people, and the risks they face, have gone through three main stages, although clearcut distinctions between stages cannot always be drawn, and different approaches may coincide or compete at specific time periods. Nevertheless, certain dominant ideas about older people seem to have roughly succeeded each other in Western cultures.

Older people first began to be defined as a discrete group with special needs at the end of the nineteenth century, in response to economic changes arising from the industrial revolution. Old age came to be seen as a justification for frailty, meriting a benevolent response. The second stage involved paternalistic protection, and was fuelled by the rise of geriatrics as a medical speciality, and by the agendas of the health and social care professions. This stage is linked to the growth of the welfare state in the post-war period. Most recently, the paternalistic approach has been challenged by those who argue that protective policies infringe the personal rights of older people. This challenge has been paralleled in other areas, for example with respect to services for people with disabilities, as ideas of normalisation and client rights have become central to debates about care for potentially vulnerable categories of people. However, an approach which insists on treating older people as no different to others runs the risk of discounting the problems experienced by those who are frail, or who have difficulty in carrying out their daily activities.

Given the inherent tension, at the extreme, between protective, custodial strategies which deny older people autonomy, and normalising strategies which ignore real problems, research which elucidates the views of older people themselves about risks seems essential.

## The 'problem' of older people

Fuller and Meyers (1941, p. 321) have argued that 'social problems' are:

> *what people think they are, and if conditions are not defined as social problems by the people involved in them, they are not problems to those people although they may be problems to outsiders or to scientists.*

Older people have not been seen as a 'social problem' demanding a collective solution until quite recently. The main concern in Ancient Greece was the tendency of older men to keep control of family finances, and therefore of their children (Minois, 1987). In this case, young people were deemed to be at risk from their elders, and suggested solutions were directed to helping them by reducing the power of the old. In Britain, the first mention of older people as a group at risk came at the end of the nineteenth century (Macintyre, 1977). Before this time, the Elizabethan poor laws had not distinguished between paupers on the basis of age. Although the needy included large numbers of older people, they were not differentiated from other groups in terms of the support provided for them or the criteria for relief.

This situation changed as policy-makers began to realise that the system of Poor Law relief, centred around incarceration in bleak workhouses, and meagre in the extreme so as to encourage people to find work, was inappropriate for older people, who were unlikely to ever return to employment. Their destitution did not result from 'fecklessness', but from ill-health, and from the increasing reluctance of an industrial society to employ older people rather than their younger, stronger colleagues (Victor, 1994). As the Majority Report of the Royal Commission on the Poor Law, published in 1909, noted, 'the practice of considering the AGED as a class by themselves for the purposes of poor relief is one of modern growth', (Part 4, paragraph 304, cited in Gray, 1979).

At one level, this development benefited older people, because it legitimated a benevolent approach to welfare, on the grounds that they could not be reasonably expected to protect themselves from poverty and hunger. Such protection could only be afforded through continuing employment, no longer available to older people (Quadrango, 1982). As society became more industrialised, employers looked for fit, younger workers. In an agricultural society, older people could perform useful tasks, but the use of industrial machinery made agility and physical fitness more necessary. At the same time, no system of pensions was universally available, and older people who could not work were left destitute unless their families could support them. As families were fragmented by moves to industrial centres, this option became less available.

Differentiation of the destitute elderly as 'deserving' poor did have negative consequences for them, however. Identifying older people as a specific group who need particular support made it easier to think of them as a class of people who face the same risks, and who cannot deal with life unaided. Older people were provided with assistance which, while ostensibly more humanitarian than other poor law relief, differed little in practice. The workhouse, with its minimum levels of comfort and dehumanising routines, was 'a legacy that was not abandoned' (Townsend, 1962, p. 32). Townsend's portrayal of life in residential homes for the elderly suggests that the identification of older people as a special group often led to their confinement in appalling institutions, supposedly 'for their own good'.

## PROTECTING OLDER PEOPLE FROM RISK

The identification of older people as a discrete group meriting particular kinds of support marked them as a social problem. Macintyre (1977) identifies two types of response to this 'problem'. The first, which she calls the *'humanitarian formulation'*, centres on concerns about the best way to protect vulnerable people who deserve help. The second, organisational, formulation focuses on finding ways to ameliorate the 'problem' in ways which causes as little administrative inconvenience and expense as possible. In response to massive projected rises in the number of surviving elderly people, the debate has become more concerned with costs than with the quality of provision.

Both approaches to the 'problem' of older people affected service provision in a context of developments in geriatric medicine and the increasing professionalisation of care. These service-driven changes had a part to play in a transition from the simple recognition of older people as a category to a concern with protecting them against risks 'for their own good'.

## THE RISE OF GERIATRIC MEDICINE

Textbooks of geriatric medicine which provide an historical introduction usually tell the story of the rise of this discipline as a humanitarian triumph of science over stereotypes. Most attribute the birth of modern geriatric medicine to Marjorie Warren, who was appointed to the West Middlesex Hospital in 1935. The conditions that she found there resembled those in the workhouse. Death and decline were accepted as inevitable, and programmes for rehabilitation or recovery had not been established. Patients developed complications as a result of being left in bed. The overall approach to care lacked therapeutic optimism. Warren instituted programmes of rehabilitation which succeeded in enabling a proportion of patients to leave hospital. Geriatric medicine became a recognised medical speciality, although one which has remained lower in status than many others.

The medicalisation of old age was fuelled by research programmes which investigated the incidence of health problems in later life, and evaluated treatments. The process of 'normal' ageing has been examined, theories about underlying mechanisms formulated, and debates conducted about how to prevent or delay these processes. Many writers have discussed the medicalisation of life, notably Szasz (1961) in relation to mental illness and Foucault (1973) more generally. Medicalisation involves the pathologising of 'normal' aspects of life which become part of the territory of the medical profession. As their terrain expands, doctors become experts to whom society looks for definitions and solutions of new 'problems'. Critics of medicalisation argue that power invested in the medical profession engenders passivity and powerlessness in the objects of their scrutiny: namely, patients. Medicalisation turns patients into non-experts who cannot be expected to know their own best interests.

The medical literature emphasises the pathology of ageing. For example, a 'useful' *aide mémoire* for practitioners presented by Bennet and Ebrahim

(1995, p. 72) describes the 'I's of old age, Immobility, Incontinence, Instability, Inability, Insanity and Iatrogenesis'. Such images of old age have a long history. Shakespeare, in *As You Like It* (Act II, Scene vii), claimed that old age:

> Is second childishness and mere oblivion
> Sans teeth, sans eyes, sans taste, sans everything.

However, we now have a medical specialism built around this view.

Although overpreoccupation with the pathology of old age can be satirised, it must be accepted that some old people, at least, have health problems which put them at risk. For example, reductions in visual acuity, hearing and mobility may reduce an older person's ability to manage environmental hazards. While neither inevitable or universal, such disabilities, leading to greater risk, are more likely to be experienced by older people. Bennet and Ebrahim (1995), for example, state that, among older people who are asked, 30 per cent report having had serious falls in the last year.

Increases in morbidity can be seen as an inevitable concomitant of survival. The longer a person lives, the more they will be exposed to environmental stressors and disease processes. Medical textbooks tend to assume that older people will suffer more illnesses, and multiple health problems (Bennet and Ebrahim, 1995). This logic can be questioned, however, given that many other factors are involved in morbidity, such as diet and lifestyle, but the image of the increasingly battered, ageing body retains its power in a youth-oriented culture.

Health-care workers, whose experience of healthy older people is often limited, learn to expect that older people will have multiple problems. This message is reiterated in geriatric medicine textbooks. Bennet and Ebrahim (1995, p. 87), for example, caution the practitioner assessing mobility problems in older people to *'make sure the patient can see. Blind people do not always tell the doctor!'* The concept of risk is employed very broadly in some medical writing. Iliffe *et al.* (1992) title their paper in the *British Medical Journal 'Are elderly people living alone an at-risk group?'* and use the notion of 'at risk' to refer to any evidence of morbidity or use of services. The term 'at risk' seems to have become a professional shorthand for 'likely to be ill and need care'.

The rise of medical interest in older people, then, has bestowed a mixed blessing on its intended beneficiaries. It has enhanced the treatment of a number of health-care problems, but can foster negative stereotypes which fail to acknowledge that many older people can manage well without professional interference. For example, Arber and Evandrou (1993) concluded, on the basis of secondary analysis of the 1980 General Household Survey, that the majority of older people enjoyed unlimited personal mobility, and could easily cope with household tasks. As argued in Chapter 2, risk analysis entails the attribution of aggregate properties of an observer-defined category to the individuals within that category, and so engenders stereotyping.

Medicalised professional perspectives legitimate paternalistic approaches to care. A striking example, discussed by Norman (1980), is to be found in the Second Reading of Aneurin Bevan's National Assistance Bill, implemented in

1948. This Bill contained a section dealing with the 'compulsory removal' of infirm old men and women into care. Such a course had been recommended by the Webbs in their Minority Report of the Poor Law Commission (Webb and Webb, 1909, p. 352) for older people who refused admission and who *'linger on, alone and uncared for, in the most shocking conditions of filth and insanitation'.*

The section was challenged by Lieutenant-Colonel Elliot on the grounds that it required only one medical certificate to deprive a person of their liberty – but his protests were dismissed, Bevan arguing that when an older person was incapable of looking after himself, *'some authority must be responsible for looking after them and someone must do something about it'.* The Act went through a third reading with only minor amendments, and Elliot's comments were described by one MP as a slur on the medical profession.

The paternalism evident in this example of policy-making was not entirely benevolent. Gray (1979), in her discussion of this episode, argues that although the debate was couched in humanitarian terms, another less publicly expressed imperative was facilitating the slum-clearance programme. By passing the Act, authorities could speed-up this programme by exercising their powers of compulsory removal where older people refused to leave their homes.

Humanitarian and organisational influences on the formulations of old age as a social problem cannot always be separated. For example, the humanitarian concern of social services to offer the most appropriate services is coloured by an awareness that a failure to recognise vulnerability and risk can lead to adverse consequences for both the service and individual professionals. Public outcry about the failure to prevent fatalities and accidents is an ever-present threat, and social services are often criticised for being too cavalier about risk. As Brearley (1979) has argued, in the case of social work, official guidelines about protecting older people are often too vague to be helpful, increasing professional vulnerability to criticism.

The expectation of a multiple, complex pathology sensitises health-care workers to vulnerability in older people. However, risk assessment requires more than the identification of physical problems, but must include consideration of the environment in which the person lives. Medical diagnosis may focus exclusively on pathology, symptomatology and the identification of appropriate medical treatment. When more wide-ranging assessments have to be made, for example to decide whether a person needs to move into a residential home, the interplay between the person, their environment and their social networks becomes critical.

Wynne-Harley (1991, p. 9) concluded that the social workers whom she interviewed had become oversensitive to the risks for older people.

> *With rare exceptions, social workers interviewed expressed concern about potential dangers in the lifestyles of normally active older people living in the community. Few of these could be judged by any reasonable assessment to be at risk. Neither would their actions be considered hazardous in preretirement days.*

Many varied protocols assessing wider risk concerns for older people can be found in the literature. Most seem designed to ensure that risks will not be overlooked or underestimated, and take the practitioner through an exhaustive consideration of potentially problematic areas. Brearley (1982), for example, discusses a vast range of 'hazards', suggesting that they be divided into 'predisposing' and 'situational' types. Even though Brearley does state that care must be taken to assess strengths as well as deficits, the sheer volume of pages on hazards tends to overshadow this message. One of the predisposing hazards that he identifies is age itself, illustrating the way in which characteristics associated probabilistically with a category can become confused with those of individuals within a category, as argued in Chapter 2.

Approaches focusing on functional ability, such as the Clifton Assessment Procedures for the Elderly (CAPE), developed by Pattie and Gilleard (1979), reflect the concerns of formal caregivers and, implicitly, the types of services which happen to be available. As Key (1989, p. 68) has argued, *'Selective assessment is orientated to the interests of the organisation from which the assessment originates.'* Marshall (1990) notes that assessment tools concentrate on impairment rather than potential. This negative bias matches that found in the modern treatment of risk as the probability of adversity (Douglas, 1990). Such tools unconsciously reproduce a medicalised view of health as the absence of disease.

The assessment tools often direct workers to perform their own tests, and to gather corroborative, external evidence in order to avoid relying on the older person's verbal reports, which are deemed less reliable. The implicit assumption that older people are incompetent and untrustworthy is built into these forms of assessment.

As long as news stories continue to highlight culpable neglect, professionals and policy-makers will go to great lengths to appear to be protecting older people. This protection may not effectively address the risks they face. For example, the risk of hypothermia has yet to be met by anything other than meagre heating allowances. As will be shown below, protective strategies may themselves create risks.

## ENCOURAGING RISK-TAKING

The value of protective strategies has been increasingly questioned in recent years. Such strategies, themselves, generate new sets of risks, through processes of reflexive recursion, as discussed in Chapter 2. For example, Poyner and Hughes (1978) found that 35 per cent of a sample of 133 fatal accidents suffered by older people occurred in institutional care, while only 4.8 per cent of the population over 65 lived in such places. Although it can be argued that those in hospital are more vulnerable, these figures do challenge the assumption that institutions provide places of safety.

The risk of other, less dramatic, forms of adversity can also be heightened through the unintended consequences of preventive strategies. Norman (1980) argues that relocation can reduce the confidence, and increase the dependency, of someone who was only just coping with life in a familiar environment. Baker (1976) presents a graphic account of an older woman admitted to hospital from her home where she was living in squalor, only to be seen some weeks later very clean and well-fed, but apathetic and despondent, her independence eroded.

The strategies used to protect older people from risk create new dangers. Their use also raises ethical issues concerning the human rights, liberty and dignity of older people, not just because protection can involve relocation to places in which life becomes routinised and personal freedom constrained, but because the intervention itself can deny an older person's right to autonomy. In cultures in which independence is valued (Victor, 1994), risk-taking becomes an expression of personal freedom. The antithesis to the position of the protection lobby is the argument that older people should be encouraged to take risks, as part of 'normal life'. Discouraging risk-taking, the argument goes, sets older people apart from the rest of adult society, in a similar position to children.

The 'pro-risk' position seems to offer an alternative to a sometimes demeaning, and often ineffective or counterproductive concern with protecting older people from risk. Norman (1980), a chief exponent of this position, has argued that professionals who manage risks on behalf of older people should acknowledge the right of the latter to accept risks. As she points out elsewhere, 'We all take risks every moment of our waking lives, weighing the likely danger of a course of action against the likely gain' (Norman, 1987, p. 16). This emphasis on the normal risk-taking of everyday life echoes the movement towards 'normalisation' in the care of people with learning difficulties and, more generally, the consumerist impetus to shift the balance of power from service-providers to users.

The encouragement of risk-taking can, however, take more extreme forms which, at one level, appear to be empowering but, in other ways, seem dismissive of older people. For example, Clough (1978) has described aggressive rehabilitation programmes for older people, and, in contrast, regimes where staff have decided that butter should be replaced by margarine in meals, because it is better for the health of the older person. This type of involuntary health promotion reduces the autonomy of older people, and discounts their own views.

A similar tendency can be seen in some of the literature on the attitudes of older people towards crime. Their responses to crime can seriously affect the life quality of older people (Cook et al., 1978). Hough and Mayhew (1993), among others, have argued that older people overestimate the threat of violent attack or robbery, since, statistically, they are less likely to experience such crime than younger people. This literature portrays older people as living defensively, and dismisses their fears as irrational. Suggested remedies include, as so often, educating them about 'real' risks, and encouraging them to use security devices. The literature, thus, appears ambivalent as to whether older people's fears are to be changed by education, or reduced through security precautions.

As noted in Chapter 1, a mode of thinking which draws contrasts between professional, expert knowledge of 'real' risks and irrational lay beliefs is commonly found in risk analysis. Such thinking is usually followed by a call for more education of the public. However, this approach discounts knowledge gaps and value judgements in the expert view, and treats the flow of information between professionals and the public as a one-way stream from the former to the latter (Bradbury, 1989).

The assumed irrationality of older people's fear of crime has been challenged on a number of grounds. Although they may enjoy a lower statistical risk of becoming victims of crime, its impact, e.g. the effects of physical violence, is likely to be greater (Mawby, 1988). Maxfield (1987) has linked fear of crime to the generalised powerlessness felt by many older people. Pain (1994) found that the older women in her study reported levels of fear which related closely to their personal experiences of violence and sexual harassment. She suggests that older women's fear of crime, far from being irrational, is based on 'accumulated knowledge'. Decontextualised research, which fails to relate risk beliefs to wider life experiences, would not detect such connections. Jerrome (1992, p. 4) has argued that:

> The methods used to acquire information are such that the subjective experience of ageing is subordinated to the objective accounts provided by youthful researchers. Very little contemporary research addresses the issues of ageing from the elderly person's point of view.

## Listening to older people

Both the 'protection' and the 'pro-risk' approaches to the care of older people are based on *a priori* beliefs. The former assumes that older people become incompetent as a result of the ageing process; the latter that they ought to be treated in the same way as younger people in terms of independence and autonomy. These assumptions are derived from 'objective' reports of morbidity in the first instance, and abstract notions of freedom in the second. The voice of older people themselves is missing from these arguments. Hearing what they have to say about risk may enable a balance between autonomy and safety to be struck which matches their own wishes.

One of the most interesting studies which has examined risk from the older person's perspective (Wynne-Harley, 1991) sought to explore the ways in which they incorporated risks into their daily lives. Interview accounts suggested that they 'trade-off' certain risks. For example, despite the danger, a woman continued to cycle through busy streets, in order to alleviate arthritis, which she saw as a greater threat to her quality of life than the risk of accidents. Trade-offs also occurred in the ways that respondents regulated the minutiae of their lives. Another women used an electric heater in her bathroom, despite the risks of electrocution and falling over the wires, because she was more concerned about the risk of dying of hypothermia if she fell in an unheated bathroom. Some people rejected safety precautions because of their perceived impact on their quality of life. For example, one woman did not want a fire extinguisher in her kitchen because she felt it would worry her, while another stressed her right to live as she wished, without interference from others.

Wynne-Harley's study suggests that older people define personal risks in their own way, and develop management strategies which involve balancing multiple costs and benefits. An older person may accept certain risks in order to avoid being patronised by professionals or younger relatives. The risk-management strategies identified by participants in this study may seem strange to an outsider, and one can imagine the negative response of professionals to some of their practices. However, the trade-offs and strategies identified in the study were adopted in a context of inadequate advice and equipment. For example, the woman who took an electric heater into her bathroom, presumably, had not been given advice or resources which would have enabled her to adopt a safer alternative. Detailed exploration of the ways in which older people define and manage risk can suggest ways in which professionals may intervene without threatening their autonomy or leaving them unprotected.

A recent study in which older people going into nursing and residential homes were interviewed about their reasons for moving (Reed and Payton, 1996) provides a counterbalance to the views of the pro-risk lobby. Professionals generally regard moving into a care home as a 'last resort' for those who cannot live in their own home with available support. The recent community-care reforms (DOH, 1989, 1990) assume that residential care should be avoided as much as possible. However, some of the older people in our study sought residential care because they saw it as a safe haven.

Research participants reported a variety of fears. They commonly worried about crime or attack, and the trigger for fear – for example hearing rowdy teenagers in the street outside, or thinking that someone was trying their door handle, could sometimes be interpreted in different ways. As one participant said:

> I couldn't stay there. One thing was the kids, they used to make such a noise outside, and I worried, you know. I mean I was on my own if anything happened, I couldn't have defended myself.

Such events, although not necessarily posing a direct threat to participants, reminded them of their potential vulnerability. Their feelings of insecurity were reinforced by television or newspaper 'horror stories' which they recounted.

Some participants expressed concern about the unavailability of immediate help in the event of an accident or health crisis. Respondents imagined themselves falling, or becoming ill, and unable to get help, or even 'lying all night on the floor', as one resident said. Those living in isolated houses, or lacking neighbours whom they could contact easily, felt most vulnerable. Participants feared two separate kinds of adversity: first that they might be in pain, but unable to obtain help; and, second, that they might die alone. These concerns were summarised by one participant who said:

> Well, if anything happened through the night, I mean no one would know, I could lie there and no one would know. I don't like to think about it, but you read about it, don't you, people being found days later, dead. That's awful.

Dying alone symbolises the uncaring side of a society in which familial ties and responsibilities have been eroded as a result of social changes.

The risks which concerned respondents involved more than simple practical contingencies. Services available in the study area, such as alarm and emergency help-call systems, could have minimised the risk of not being able to get help when needed. However, the provision of such safety devices would probably not have prevented these participants from feeling uncomfortable about living alone. Their concerns and feelings of insecurity were much more diffuse.

## Discussion

Adequate understanding of older people's feelings about risks does not just require the consideration of specific threats which concern them, but needs to address their more general feelings of loneliness and neglect. Care which simply involves the identification and provision of appropriate services will not meet these wider concerns. Ideally, a reconstruction of society so that it respects and cares for its older members is required. Professionals working in a less than Utopian society must become more critical of attitudes to older people, embedded in service provision, which colour the ways in which they perceive and manage risks. A commitment to listening to older people should be a fundamental component of good practice.

Much of the material concerned with risks for older people is produced by professionals, researchers and policy-makers, and reflects their perspectives. Images of frailty and vulnerability predominate. Responses to these images express either paternalistic concern with protection, or an equally paternalistic promotion of risk-taking. Both positions fail to take into account the ability of older people to make their own decisions. The former overemphasises their vulnerability, while the latter dismisses it. Listening to older people, and finding out how they perceive and respond to risk, seems to offer a way forward. Work of this kind is now beginning to be produced. Listening to older people, however, is not something that we, as a society, have done very much of in the past. Our culturally derived stereotypes of older people as incapable and incompetent provide powerful disincentives to taking their views seriously. Possibly, we might not like what we hear. Providing the support which older people want may seem too onerous or too challenging to professional ideas. Until we do so, however, we will fail to live up to the rhetoric of community care.

# 13 Risk as an integral part of nursing

Jacqui Russell and Ann Smith

| |
| --- |
| Introduction |
| Methodology |
| Data analysis |
| Discussion |

## Introduction

Risk management in health care has traditionally focused on the prevention of unwanted consequences for patients. However, the nature of organisational concern with risk has changed as public attitudes towards health care have become more consumerist, claims for litigation have risen, financial management has been devolved to Trusts, and Crown immunity has been abolished (Healthcare Service Commissioner, 1994; Roy, 1996).

Risk has become an organisational priority, and various management strategies have been developed. Wilson (1995a) describes the main aspects to be considered as the systematic identification and assessment of risks to patients and staff; their reduction through the provision of appropriate, effective and efficient levels of patient care; the prevention of untoward incidents; and comprehensive, accurate communication about, and documentation of, care. Although we agree in principle with this analysis, Wilson seems to assume that risks can be clearly identified, and that risk reduction for staff and patients are necessarily compatible. We question both these assumptions.

Formal risk-management strategies attempt to reduce the likelihood of adverse consequences through the utilisation of 'expert' knowledge, and the promotion of adherence to safety policies, protocols and standards. However, as Grinyer (1995) has argued, policy-makers sometimes see risks as one-dimensional, rather than as part of multidimensional, socially embedded processes. Some less obvious risks may not be recognised, for example emotional risk to nurses from encounters with dying patients, and, therefore, may not be included on the management agenda.

Nurses are faced with a rapidly changing professional scene with respect to professional boundaries, community care, length of hospital stay, technological advances, new forms of drugs and investigative procedures, risks from infection, handling and moving patients, managing violent or confrontational behaviour, informatics and patient rights. The organisational response to such changes has been expressed in a plethora of directives and protocols aimed at reducing problems, complaints and litigation. These developments have had important implications for professional education. Nurses are bound by the UKCC Code of Professional Conduct (1992a, p. 2) to *'acknowledge any limitations in knowledge and competence and decline any duties or responsibilities unless able to perform them in a safe and skilled manner'*. The difficulties involved in upholding this principle in practice should not be underestimated, for example, when nurses are faced with an emergency, or a shortfall in staffing levels. Although officially encouraged, 'whistle blowers' have risked professional isolation and stress (Samuels, 1993).

Their work situation puts nurses at risk of suffering heightened stress levels. The seminal work of Menzies (1970) identified ways in which nurses' use of individual and collective defence mechanisms to reduce the risk of stress resulted in the depersonalisation of patients. Although her psychodynamic framework can be criticised for its lack of recognition of the effect of organisational factors such as interprofessional power structures and norms about 'work' (Chapman, 1983), it has greatly influenced contemporary nursing. The current emphasis on individualised, holistic care within primary nursing may produce an improvement in the quality of care, and in job satisfaction. But, without adequate support, or recognition for factors outside the internalised world of the nurse's psyche, an emphasis on individualised care can lead to feelings of failure and to an increase in *'the emotional labour of nursing'* (Smith, 1992).

Because nurses operate in an uncertain world, their role, inescapably, involves both risk management and risk-taking. They have to make predictions about the likely impact of differing approaches to the implementation and organisation of care, often in circumstances where rapid responses are essential. The research discussed in this chapter focuses on such judgements.

## Methodology

For a number of years we have gathered written records of critical incidents reported by registered nurses and students, in order to explore their perceptions of risk-taking and other aspects of nursing practice. Most of these critical incidents have been written for reflective workshops (Smith and Russell, 1991, 1993). The following strategy has been adopted.

- Participants are asked to write about incidents from clinical experience which have made a particular impression on them, noting the context in which the incident occurred, and what they could remember thinking or feeling at the time.
- The incidents are collected from the students and categorised by the teachers, who look for common themes.
- During the workshops, a process of reflection is stimulated by asking participants to consider the incident both descriptively and analytically.

The data from the workshops has been recorded, transcribed and utilised, together with the reports of the critical incidents, in an ongoing research study. The sample contained a mix of student and qualified nurses and midwives. All participants agreed that their responses could be used for research purposes. This chapter focuses on incidents involving issues of risk.

Reflection itself can involve risk, may challenge deeply held assumptions and values, and can cause problems if not conducted within a supportive environment (Brookfield, 1990). But, used sensitively and carefully, reflection can contribute to a culture of learning which helps individuals to cope with the uncertainties of practice (Schon, 1983, 1987; Kolb, 1984). The critical incidents have provided us with a rich source of material concerning nurses' experiences, views, beliefs, preoccupations and values. Although we have not asked them to focus particularly on risky situations, we have been able to draw on a number of these incidents to illustrate and illuminate some of the key notions associated with risk.

## Data analysis

### RISK AND PERSONAL ACCOUNTABILITY

Their training, vocation and organisational culture can give nurses a heightened sense of personal responsibility for patient outcomes.

> I was working in a clinic and removing sutures from a boy's leg. He was accompanied by his father, who chatted to me and seemed quite relaxed. As I was removing the sutures, talking to the child to put him at ease, I saw the curtains around the cubicle move and heard a loud crash and looked round to see the father lying on the floor, unconscious. The child was very distressed and began to cry. It was found that the father had a fractured skull and had to be admitted. Although the father told me later he had no warning of the faint and so had no chance to tell me, I worried that I should have noticed and done something to prevent the fractured skull. (Qualified nurse)

The nurse's response to this real-life incident illustrates the hindsight effect: a psychological process which has been experimentally demonstrated in a variety of hypothetical situations (see Chapter 5). The effect may be amplified in roles such as nursing which encourage a strong sense of personal responsibility (Grinyer, 1995). Nurses often seem to assume implicitly that risks can always be identified and prevented. As Holden (1990) has argued, professional intolerance of uncertainty itself creates problems.

Some more recent incidents reflect concern about risks arising from the creation of the NHS internal market through the NHS and Community Care Act 1990, for example pressure on staff to increase the rate of patient turnover through hospitals.

> I felt that it was inappropriate for the patient in such an unstable condition to be transferred from ICU when intensive care was required. Would she still be alive now if she had stayed there? (Staff nurse)

## RISK AND PATIENT BEHAVIOUR

While carrying a strong sense of individual responsibility for patient out-comes, nurses have to deal with behaviour which appears irrational, self-destructive or offensively non-compliant, or which does not conform to the traditional medical model.

### Risk and the maintenance of nurse/patient relationships

As pointed out in Chapter 1, an adequate concept of risk needs to be multidi-mensional. McKie *et al.* (1993) argue that emphasis has shifted within health-care systems from 'at risk' groups (those likely to be at risk of particular diseases or complications), to those judged to be engaging in risky behav-iours, such as illicit substance abuse.

Potentially risky behaviours and environmental hazards may be identified from morbidity and mortality data, but a purely epidemiological approach fails to address crucial questions concerning lay beliefs about health. Nurses who have to sustain trusting relationships with patients cannot simply dismiss opinions which may be judged irrational from a purely medical perspective.

> *The nurse tactfully asked N if she was aware of the harmful effects to herself and that her baby would be damaged if she was constantly exposed to passive smoking. N's reply was that 'I don't believe in any of that rubbish about damaging your health. My husband's father smoked all his life and when the doctor told him he had bad circulation in his legs due to his smoking and that he must stop, he did but he still died of gangrene in his legs, nothing to do with smoking. Anyway, I'm not daft, how can smoke you inhale in your lungs affect your legs? It's just another fad it'll blow over.' The nurse tried to explain the connection but N wasn't having any of it so we left. Afterwards, the nurse said 'I didn't push those touchy issues too far this time for fear she won't let me in next time and my relationship is damaged permanently.'* (First-year student nurse, observing commu-nity nurse, quoted in Smith and Russell, 1993, p. 123)

Some adversities can be prevented. The following incident illustrates the way in which a trusting nurse–patient relationship can prevent risk escalation.

> *Sarah was nineteen, unpredictable in mood and behaviour ... One evening the enrolled nurse found her by her bed, emptying the contents of her locker on to the floor. She then picked up some of the heavier objects and threw them at the window. She ignored other patients when they asked her what was wrong. On seeing the enrolled nurse, Sarah became hysterical, screaming at her to get out and continuing to throw things. She would not talk to the enrolled nurse and warned her to 'stay away' or she would 'regret it'. Several windows were cracked or broken at this point. The student saw what was happening and came and fetched me ... I asked the student and the enrolled nurse to qui-etly withdraw and then went to Sarah. I asked her if she would stop throwing things as I was concerned for the safety of other patients. I said that if she did that I could talk to her about what was upsetting her. We then sat on her bed and talked. During the course of our conversation, I noticed that her hand was constantly closed as if gripping some-thing. After much persuasion, she revealed that she was holding 14 temazepam capsules. She said she had been pretending to take these at night and had hidden them one at a time under her tongue. She reluctantly handed them over to me ... At the time of the incident, I had a number of concerns: the safety of Sarah, the safety of the other 32 patients, the safety of staff. What if?? ... I was reassured by the relationship I had worked*

*hard at establishing with Sarah prior to the incident. This enabled me to be honest and direct with her and I was able to predict her response and behaviour.* (Qualified mental health nurse)

## Responding to self-harm

Nurses involved in emotionally stressful situations need to find ways of managing feelings of frustration, anger, sadness and inadequacy when faced with patients who, from a purely medical perspective, seem to put themselves needlessly at risk. Sometimes nurses expressed negative moral judgements about what they saw as weak reasons for drastic actions.

*I felt very angry with this young girl of 16 who took panadols and alcohol because she had had a row with her boyfriend, and she'd only known him a few weeks. How could she put herself so much at risk! She was lucky not to get permanent liver damage.* (Student nurse)

Other accounts of such incidents show how nurses can learn to see acts of self-harm from the patient's viewpoint, rather than purely from a medical perspective.

*I was surprised at the number of people who put their lives at risk by taking overdoses ... Also I thought how pathetic they seemed to begin with until you really got to talk to them and discovered why they had tried to kill themselves. How young they all appeared to be!* (Student nurse)

The following example illustrates the dilemmas which nurses face when they have to balance risk to patients against their own safety.

*While I was on duty, a young girl came in who had been slashing her wrists with a razor blade ... She had come in with police who said they had removed all razor blades. We went into the suture room, everything seemed OK, she was being very co-operative but then all of a sudden she produced a razor blade and threatened to slash her wrists again. At this time apart from feeling really shocked and unprepared I also felt inadequate. I did not know what to do. I didn't attempt to take the razor blade because to be honest I thought I might be hurt in the process. I was asked to get the policeman who was in the corridor but by the time we returned the staff nurse had managed to retrieve the razor blade.* (Student nurse)

Such dilemmas do not have optimal solutions, and require nurses to make rapid life-and-death decisions. Nurses may then reflect lengthily on their actions, and be at emotional risk. Managers and educationalists need to appreciate the importance of developing effective support mechanisms, such as debriefing exercises and clinical supervision (Butterworth and Faugier, 1992; Kohner, 1994).

## Responding to conflict and violence

Nurses also had to deal with potentially dangerous disputes between patients and their relatives. Second-order uncertainty arising from the unpredictability of patient violence appears to have particularly disturbed the student nurse quoted below.

*A young lady was admitted who was having a miscarriage. Her husband accompanied her and they were upset because it was their first baby. The husband seemed to me to be very protective and concerned. During the doctor's examination, the lady's father arrived and asked to see his daughter but her husband made it quite clear that he did not want to see his father-in-law. When the husband saw him talking to the staff nurse in the corridor, he became very angry, swearing at his wife and threatening to do all sorts to the father. He was eventually calmed down by members of staff and left peacefully ... apparently, he had a history of beating his wife. It frightened me because I have never seen someone change so quickly from being caring and gentle to being aggressive and violent.* (Student nurse)

## Responding to rejection of the medical model

Although patient autonomy is widely advocated, tolerance may wear thin when nurses see patients as taking unwarranted risks.

*A 25-year-old woman was admitted following a minor elective surgical procedure. She was divorced and had custody of her two children. Although this type of surgery would not normally result in an admission to the intensive care unit, on this occasion it did, the reason being that the patient was a Jehovah's Witness who was severely anaemic as a consequence of her operation. During her stay, she refused any treatment with blood products, despite her continuing deterioration. Her father maintained a bedside vigilance and was extremely angry and distressed by her refusal to agree to treatment. Despite alternative therapy, the patient's condition worsened; this eventually resulted in her transfer to the ward where she died three days later. Generally the staff involved in caring for this lady were very distressed and angry and felt extremely upset for the parents and the children involved.* (Staff nurse)

Nurses sometimes have difficulty dealing with the idea that a person has chosen to die.

*I felt very angry with Alan for losing the will to live and giving up the fight and I felt guilty for feeling like that too.* (Student nurse)

The language used in caring for dying patients often takes the form of military metaphors (Martin, 1994), with the implication that giving-up involves a cowardly surrender. In other incidents, nurses have used the terms *'fighting for her breath'* and *'battling against cancer'*. Patients who *'never gave up hope'*, were *'clinging on to the end'*, or *'struggling against the odds'* were viewed positively. Those *'giving up'* were, perhaps, seen as less brave, and as guilty of putting themselves at risk of dying earlier than necessary.

*We were starting to get despondent about an elderly lady who wouldn't eat ... Her husband asked us to make an extra effort to make her eat, even by bullying her into eating. After his plea, we all became even more involved but after a while it became evident that she was not going into remission from her leukaemia. I could not help myself from feeling angry with her for not co-operating and letting herself die. I saw her the night before she died and it upset me to think that someone would give up without a fight.* (Student nurse)

Nurses often turn to humour to reduce tension in difficult situations.

*I was sitting at the triage desk when a car screeched to a halt outside, somebody was bundled into a wheelchair and pushed through the department doors. The car then sped away. I was presented with a young man who was navy blue and not breathing. He was approximately 25 years old. I quickly wheeled him into the resuscitation room and commenced emergency treatment ... It transpired that the young man had injected a large amount of heroin. Once this information had been obtained, IV narcon was adminis-*

*tered. This resulted in the young man gaining consciousness very quickly and in strong language expressing a wish to leave the department. He leapt off the trolley and ran out of the department with me running after him asking for the BP cuff back. This he threw to the ground but kept on running. I returned to the triage desk. The receptionist commented that if she was brought in unwell, she hoped I would be there to 'triage' her as that was the fastest recovery she had ever seen.* (Staff nurse)

A number of risks can be identified in this incident. The friends risked being identified, and the patient faced the health and legal risks associated with taking heroin. There was a professional risk to the nurse in 'allowing' a patient to leave against advice. But the nurse, in collaboration with his colleague, turned a potentially stressful incident into a humorous one.

## RISKS TO NURSES

### Nurse abuse

Periodically, nurses have to contend with sexual harassment and insults.

*Around 11.30pm I was asked to do a dressing so I collected the patient from the waiting area after he had been seen by the casualty officer. The person was clearly worse for wear from alcohol. He was noisy, rude and slurring his words. I tried to be assertive but kind and he sat while I completed the dressing without interruptions. As I was giving him information for his GP, and telling him about keeping his dressing clean and dry, he began to get agitated and stood up from the chair and demanded a kiss. I quite calmly opened the door for him and said 'I think you'd better go now.' He said 'OK, love,' and walked off. At this point I felt very nervous (the shock really hit me then) and I watched the particular patient until he left the department.* (Student nurse)

The following quotation illustrates the inner conflict which a nurse could experience between her professional role and her personal response to insults.

*A young man was brought in by ambulance and was wheeled in to a cubicle to have a cut on his head cleaned. As he was quite drunk, we sat him in the waiting area so we could keep our eye on him. I went into the dressing-room and when I came out found that the lad had vomited large amounts of lager all over the floor. This wasn't a problem but as we began to clear it up he and his friend began laughing and giggling at us for having to clean up his vomit. Although the staff nurse told him he was very rude, he seemed totally unbothered. I felt angry, very small and like a little cheap dogsbody. It may sound very unprofessional but I thought that if I was on duty when he came back to have his sutures out, I would like to gently remind him of his rude behaviour by being a little bit rough when removing them. I know my anger was justified but I also know that I shouldn't have wanted revenge on him for making me look a fool.* (Student nurse)

A sense of guilt arising out of high expectations of oneself can be seen as part of the *'emotional labour of nursing'* (Smith, 1992).

### 'Sticking your neck out'

Both students and qualified nurses often referred to professional risks arising out of their patient-advocacy role. Advocacy may mean challenging more senior colleagues in the institutional hierarchy. The incident described below concerns a couple who wanted to have their first baby at home, despite the risks perceived by both the obstetrician and the midwife's supervisor.

*As the pregnancy goes to one week post-mature I visit daily to assess. R agrees to foetal monitoring – alternative days – not daily as medical staff want. I discuss the home situation with my supervisor. She does not support home births, particularly in the first pregnancy. I am being pushed into suggesting a hospital induction, but on what grounds? Post-maturity by itself is no indication.*

*Friday 4am: Thank God R is in labour, C rings me at home, I go to the house. The labour is lovely, relaxed, happy normal, natural. A beautiful girl, 7 lbs 6ozs. Both grandparents and the dog are there. As we sip champagne and nibble home-baked cookies, I reflect. This is midwifery. I was with them. I stick my neck out against supervisor and medical staff. I acted professionally. I used research to back-up my practice. I was an advocate for R and C. The most positive experience of my career to date.* (Qualified midwife)

The midwife was helped in her advocacy role by the relationship she had built-up with the couple. In addition to assessing the risks for mother and baby, she had to appraise the professional risk involved in standing-up for good practice, as she saw it. If a problem had arisen with the birth, she could have found herself in a difficult position, both professionally and in terms of her own sense of responsibility. It would have been easier to shelter under the safety net of institutional protection rather than adopt an autonomous stance.

In contrast, the nurse quoted below questioned a patient's medical treatment, but felt reluctant to communicate her view of the costs and benefits involved to either the patient or the medical staff.

*A gentleman in his late seventies was given the option of long-term dialysis. He was informed by the medical staff that it would save his life and make him feel much better. He was one month into the treatment and making twice-weekly visits to the hospital, each journey taking nearly two hours due to the distance. The patient was exhausted as he took an hour to get ready prior to the ambulance arriving which meant rising at 6am. He asked me why he was not told how tiring his treatment would be and now he felt much worse. He said he would like to stop the treatment but the family would be very upset. Because of my experience I was well aware at the onset of the patient's illness what his prospects of coping with the treatment were, particularly since he lived many miles from the hospital. I felt that the medical staff's view was unrealistic but I was unable to say so.* (Qualified nurse)

Such incidents raise questions about whether nurses are gaining confidence in their ability to assert themselves within multidisciplinary teams in order to act as patient advocates. Although this nurse's view of the situation can be debated, it is interesting to consider why she felt unable to give it expression. What risks did she feel she would have taken in questioning the decision? How would the family and medical staff have responded if she had done so? Did she think it was not her place to challenge the decision?

In workshop discussions, nurses often express concern about the difficulty they have in asserting themselves. As one nurse put it:

*I was educated to obey the establishment and authority and this in addition to my natural non-assertive personality causes me many unhappy moments because I am worried that to question or show disapproval will result in me being told that my opinion is of no value.* (Qualified nurse)

Non-assertiveness may stem from a person's lack of confidence in their ability and knowledge, making personal risk-taking more difficult. Feminist theorists have linked the oppression of women to their socialisation into passive and subordinate roles, with a consequential loss of self-esteem (De Beauvoir, 1960; Friedan, 1977). The low status attached to caring and the 'dirty work' of nursing (Lawler, 1991) may influence the way nurses see themselves, within a profession which has had a history of subservience to authority, usually medical. Pascall (1986) refers to the increasing male control of female work in general, and Thompson (1995) notes the insidious nature of social power based on the ability to prevent contentious issues from being openly discussed.

There are dangers, however, in concluding that nurses do not challenge authority primarily because of personal diffidence. Critical incidents illustrate the complex social repercussions of challenging the system, as well as the personal guilt which nurses can experience when they feel powerless to help patients.

> *Over the three days a patient had expressed his concern and anxieties to me about not receiving any information at all about why he couldn't go home as he felt perfectly well. Several times I told qualified staff about how this patient was feeling worried about not knowing what was happening. All they could tell him was that they were awaiting the results of an X-ray to come back. This still left him feeling very frustrated. Maybe I was wrong in doing so but I told him that he should perhaps ask the consultant next time he came on to the ward as to why he hadn't been told anything ... He seemed very hesitant and anxious so I stood beside him as the consultant came by. The patient stood up and began to explain how he hadn't been told anything. The consultant interrupted and told him that he had only been on the ward for two days and that he would get one of his house officers to see him and walked off. During this brief interaction, the consultant only made eye contact with the patient twice and the rest of the time he kept his head down and spoke down as if to the patient's slippers. The patient was left standing open-mouthed. I will never forget the look of despair on his face. He walked back to his bed shaking his head. I felt guilty as I was the one who had encouraged him to ask.* (Student nurse)

When nurses do 'stick their necks out', they may face immediate problems not only with other professionals, but with members of the public, and become more reluctant to take personal risks in order to protect a patient.

> *This young girl was admitted to our ward following a large paracetamol overdose. She had refused to accept medication, saying that she just wanted to see her boyfriend. I tried to convince her of the seriousness of her condition and the outcome if she continued to refuse any medication such as activated charcoal, parvolex, etc. Up to this moment nobody had mentioned the word 'death' and when I said to her rather bluntly that she would be dead by the weekend, she changed her mind and accepted the medication. A few days later, on discharge, she came up to me with her boyfriend and was verbally abusive to me while her boyfriend and family tried to assault me physically for 'upsetting her' by telling her that she may die. After this incident I was rather reluctant to tell any other person who had taken an overdose of the possible outcome.* (Qualified nurse)

## RISK AND PROFESSIONAL IDENTITY

### Behaving professionally

Nurses are constantly concerned to act professionally. This requirement may lead them to take perceived risks which, personally, they might avoid.

*When it came to standing on his doorstep my fear began to set in. Once inside and faced with him I felt like I could walk out of the house, not knowing whether I had caught it or not, even though I had the knowledge that AIDS cannot be caught on the contact that I would be having with him. His mother offered us cups of coffee when we visited, but the thought struck me, 'Has he had a drink from this cup?' However, at the same time and as a reassurance to his parents I felt obliged to have one to show that I was not concerned. They drink out of them every day, don't they!* (Student nurse)

This student experienced an uncomfortable conflict between her sense of danger, perhaps based on wider cultural terror about AIDS, and beliefs derived from formal knowledge. However, because she wanted to act professionally, she was prepared to ignore her fears. The quote illustrates one of the main themes of Chapter 1: the gulf between personal and professional engagement with risk.

## Getting involved

The emotional risks, for nurses, of becoming personally involved can be seen in the following account of a nurse's extended distress following the death of a patient.

*B was 72 years old, debilitated and dying. I entered her room one Friday morning as usual. She appeared particularly low in mood. I chatted inconsequentially about my going on holiday the next day. I said I hoped B would be feeling better when I returned. B had enormous brown eyes and a steady gaze. From half-closed lips and with a slightly guarded expression she verbalised what we were both thinking. 'I won't be here when you get back from holiday.' I knew she meant that she was going to die. She then directed her full gaze on to my face. I immediately avoided eye contact and found myself straightening her sheets again. The urge to dismiss her statement and leave the room was overwhelming. I couldn't move. The lump in my throat increased and my eyes filled with tears – still I avoided her. She continued gazing at my face – waiting ... Finally I turned to B looked directly into her eyes and simply nodded. I took her in my arms so she wouldn't see my tears  The atmosphere in the room had changed from tension to peace ... I knew I wouldn't see her again. I went on to the sluice and broke my heart. B died the next day. Nurses are human and in providing human-to-human contact with dying patients, they often experience pain and suffering themselves ... I am still afraid four years after the incident of my feelings. I almost feared emotional disintegration by examining the incident too deeply. This suggests that my grief following this lady's death remains unresolved. It is my belief that if the support had been available at the time, then my feelings related to this lady may have been better reconciled.* (Newly qualified staff nurse, reflecting on an experience she had had as a student)

A student nurse expressed his feelings at not being able to end a relationship in a satisfactory way.

*A little boy of five years old was admitted with bruising to his face and body, who it was suspected had been abused by his parents. At first I was angry at the parents, even what could be described as mad but also a little afraid to get involved ... and although at first I felt a little embarrassed and stupid I suspect that he began to see me as a father-figure. Towards the end of my stay when I had to leave I found it difficult to just walk away, feeling that I had not enough time to say goodbye and to prepare myself properly for leaving. I also felt a little embarrassed, not knowing what to do, who to talk to and express how I felt. I felt helpless and trapped in a situation which I did not understand. I felt it was difficult to accept this as part of the role of the nurse and at the end of the day I could not close my mind to it. I felt I should do more, but what? I did not know, but as a result I felt guilty and helpless at not being able to do more for the sake of my own peace of mind.* (Student nurse)

The above incidents suggest that 'distancing' occurs during nurse socialisation not as a result of an uncaring attitude on the part of the nurse, but as a means of coping with the risk of getting involved.

The final example reminds us that nurses have to take account of being a potential source of risk to patients.

*While on the paediatric ward, there was a young girl of 14 suffering from anorexia. She was difficult to communicate with at times but I, like the other staff, spent a great deal of time talking to her and encouraging her to eat. After a while we built up a good relationship and I think she began to trust me. One morning I found her in the corridor in some distress, sobbing, and I did what I thought was something very natural, I put my arms round her to try and give her some support and find out why she was crying. Afterwards the staff nurse took me aside and very gently told me that I was putting myself at risk by hugging a teenager even though I might be doing it with the best of intentions.* (Male student nurse)

## Discussion

The changing face of health care, with a growing emphasis on consumer rights and expectations, competitiveness, quality assurance and accountability, provides a challenge for nurses who have to manage complex risks, both for patients and themselves. Risk-taking can be stimulating and rewarding, and good management can reduce the probability of adverse effects. We have argued, however, that many of the risks involved in nursing practice are hidden, unexpected and likely to engender emotional distress.

Nurses need support in dealing with risks if advocacy, autonomy and professional accountability are to become more important elements of advanced practice (UKCC, 1992b). Peters (1987, p. 485) reflected that:

*brave acts of creation must begin with a vision which not only inspires, ennobles, empowers and challenges but at the same time promotes confidence enough in the midst of a competitive hurricane to encourage people to take day-to-day risks in extending the vision.*

However, critical incident analysis shows clearly that risk management often involves moral dilemmas which lack easy solutions, and that nursing autonomy is affected by organisational as well as personal constraints.

A great deal of attention has been paid, quite rightly, to the nature of health-care-related risks for patients. The risks to the physical and emotional wellbeing of nurses should not be underestimated. Formal recognition of the need for adequate support mechanisms and educative strategies is required in order to ensure that risky situations are managed as well as possible, and that effective support is given. Unless such measures are taken, nurses will not become truly autonomous, confident practitioners in a complex world.

# Risk and blood-pressure measurement

## David O'Brien and Maria Davison

## Introduction

This chapter aims to critically analyse the ways in which nurses and midwives approach the problems associated with blood-pressure measurement. It draws on physiological and behavioural science literature, and empirical research completed by the authors.

Blood-pressure measurement can be viewed in two ways: first, as a risk-management procedure based on scientific rationality, physiological principles and the application of a relatively simple, reliable technology; and second, as a form of reassuring ritual, undertaken routinely, irrespective of clinical need or the use to which blood-pressure information is put. According to Walsh and Ford (1992, pp. ix–x)

> Ritual actions imply carrying out a task without thinking it through. The nurse does something because this is the way it has always been done ... the nurse does not have to think about the problem and work out an individualised solution; the action is ritual.

The scientific status of blood-pressure measurements in nursing and midwifery practice is predicated on the assumption that such measurements are reliable and valid. One objective of this chapter is to question this assumption. A second objective is to consider the use of blood pressure information in clinical practice. It is argued that such information needs to be understood in the context of individuals' physiological, psychological and social condition. The chapter considers the following four topics: pathophysiological and epidemiological evidence of the risks associated with blood-pressure deviations; the risk of errors in blood-pressure measurement; the potential consequences of such errors; and the use, by nurses and midwives, of blood-pressure measurements in the management of risks to the health of patients.

## Pathophysiological and epidemiological perspectives on blood pressure

Medically, blood-pressure measurement has the status of a clinically significant observation. Deviations from the norm have been associated with increasing risks of morbidity and mortality (Krakoff, 1994; Scanlon and Sanders, 1995). Hypertension (elevated blood pressure) leads to increased risk of cerebral and subarachnoid haemorrhage, thrombotic strokes, heart failure, aortic aneurysms and progressive renal failure (Krakoff, 1994). Hypotension (low blood pressure) can be caused by hypovolaemic and toxic shock and anaphylaxis due to massive allergic reactions (Scanlon and Sanders, 1995). Normal blood pressure is maintained through a variety of complex mechanical, neurological and chemical processes involving blood volume, heartbeat, elasticity of the arterial walls, peripheral resistance and venous return. Chemical influences include concentrations of potassium, sodium and calcium. An example of a mechanical influence is the sensitivity to pressure changes of baroreceptors located in some large arteries.

Clancy and McVicar (1995) distinguish short-term homeostatic blood-pressure mechanisms, designed for rapid response situations, and long-term control mechanisms. A large number of social, psychological, demographic and genetic factors have been linked with blood-pressure variations in populations. Alderman (1988) discusses associations of blood pressure with gender, age and ethnicity. Women have a lower mean blood pressure than men of a similar age until the time of the menopause, when the positions are reversed. Blood pressure increases with age, and is higher, on average, among Black American men than among their White equivalents.

Heredity, climate, diet, personal wellbeing and disease are correlated with blood-pressure variations. Elford et al. (1990) found that, in the UK, systolic blood pressure increases on a south-to-north gradient. This study concluded that the time spent in a geographical area predicted systolic blood pressure better than place of birth: a finding which attests to the importance of environmental influences. The precise reasons for this north/south divide are not known, but Elford et al. suggest that differences in the patterns of alcohol consumption, variations in physical activity and socioeconomic factors may be involved. The seasons also affect blood pressure which increases in the winter months (James, Yee and Pickering, 1990). Lewis and Timby (1993) link individual variations in blood pressure with emotional arousal, pain, smoking and alcohol consumption.

# Accurate blood-pressure measurement: Reality, myth and risk

Within nursing and midwifery clinical contexts, blood-pressure measurement is generally regarded as an essential indicator of the health status of the individual, and as a key variable guiding decisions about clinical interventions. This view assumes, implicitly, that blood-pressure can be easily recorded with a high level of reliability and validity. Educationally, blood-pressure measurement tends to be treated as a task which nurses can master easily in the early weeks of their training. Contemporary research suggests, however, that, far from being unproblematic, the taking and recording of blood pressure is a complex nursing activity which draws on knowledge of the physiological, psychological and social sciences, and requires a considerable level of skill. The discussion which follows focuses upon two key issues: sources of measurement error and their implications for risk management; and blood-pressure measurement as a form of ritual.

## THE REQUIREMENTS FOR ACCURATE BLOOD-PRESSURE MEASUREMENT

Most major introductory nursing texts at least mention the importance of blood-pressure measurement in nursing assessment (Hinchliff, Norman and Schober, 1993; Brunner and Suddarth, 1992) while others contain more substantial discussion (Sorensen and Luckmann, 1986; Boore, Champion and Ferguson, 1987; Royle and Walsh, 1992). Similarly, several journal articles have been written with the aim of promoting the accurate measurement and recording of blood pressure (Petrie *et al.*, 1986; Draper, 1987; Jewell, 1987; Hill and Grim, 1991; Jolly, 1991). The literature identifies a range of factors on which the accuracy of blood-pressure measurement and recording depend. These are listed on page 266 in Table 14.1.

Blood-pressure results from the lateral force caused on the walls of arteries by pressure from the heart. Blood flows throughout the circulatory system, from an area of high pressure to one of low pressure, because of pressure changes. The heart's contraction forces blood under high pressure into the aorta. The peak of maximum pressure when ejection occurs is the systolic blood pressure. When the ventricles relax, the blood remaining in the arteries exerts a minimum or diastolic pressure. Diastolic pressure is the minimal pressure exerted against the artery walls at all times (Potter and Perry, 1995).

### Auscultatory measurement technique (stethoscope and sphygmomanometer)

The recommended technique for measuring blood pressure is as follows. The cuff should first be inflated for 3–5 seconds until brachial pulsation ceases, and an initial estimate of systolic pressure noted. A stethoscope should not be used to detect pulse cessation at this stage. The cuff is then deflated, and the stethoscope placed over a marked site. If the stethoscope is pressed firmly, or the cuff is touched, diastolic pressure may be greatly underesti-

**Table 14.1**    Measuring and recording arterial blood pressure accurately: Some key variables

### 1 The patient

| | |
|---|---|
| 1a | Sitting or lying for at least 3 minutes |
| 1b | Remove clothing from arm |
| 1c | Psychologically calm |
| 1d | Arm supported level with heart |
| 1e | No recent smoking or alcohol consumption |

### 2 The equipment

| | |
|---|---|
| 2a | Bladder cuff at least 80% of arm's circumference |
| 2b | Sphygmomanometer calibrated 6 monthly |
| 2c | Sphygmomanometer and stethoscope regularly maintained |
| 2d | Stand mounted sphygmomanometer preferred (mobile with a vertical mercury column) |

### 3 The observer

| | |
|---|---|
| 3a | No hearing deficit or special stethoscope |
| 3b | Good initial education |
| 3c | Good understanding of measurement principles |
| 3d | Opportunities for updating and practice |

### 4 The technique

| | |
|---|---|
| 4a | Patient's arm adequately supported |
| 4b | Point of maximum pressure over brachial artery detected (may be marked lightly with a felt pen) |
| 4c | Cuff fitted firmly and comfortably, and well secured |
| 4d | Centre of cuff bladder placed over brachial artery |
| 4e | Lower edge of cuff bladder 2–3 cms above marked site |
| 4f | Cuff inflated for 3–5 seconds until brachial pulsation ceases to estimate systolic pressure (do not use stethoscope) |
| 4g | Cuff deflated at 2–3 mm Hg per second until Korotkoff sounds detected (see below) |
| 4h | Blood pressure recorded to the nearest 2mm |
| 4i | If necessary, measurement repeated after at least 1 minute has elapsed |

mated. The cuff should be inflated rapidly to 30 mm Hg above estimated systolic blood pressure, and then deflated at the rate of 2–3 mm Hg per second. The point at which clear repetitive tapping sounds first appear for at least 2 consecutive beats (Korotkoff sound 1) indicates the systolic pressure. The point at which these sounds finally disappear (Korotkoff sound 5) gives the diastolic blood pressure. If these sounds do not disappear, the point of muffling (Korotkoff sound 4) should be used, as is done routinely in pregnancy. The blood pressure should then be recorded to the nearest 2mm Hg.

## Potential sources of variation and error

Errors may be associated with characteristics of the observer, the patient, the technique or the equipment (Boore, Champion and Ferguson, 1987; Jewell, 1987). The observer may have hearing deficits, or a poor understanding of the rather complex principles of blood-pressure measurement.

Certain temporary patient characteristics can lead to errors in the estimation of their normal blood pressure. Physical and physiological variables include excessive heat, cold, constrictive clothing, having a full bladder and recent behaviours which affect blood pressure, such as smoking, alcohol consumption or brisk physical activity. Psychosocial variables include states of anxiety and excitement (Jewell, 1987).

Poor technique provides another potential source of measurement error. Possible failings include excessive stethoscope pressure (giving an artificially low diastolic pressure), excessively fast or slow deflation of the cuff, non-support of the patient's arm (leading to systolic pressure overestimation), repeating blood-pressure measurement before one minute has elapsed, and not applying the cuff firmly and evenly in the correct position.

Accurate measurement requires the correct calibration of sphygmomanometers. Conceicao, Ward and Kerr (1976) found that sphygmomanometers in a group of teaching hospitals were poorly maintained, and that almost half had defects. The author also suggested that aneroid are less robust than mercury sphygmomanometers. Too short cuffs (see above) are associated with an overestimation of blood-pressure in obese patients (O'Brien and O'Malley, 1981).

Inaccurate blood-pressure measurement can give rise to considerable risk, especially for hospitalised patients undergoing clinical treatment. It might be supposed that care would be taken to make measurement in these contexts as accurate as possible, but the research outlined below suggests that this does not always happen. Accurate measurement is most critical at the margin between a normal blood-pressure level and one which should cause clinical concern. For example, an increase in a pregnant woman's baseline diastolic blood pressure of more than 10mm Hg would warrant further investigations. Similarly, in surgical settings, the assessment of hypovolaemic (blood loss) shock reactions depends on knowledge of blood-pressure levels, particularly diastolic pressure. Blood-pressure measurement influences clinical decisions about whether, for example, to give blood transfusions, narcotic pain relief, or early resuscitative interventions. Inaccurate measurement will lead to a risk both of needless interventions, and of failure to detect real problems.

## BLOOD-PRESSURE MEASUREMENT AS RITUAL

The requirements for accurate blood-pressure measurement are instrumentally and physiologically determined. However, blood-pressure reading also involves a symbolic social act which helps nurses to display their concern for patients' safety, and to demonstrate their contribution to scientifically grounded care. This concern is conveyed in ritualistic and routinised behaviours unconnected with direct clinical needs (Menzies, 1970; Chapman, 1983; Kilgour and Speedie, 1985; Walsh and Ford, 1992).

Ritualistic actions, based on traditional routines, appear incompatible with modern problem-solving, holistic, research-based philosophies of nursing care. The existence of a custom of assessing blood pressure at fixed and predetermined times, without reference to the clinical status of individual patients, suggests that clinicians lack judgement and insight. However, the taking and recording of blood pressure has psychological and social, as well as clinical, significance. Menzies (1970), for example, using a psychoanalytic approach, proposed that such routines served the function of protecting individual nurses against anxiety. The routinisation of procedures such as blood-pressure-taking contributed to the establishment of social systems based on task allocation. Such systems, she argued, protected practitioners from stresses which might arise from closer engagement with patients in more holistic nursing care. At the time that Menzies was undertaking her research, student nurses were not prepared for individualised patient care. They were advised not to get closely involved with patients' problems, but to adopt a task-orientated approach to care. Elements of this approach can still be found in contemporary clinical practice, as evidenced by the routine monitoring of vital observations, and the ritualisation of blood-pressure measurement and recording.

Using a social action perspective, Chapman (1983) has suggested that practices which cannot be justified on direct therapeutic grounds, including the routinised taking of blood pressure for no demonstrable clinical purpose, have strong symbolic significance, communicating to both patients and significant peers the nurse's caring commitment. These symbolic practices are picked-up during professional socialisation and, like all learnt behaviours, are resistant to change. To illustrate with a hypothetical example: a patient admitted to a medical ward for investigation of a duodenal ulcer might also be hypertensive. Normally, such a patient would have their blood-pressure recorded at six-monthly intervals by their GP. But, in hospital, blood pressure will be recorded daily or more frequently, even though it is unrelated to the clinical problem for which the patient has been admitted. Such practices disrupt patient routines and provoke anxiety. But, paradoxically, patients with considerable experience of hospital life often believe that such ritual practices are necessary, and may well become concerned if they are not carried out.

The organisational origins of hospital blood-pressure measurement practices often cannot be identified clearly. Burroughs and Hoffbrand (1990) found that, despite the absence of specific policies, 78 per cent of nurses in their survey believed that guidelines did exist which required that all new admissions should have their blood pressures recorded at four-hourly intervals, and that all postoperative patients should have their blood pressures checked every half hour. These practices can be seen as part of a 'worst-case' risk-management strategy which is justified on rare occasions, for example when a patient suddenly and unexpectedly deteriorates. Such worst-case scenarios strongly influence nursing and midwifery practice. They are reinforced by a professional socialisation which stresses the need to avoid allegations of patient neglect, and possible litigation. Paradoxically, minimising one hypothetical risk by recourse to almost obsessional behaviour may increase the overall risk, since time can only be devoted to one activity at the expense of others.

## An empirical study of blood-pressure measurement

In order to further explore issues of technique, sources of error and the management of risk in blood-pressure reading, an empirical study, undertaken by the authors, will be briefly described below.

## METHODOLOGY

### Sample

The study sample included 17 ward-based qualified nurses and midwives with at least six months post-registration experience, and 15 student nurses and pre-registration student midwives at various stages of their nurse or midwifery education. Research participants worked in general medicine, general surgery or midwifery in the same District General Hospital. The sample was a convenience one, with respondents volunteering to take part in the research, following explanation by one of the researchers. Such a sample does not necessarily represent the population from which it is drawn, and any generalisations made below should be treated with caution.

### Methods

The knowledge and practice of the sample were investigated through questionnaires, observation and interview methods. In order to assess the knowledge base of the practitioners, a structured questionnaire was designed and administered. The items contained in the questionnaire were based on a literature review, and their content is summarised in Table 14.2, below. An observational study of the ways in which nurses took and recorded arterial blood pressure on the ward was undertaken. The observational criteria were derived from the literature review, and are summarised in Table 14.3. Semi-structured interviews were used to explore nurses' and midwives' views about the routine taking and recording of blood pressure, and about the ways in which decisions to start and stop such observations were made.

### Results

As no statistically significant differences were found between the qualified staff and students, all results are reported for the total sample.

### The questionnaire

The topics covered in the questionnaire are summarised in Figure 14.1, below.

| Items assessed |
| --- |
| Previous teaching (90%) |
| Opportunities to practise (90%) |
| Opportunities for updating knowledge and skills (30%) |
| Correct cuff-deflation rate (30%) |
| Routine estimation of systolic blood-pressure (30%) |
| Potential sources of error (11%) |
| Identification of Korotkoff sounds (6%) |
| Physiological determinants of blood pressure (6%) |
| Psychosocial factors influencing blood pressure (6%) |

**Figure 14.1**   Taking and recording of arterial blood-pressure: Questionnaire assessment of knowledge. Percentages obtaining maximum scores in parentheses (N=32)

Over 90 per cent of respondents reported receiving formal instruction in the taking and recording of arterial blood pressure, and had been given the opportunity to practise the technique prior to clinical placements. However, less than 30 per cent had updated their skills and knowledge. Since initial teaching typically occurs early in nursing and midwifery programmes, students as well as qualified staff need this updating.

In relation to the technique itself, almost 70 per cent, could not identify the correct cuff deflation rate (2–3 mm per second). Only 31 per cent claimed to routinely estimate systolic blood pressure using the correct technique. The theoretical clinical risk in not estimating systolic blood pressure arises from the possible presence of an intra-auscultatory gap, i.e. a failure to detect real systolic pressure because of non-audible Korotkoff sounds when using a stethoscope. Initial estimation of systolic pressure without the use of a stethoscope would offset the possibility of this type of error. However, the authors have been unable to find any empirical evidence of the seriousness of this risk.

Only two respondents could correctly match descriptions of Korotkoff sounds to their appropriate Korotkoff number. These sounds can be heard while the bladder of the sphygmomanometer is being deflated, with the aid of a stethoscope placed over an artery (most commonly the brachial artery). The first sound is a clear tapping, and systolic pressure can be recorded at this point. The sound then softens, in phase 2, and a sharper sound returns, in phase 3. Phase 4 occurs when there is abrupt muffling, and phase 5 when sound disappears, at which point diastolic blood pressure can be read (Boore, Champion and Furguson, 1987).

Only one respondent could identify four physiological determinants of normal arterial blood pressure, the maximum score possible in this research, and 53 per cent could name only one determinant. With reference to psychosocial factors influencing blood pressure, nearly 90 per cent identified two factors, 34 per cent mentioned three factors, and 6 per cent named four factors, the maximum score possible. At least one source of error in the measurement and recording of blood pressure was mentioned by 91 per cent of respondents, but only 34 per cent could identify four, the maximum score.

## The observation schedule

As can be seen in Figure 14.2, nurses' and midwives' blood-pressure measurement technique deviated substantially from recommended good practice.

No nurse or midwife met all the criteria contained in the observational schedule. While generally good results were obtained for a number of items, the low scores obtained for adequate support of the arm, correct deflation rate and being at eye level with the sphygmomanometer, and the very low score for estimating systolic pressure, suggest considerable potential for inaccuracy.

## The semi-structured interviews

The semi-structured interviews (N=32) were concerned with respondents' accounts of why arterial blood pressure were routinely taken; who makes

| Percentage sample meeting criteria for good practice |
| :--- |
| Prompt recording of blood pressure (91%) |
| Maintaining sphygmomanometer in the vertical position (88%) |
| Removal of restrictive clothing from the arm (81%) |
| Good initial approach (78%) |
| Good final communication (72%) |
| Correct cuff application (smooth, firm , without wrinkles) (63%) |
| Sphygmomanometer level with heart (63%) |
| Correct cuff position (50%) |
| Adequate support of the arm (44%) |
| Nurse at eye level with sphygmomanometer (44%) |
| Correct deflation rate (41%) |
| Estimation of systolic blood pressure (6%) |

**Figure 14.2**   Taking and recording of arterial blood-pressure observation schedule (N=32)

decisions to stop routine blood-pressure measurements; whether blood-pressure measurements were performed by a named nurse (or associate) or as part of a task-allocation system; and their opinions about whether blood pressure were taken unnecessarily. The respondents were able to identify, between them, 25 circumstances in which routine blood-pressure monitoring would occur, the most common being pre- and post-operative observation, hospital admission, chest pain, hypertension and pregnancy.

Over 80 per cent of the sample had taken routine blood pressures which, in their opinion, were unnecessary. The reasons given included blood-pressure reading being part of the normal routine; being instructed by a sister or doctor; being afraid to make the decision to stop; having to complete a form which had space for recording daily blood pressure; and resistance to change.

Over 80 per cent of respondents believed that qualified nurses or midwives should decide when to stop routine recordings, while only 13 per cent considered that doctors should take this decision. Half of the sample considered that blood-pressure reading and measurement should be done by the named nurse, while 25 per cent believed it would be a delegated task. A further 25 per cent had an intermediate position, believing these tasks should be carried out by a named nurse in the morning, but as a delegated task in the afternoon and at night.

## Discussion

The results obtained in this study indicate that the techniques which nurses and midwives use to read and record blood pressure create a substantial source of potential errors. These deviations from good practice are associated with considerable gaps in practitioners' knowledge of the principles of blood-pressure measurement. Measurements of questionable accuracy feed into clinical decision-making and the management of risk by nurses and midwives. The doubtful reliability and accuracy of routine blood-pressure readings suggests that they have a ritualistic function, providing a display of concern for patient safety.

The lack of formal education for health-care professionals in the taking and recording of blood pressure has been cited by several authors as a possible cause of erroneous practice, in medicine as well as in nursing and midwifery. For example, Feher, Harris-St John and Lant (1992) found that 43 per cent of a sample of qualified doctors did not know the extent to which the arm should be covered with the cuff bladder; that 61 per cent could not identify the situations in which Korotkoff 4 sounds should be used in the measurement of diastolic blood pressure; and that 59 per cent were prepared to round the reading to the nearest 5–10 mm Hg. Similar problems were noted by Kemp, Foster and McKinlay (1993) in a study of clinical staff which included 100 nurses. They found that 40 per cent of the sample claimed to have had no formal training in the technique; that 75 per cent had had no further update in the technique since qualification; that only 4 per cent had received updates within the past year; and that 85 per cent considered their readings accurate, although 50 per cent admitted to occasional estimation of blood pressure without recourse to the full formal procedure. The authors concluded that knowledge of blood-pressure measurement and technique is poor, probably as a result of inadequate training.

With respect to the routinisation of blood-pressure measurement, Kilgour and Speedie (1985) found that a significant number of patients had their postoperative blood pressure assessed beyond the period of clinical stability. Burroughs and Hoffbrand (1990) found, as already noted, that nearly four out of five nurses in their sample wrongly believed in the existence of hospital policies requiring blood-pressure reading at four-hourly intervals for new admissions. Nurses felt that their continuance with observations which had been stable for some time gave patients a sense of security, minimised the danger of something being missed, and protected them from possible medico–legal complications. The above researchers argue that recording errors are likely to increase sharply with the number of observations made, especially in the absence of a clear rationale for undertaking them.

The present study highlights several issues relevant to risk and its management in relation to blood-pressure measurement. The suspect reliability and validity of such measurements brings into question the notion that the procedure is a relatively unproblematic activity, easily delegated to nursing and midwifery students.

During the past two decades, nursing has evolved from a profession which characteristically emphasises routines, rituals and procedures to one which attempts to found its practice on individualised, problem-solving and research-based approaches to care. This approach has presented considerable challenges to a profession little used to justifying the rationale for current practices. The skilled assessment of physiological parameters, including the taking and recording of blood pressure, remains crucial to the practice of nursing. Such observations must have a clear rationale. The data presented in this paper illustrate the way in which a common, apparently unproblematic, nursing activity can be called into question.

The ritualistic elements in blood-pressure measurement have their origins in an era of nursing in which critical thought and careful reflection were not highly valued in mainstream nurse education. Nursing activities were guided by a reliance on set procedures which were unproblematically applied to most nursing situations. Once established, such rituals readily become part of the culture of nursing, and provided comfort and certainty to nurses in their everyday work. Given this history, it is not surprising that there has been a marked reluctance to critically challenge cherished and established approaches to practice, especially when the alternative demands individualised risk management, and raises questions about appropriate clinical decision-making and professional accountability.

# PART THREE

# Dilemmas in health-risk management

MERTHYR TYDFIL COLLEGE
LIBRARY

# Risk: A nursing dilemma

## Glenda Cook and Susan Procter

Introduction

The dilemma of safety versus autonomy

Respect for autonomy

risk-taking in rehabilitative care: a moral dilemma

A dilemma for nursing theory

Discussion

*I think, because of the nature of nursing in particular rehabilitation ... you wouldn't gain an inch if you didn't take a risk in the delivery of care. For example, a patient may be desperate to go home. They may manage, or they may not manage. We just don't know. We can put every kind of service in, we can get rails, commodes, etc. We can do everything, but at the end of the day the patient may be at risk of falling, and may not manage. On the other hand most patients manage far beyond your expectation.* (Staff nurse, elderly rehabilitation, quoted in Cook, 1994)

## Introduction

The above statement illustrates the uncertainty implicit in many areas of nursing practice, and epitomises the pervading atmosphere of risk (Annandale, 1995). Traditionally, health care activity has mainly focused on the repair of the body through surgery and drug treatments, and much of the debate on risk-taking in health-care has centred on such interventions. However, more recently, additional sources of risk in health-care practice have been highlighted in the psychosocial domain. Nurses and other professionals allied to medicine confront these issues during their daily activity with patients and clients.

Discussions of the uncertainties associated with health-care practice have been primarily concerned with the identification and management of negative outcomes. This orientation matches prevailing conceptions of risk. For example, the 1986 *Oxford Dictionary* defines risk as a situation involving a chance of danger, loss or harm. However, the term risk was first introduced to the English language in the seventeenth century in the context of gambling (Hayes, 1992). It referred to the probability of losses **and** gains. Originally a neutral term, risk has acquired solely negative connotations in the modern era. Health-care professionals need to rediscover the original, wider connotations of risk, and to balance the possibility of negative outcomes against potential gains from risk-taking activities.

Risk-taking is a normal part of daily living at all stages of life. For example, allowing young children to climb stairs with minimal supervision enables them to explore their environment, and to take their first steps towards independent living, but exposes them to the risk of falling. Similarly, elderly patients who use the commode, or go the toilet independently during the night, may re-establish skills which enable them to be discharged. If an accident does happen, the nurses involved may face an onslaught of complaint and investigation, but their skilled management of risk in successful cases is rarely recognised.

There have been calls to recognise risk-taking as an inescapable component of both health behaviour (Josephs, 1993) and professional practice (Counsel and Care, 1993). Rehabilitation programmes involve activities which necessitate a degree of risk. Practitioners make decisions, for example, about the supervision levels needed for patients who are regaining the ability to walk with or without the assistance of walking aids; how much freedom to give to patients to walk independently in the hospital grounds; whether to comply with a patient's request to be given a hot cup of tea; or whether to support a patient who wishes to be discharged to their own home.

Nurses planning care have to choose between various possible courses of action which may or may not aim to maximise patient safety. Patients may be supervised when walking, given tepid drinks or, in the longer term, placed in institutional care for the remainder of their lives. Alternatively, nurses can offer patients programmes designed to give them choices about the risks they wish to accept. This second course of action may benefit patients by promoting their self-awareness, emotional and physical independence, ability to make choices, confidence and capacity for further personal growth. A study of adults with learning disabilities living with relatives (Heyman and Huckle, 1993b) found that individuals cared for by more risk tolerant families appeared to achieve more of their potential in acquiring everyday living skills. Rehabilitative strategies do, however, expose both nurses and patients to uncertainties which would have been avoided if they had adhered to risk avoiding approaches to care.

## The dilemma of safety versus autonomy

This chapter discusses the dilemmas faced by nurses who try to implement care which balances the maintenance of safety and the promotion of patient autonomy. The importance of risk-taking as an element in therapeutic activity has been recognised in a number of fields, including service provision for people with learning disabilities (Chapters 9 and 10) and mental health problems (Chapter 17), and the care of older people (Chapter 12). In the context of institutional care for older people, therapeutic benefits have been ascribed to self-medication (Webb *et al.* 1990), participation in outings (Parkinson, 1990) and increased personal mobility (Goodwin and Managan, 1985).

However, nurses who incorporate risk-taking into care plans may feel vulnerable and fear litigation. While UK law does not prohibit the use of strategic risk-taking, it does forbid the acceptance of unreasonable risks. Practitioners' problems in this situation centre around interpretation of the contentious, context-specific notions of reasonable and unreasonable risk. Nurses have a duty both to minimise potential harm to patients, and to maximise positive outcomes. For example, patients who are given responsibility for their own medication may overdose, underdose or non-comply with the treatment regime. Nurses must be concerned that patients might be harmed, or that they might be accused of negligence. A balance between patient freedom and safety needs to be struck. In the case of self-medication, Ryan (1993) suggests that spot checks should be included in the programme. Patients would not be given total autonomy, but would retain some sense of responsibility for their own care.

Nurses receive only vague professional guidance about reasonable risk-taking. The United Kingdom Central Council for Nursing, Midwifery and Health Visiting's Code of Professional Conduct (UKCC, 1992a, clause 1) states that nurses, midwives and health visitors should *'always act in such a manner as to promote and safeguard the interests and well being of the patients and clients'*. This instruction can be interpreted as an exhortation for nurses to maximise the safety of the patients in their care. However, it also justifies the incorporation of risk-taking into clinical practice if the intended outcome is in the patient's best interest. The above clause provides a justification for essentially incompatible clinical decisions. For example, it can be used to justify maximising supervision for patients who are attempting to reacquire their mobility, in order to guarantee their safety, and minimising supervision, so as to enhance their independence.

Judgements about the costs and benefits of alternative care strategies involving different degrees of risk are made in a wider social context. Patients and relatives are most concerned with the anticipated impact of therapeutic options on their lives. Nurses have to take into account organisational and resource constraints on the provision of optimal solutions, as well as considering the accountability issues discussed above. The impact of these wider concerns on clinical decision-making is illustrated in the following case study (see Figure 15.1), based on work the authors have undertaken with a local nursing development unit.

---

### A case study of nursing risk management

A patient who had suffered a major heart attack subsequently experienced recurrent episodes of congestive cardiac failure for which she was periodically admitted to hospital. She lived in a small village, at some distance from the hospital. Her husband had Alzheimer's disease, and became very agitated when she was admitted. He would wander around the streets looking for her, causing considerable problems for neighbours and local services.

---

**Figure 15.1** A case study of nursing risk management

The patient whose circumstances are summarised in Figure 15.1 had had to come to terms with her recurrent attacks of congestive cardiac failure, and could not understand why she needed to be admitted to hospital, as she was very worried about her husband. She felt that if she could be looked after at home, her husband could always be directed to her when he became agitated. She was prepared to accept the greater risks to her health associated with care at home, where she would not receive 24 hour surveillance, in order to reduce the risk to her husband arising from his wanderings, and the resulting stress for family, friends, neighbours, local police and social services. Unfortunately, this patient could not be looked after at home because the necessary health care services could not be provided locally, a reflection of the historical emphasis on hospital provision.

This case study highlights the central theme of an Audit Commission Report (1992). The Report challenged the existing provider-oriented approach to health-care provision which, it argued, emphasises smoothly running routines and catering for people who meet the criteria for existing services. The Audit Commission (1992) presents alternative models of service provision which focus on the needs of individual service-users. They suggest that each person should be assessed as an individual, and that services should adjust to meet the needs of the individual, who should be provided with a greater degree of choice.

This approach, and the consumerist emphasis in recent policy initiatives, for example the NHS and Community Care Act 1990, on promoting patient choice and autonomy can be questioned, and subjected to ethical debate. Preserving or lengthening life, or reducing the incidence of injury to self and others resulting from autonomous action, may be valued more highly than autonomy which might result in injury or risk to the patient's life. Relatives and professional carers may feel justifiably concerned about the welfare of patients who insist on living alone despite difficulty in undertaking daily living activities. Under these circumstances, the patient may place a higher value on their independence than on their lives – but others may not support this position, or the patient's right to make life-threatening decisions.

This dilemma surfaces in risk-management decisions taken within a specific therapeutic context, as well as in those about the appropriateness of alternative environments. For example, individuals in receipt of care in a nursing home have given up the independence associated with living in their own home, but do not necessarily have to surrender all other aspects of their autonomy. Nursing can be directed towards maximising opportunities for independence within the allegedly 'safe' environment of the nursing home. However, in this context, as in any other, the value of minimising the risk of injury or loss can take precedence over the promotion of independence. For example, restrictions may be put on residents' independent social activity. They may be required to use a lift rather than the stairs, or their access to their own financial resources may be limited.

Nurses frequently make choices between two or more alternative courses of action which can be judged, depending on the observer's values, to have varying merit. The individuals involved in the situation (patients, relatives, nurses, other professionals) may or may not share similar priorities. Decision-making in these circumstances requires the nurse to identify the values and ethical principles which underpin each potential action, and to choose between options. Veatch and Fry (1987) suggest that differences in value orientation centre around issues of physical safety, psychological wellbeing and the maintenance of standards of ethical behaviour which derive from the wider culture.

Nurses, in the role of expert, may claim to know the 'real' risks facing patients, for example, that a patient who frequently falls when mobilising unaided is unlikely ever to be capable of moving around safely enough to be able to live independently. The patient, in contrast, might be determined to live independently, or to avoid reliance on equipment. Nurses who increase the level of supervision of the patient, or insist on the constant use of the zimmerframe against the patient's wishes, act on the traditional paternalistic principle of providing care which, they assume, serves the patient's best interests.

On the other hand, nurses who act out of respect for others' autonomy will follow care plans which allow patients the freedom to choose not to use the walking aids which have been provided, or to mobilise them when they choose. A nurse who acts in this way faces the ethical problem that they *'temporarily abandons her commitment to the health, welfare and safety of the patient'* (Veatch and Fry, 1987, p. 19). Conversely, the nurse who does *'what she thinks is in the interests of the patient's health, welfare and safety'* (Veatch and Fry, 1987, p.19) may challenge patients' autonomy if convinced that they are not acting in their own best interests. This dilemma can be considered, for the sake of the argument, on the basis that the nurse's knowledge of the patient's best interests is itself unproblematic. However unrealistic, its use permits analysis of the dilemmas which nurses would face even if risk knowledge was uncontestable, rather than predicated on embedded values, and on assumptions about the ways in which aggregated statistics should be applied to individuals.

## Respect for autonomy

### THE PRINCIPLE OF AUTONOMY

The concept of autonomy refers to an individual's ability to make rational decisions, and put them into practice. Autonomy, thus, requires a combination of personal attributes, for example comprehension of the situation, and social power to obtain relevant information and implement decisions. Diminished autonomy may result from symptoms such as the disruption of cognitive functioning, depression or severe pain, changes in social status, for example the stigmatisation of old age or disability, or from the withholding of essential information.

Debates about the extent of a patient's capacity to act autonomously often arise in health care. For example, advanced age is associated with an increased occurrence of multiple pathology and diminished cognitive functioning which may impair an individual's ability to think rationally.

However, many older people are healthy and capable of making rational decisions. Decisions about giving a patient choice require a prior judgement that they can reason rationally. However, judgements about rationality are underpinned by problematic notions of what is 'real', and are often based on prejudiced stereotypes. It would be unethical to dismiss the rationality of individuals simply because they belong to a particular social group. The clinical judgement that a person is not capable of acting autonomously, therefore, raises theoretical problems, although, in cases of severe disability, for example for the people with dementia discussed in Chapter 11, nurses may feel safe about making such judgements in practice.

Being autonomous and being treated autonomously cannot be equated. The former involves making, and putting into practice, informed decisions about one's own life. The latter refers to a moral obligation to respect the autonomy of others (Gillon, 1985). The principle of autonomy upholds the inviolable right of every individual to make decisions about matters affecting their own life. This principle does not give rise to rampant individualism, but places stringent limits on the transactions which ought to occur between individuals. Beauchamp and Childress (1994) argue that treating others autonomously requires both an attitude of acceptance of their choices and perspectives, and behavioural responses which help them to put their choices into practice. Unfortunately, in most human disputes, the autonomy of one party conflicts with that of the other, making the practical application of this moral principle problematic in the absence of consensus.

## AUTONOMY AS A HEALTH BENEFIT

Autonomy can be defended not only as a moral entitlement of persons, but as a powerful therapeutic agent in its own right, at least in Western cultures which cherish individual self-expression. The positive medical impact of creating conditions which enhance an individual's sense of autonomy have been highlighted in a study of elderly nursing-home residents (Rodin and Langer, 1977). In a field experiment, residents' perceived levels of control over their environment were manipulated. Two groups in the study were exposed to different pep talks about control and personal responsibility. Otherwise, both groups received similar care. The group urged to take more responsibility were found to be in significantly better clinical condition than the control group after three weeks, and after 18 months. Over this period, 15 per cent of the 'responsibility' group died, compared to 30 per cent of the comparison groups.

The causal mechanism underlying this striking long-term effect of enhancing individuals' autonomy cannot be identified clearly. Since the experiment was not 'blind', the beneficial effect of giving residents more autonomy may have resulted from subtle changes in the interactions between staff, patients, relatives and others. As argued above, autonomy can be considered as either an individual or a social attribute. Regardless of the cause, the results indicate that enhancing an individual's autonomy can benefit their health.

## RESTRICTING AUTONOMY

Respect for another's autonomy must sometimes be restricted. Unless this principle is accepted, all actions would have to be sanctioned regardless of their consequences. Patients' choices may harm themselves or others. For example, facilitation of independent living for an incapacitated older person in their own home might result in additional stress being placed on family carers. Situations involving conflicts of interest provoke debates about whose wishes should be upheld. Beauchamp and Childress (1994, p. 126) state that the justification for restriction *'must rest upon some competing and overriding moral principle'* such as beneficence or justice.

The judicial metaphor raises questions about how 'cases' are identified and decided. For instance, the family carers of people with dementia discussed in Chapter 11 were sometimes distressed by a professional's unsolicited suggestion that they should have their relative institutionalised in order to protect their own health. In such examples, the specification of a conflict of interests is itself disputed, and professionals, in effect, claim superior knowledge of clients' 'real' needs. Professionals who make such claims lay themselves open to the charge that they are biased, or influenced by organisational interests. They may be accused of blindly following the medical model, or of wanting to return vulnerable people to 'the community' in order to free-up hospital beds. Hence, professional claims to beneficence can themselves be questioned, and may be challenged particularly sharply by those whose autonomy they seek to curtail.

## AUTONOMY AND BENEFICENCE

The principle of beneficence lays an obligation on the individual to positively contribute to the welfare of others. This principle is unchallenged in healthcare ethics. Nurses and doctors are exhorted in their codes of professional practice to contribute positively to their patient's health and welfare. For example, clause 1 in the nurses', midwives' and health visitors' Code of Conduct (UKCC, 1992a) discussed earlier, emphasises their overriding obligation to promote patients' welfare, rather than merely to protect them from harm.

Beauchamp and Childress (1994) identify two principles of beneficence. The first involves an obligation to produce benefit within an interaction, and the second a requirement to balance benefit against harm. Their analysis focuses primarily on the outcome of such interactions. Other writers have argued that the obligation of beneficence derives from the nature of the relationship between individuals. Englehardt (1986) treats beneficence as a property of social relationships, arguing that they are based on the development of implicit contracts which create frameworks of obligation. Nurses' obligations to patients include making a positive contribution to their psychological welfare through empathic responses, and attempting to minimise their pain, promote their health, and protect them from foreseeable harm. At the same time, patients are expected to positively contribute to their health status, and comply with planned care. Kelly and May (1982, p. 154) have argued, from a symbolic interactionist perspective, that *'The good patient is one who conforms to the role of the nurse: the bad patient denies that legitimation.'* Patients who stray too far from the behaviour required by nursing staff risk becoming unpopular.

Both professionals and patients may make decisions which infringe the autonomy of others. Such decisions are fraught with potential for conflict between those affected, because their perceptions of the situation may vary, and may be underpinned by different values and beliefs. Nurses who make decisions which override patients' own wishes may be accused of acting paternalistically. The following discussion attempts to further explore the dilemma of autonomy versus beneficence in relation to the care of the elderly.

## Risk-taking in rehabilitative care: A moral dilemma

Nurses devising a programme of rehabilitative care need to assess its costs, benefits and limitations, and any risks entailed. In the absence of definite contraindications, such as cognitive incapacity, the nurse is clearly obliged to produce a care plan in collaboration with the patient. To the extent that they ground care plans in patients' wishes, nurses actively enhance their autonomy. In some, straightforward, cases, the nurse can simply do what the patient wants, and does not have to consider conflicting interests.

However, the nurse and the patient may disagree in their assessment of the situation, and disagreement may be underpinned by fundamental differences in values and beliefs. Both nurses and patients are influenced by their past socialisation and present social situation.

Before such questions are explored further, the patient's competence to make rational decisions must be established. However necessary, judgements about an individual's rationality raise notorious problems because of the difficulty of disentangling them from the judge's own belief system, as already noted. Moreover, where a person is deemed incapable of making rational decisions, the next of kin may act as a surrogate decision-maker. Legal requirements for surrogate decision-making vary, and this arrangement is not required in English law. (For an examination of the relevant case law, see Brazier, 1992). The use of surrogate decision-makers raises a number of concerns because it is almost impossible to separate the interests of the decision-maker and the individual who will be affected by the outcome of the decision. One approach to the difficulties involved in decision-making for incapacitated adults has been proposed by the Law Commission in England. The principles underpinning the proposal can be summarised as follows:

1.  Individuals should be encouraged to make decisions when they are able to do so.

2.  When others must make decisions on behalf of another, their interventions should be as limited as possible, and should attempt to achieve the desires of the individual

3.  The incapacitated individual should be protected from exploitation, neglect and abuse.

This framework attempts to maintain individuals' right to self-determination. However, significant difficulties remain about making decisions in the patient's best interest. In cases where the patient's rationality is not dismissed *a priori*, nurses face a dilemma if a patient makes a choice which they believe to involve an unacceptable level of risk. In these circumstances, do nurses uphold the patient's choice, thus respecting their autonomy, despite the risks involved? Or do they attempt to override the patient's choice and uphold the principle of beneficence?

Philosophers offer various strategies to resolve this dilemma. The strategy of lexical ordering (Veatch and Fry, 1987) asserts that when two principles conflict, one should be upheld at the expense of the other. For example, The President's Commission for the Study of Ethical Problems in Medicine and Biomedical and Behavioral Research (1983, pp. 26–7), concluded that:

> *when the conflicts that arise between a competent patient's self-determination and his or her apparent well-being remain unresolved after adequate deliberation, a competent patient's self-determination is and usually should be given greater weight than other people's views on that individual's well-being.*

Pellegrino and Thomasma (1988), however, maintain that the patient's best interests should be given moral priority, and that beneficence overrides autonomy where the patient wishes to act unwisely. Baumgarten's (1980) exploration of the concept of competence can be drawn on to support this position. He argued that the patient's voluntary decision to enter into an implicit contract with the doctor justifies the latter's paternalism. A similar argument could be applied to the nurse–patient relationship. This position entails the problematic assumption that, in some cases at least, professionals know more about patients' best interests than patients do. And, given that a sense of autonomy, itself, benefits health, as shown above, it implies that the harm done by restricting the patient's freedom is sometimes outweighed by the benefits of preventing them from acting unwisely.

Beauchamp and Childress (1994) treat these two positions as extremes, and recommend a midline proposition: that moral principles can never totally outrank each other. They argue that the principles of beneficence and autonomy need to be balanced, and that the relative priority given to each will depend upon the circumstances of particular cases. Unfortunately, this compromise provides limited guidance for nurses who are left having to reason about complex problems on a case-by-case basis. Husted and Husted (1991, p. 114) summarise the position for nurses as follows:

> *The recognition of a patient's autonomy and the motivation of a nurse's beneficence do not lead to one exclusive and justifiable decision. This is because the bioethical standards ... do not themselves, inspire a feeling of perfect confidence in any decision.*

Analysis of interaction between patients and nurses must take into account considerations of perceived power. The dilemma of autonomy versus beneficence only arises for professionals in so far as they believe that they **can** take decisions on behalf of competent patients. Nurses and other professionals may be able to control patients' and relatives' choices in various ways. First, they may control caring resources directly. For example, a purchaser decision not to provide community services, or a professional decision not to refer to community services, might preclude a patient with a disability from returning to their own home. Second, they may persuade the patient to comply with their advice through forceful advocacy, drawing on the cultural credibility of medicine. Third, in extreme cases, they may invoke legal constraints.

However, patients can often draw on personal resources to inform their decision-making. The credibility of all forms of expertise is tarnished, as argued in Chapter 1. In consequence, the authority of health professionals has become considerably eroded in the late modern era. Professionals who naïvely assume that they can take charge of decision-making may simply provoke reactive responses from patients whose determination to take unacceptable risks, as the professionals see it, is strengthened by the need to assert their autonomy.

Most bioethical dilemmas derive from the limits of medical efficacy. If medicine could provide a perfect, affordable, side-effect free cure for each consensually defined health problem with which it was presented, then most patients would happily agree to surrender their autonomy during treatment, as recommended by Baumgarten (1980). (Difficulties would still arise in the absence of consensus about the definition of a health 'problem', as in certain cases of 'mental illness', and, historically, in the treatment of homosexuality as a disease.) Health-risk management dilemmas about agreed 'problems' stem from the limitations of medicine.

## A dilemma for nursing theory

Where disability remains even after medical interventions, nurses, and other professionals concerned with wider aspects of health have to work with patients and relatives in order to help them to live within the restrictions of their remaining residual capacity. This issue is currently being addressed in the development of nursing theory. Modern nursing philosophies emphasise individualised care, and the creation of partnerships between care-providers and recipients. These philosophies have been explicated in the form of nursing models based on a wide range of ethical premises.

Drawing on the work of Fawcett (1989), Leddy and Pepper (1993) grouped the assumptions about change encompassed within each of 10 contemporary nursing models, into two categories, outlined below:

- Change theories based on the idea of homeostasis assume that human beings naturally seek stability. Change, within these models, is seen as a temporary deviation from a steady state, and the desired end point of any change process is the re-establishment of stability, albeit in a new state.
- Change theories based on the idea of inherent instability assume that individuals' internal and external environments alter continually. People change physiologically and psychologically throughout their lives, as do

the social environments in which they live, particularly in rapidly evolving modern societies. Change should be viewed as providing valuable and positive experiences for individuals.

Nursing models based on the assumption of stability, which Leddy and Pepper see as underpinning nursing models such as those of Roper, Logan and Tierney (1980), Orem (1980) and Roy (1980), assume that nurses should establish agreed and negotiated outcomes for each patient. The assumption that a steady and stable state can be achieved and maintained violates patients' lived experience of the disease process. A growing body of evidence highlights daily and cyclical changes in the physical, psychological and social processes associated with long-term disability (Anderson and Bury, 1988). A steady state is often maintained at considerable cost to the patient's autonomy, for example, in the institutionalisation of the elderly (Chapter 12), psycho-pharmacological treatment of those with mental health problems (Chapter 17) and blood-sugar regulation in diabetes (Chapter 8). Maintaining stability for patients in an uncertain and changing environment also places enormous demands on health-service resources, as staff are required to continually monitor patients' health, so as to eliminate small deviations and bring patients back to the agreed steady state.

However, nursing models which treat instability and continuous change as inherent elements of the human condition – a view which Leddy and Pepper see as underpinning nursing models such as those of Rogers (1970), Parse (1981), and King (1981), favour patient autonomy, as they suggest that only the patient can respond to continuous internal and external change. If change is assumed to be continuous, there are no fixed targets to aim for, and nurses and patients need to learn together, renegotiating and modifying their everyday interactions in order to accommodate changes, for example in emotional state, social circumstances or knowledge.

The nursing literature contains assumptions about change which, although implicit, powerfully influence professional responses to care dilemmas. Explication of these assumptions may help nurses to understand the forces shaping their practice, and may provide a framework for the ongoing negotiation of health-care interventions. The adoption of models which assume continuous change requires the extensive devolution of power and autonomy to practitioners, patients and family carers, and so challenges the hierarchical structure of health-care organisations.

Historically, health-care professions like nursing, faced with considerable uncertainty about most aspects of their work, have tended to err on the side of organisationally managed safety. This approach has resulted in the production of seemingly endless procedures and policies. More recently, evidence-based clinical guidelines (National Health Service Executive, 1996) have been produced in an attempt to increase the amount of information available to health care practitioners engaged in clinical decision-making. Abiding by policies, procedures and guidelines minimises the risk to the organisation of being held responsible for negligence in the event of an unsatisfactory outcome in an inherently uncertain environment (Tingle, 1996). In consequence, beneficence becomes equated and confounded with risk-avoidance.

However, professional beneficence, in this sense, is being increasingly challenged by substantive changes in the epidemiological and demographic profiles of advanced industrial nations. As the incidence of acute, deadly infections has declined, and living conditions have improved (Marmot and Elliot, 1992), emphasis has shifted towards the prevention, treatment and management of chronic diseases for which curative options are limited (Strauss and Corbin, 1988). Most *Health of the Nation* targets (DOH, 1992) are concerned with conditions such as coronary heart disease, cancer, stroke, mental illness. Managing the long-term trajectories of these long-term disabilities requires health care professionals and institutions to respond to the instability which characterise patients' attempts to accommodate their experience of these conditions within the changing patterns of their everyday lives.

Nurses may disagree among themselves, with patients, with relatives and with managers, about the relative emphasis to be placed on maintaining stability in the management of illness, or recognising instability and the processes arising from continuous change. All may oscillate between these two poles in response to changing events and circumstances. A health care organisation may support the promotion of patient autonomy until an accident occurs, and then revert back to an emphasis on safety policies. Following an accident, the nurses held responsible may find they are blamed by the patient, carers, colleagues and the host organisation. Conversely, nurses who play safe may be criticised for unimaginative nursing care which infantilises the patient, increases dependency and still fails to eliminate risk. Even in the apparently safest of environments, patients can still fall and sustain an injury, thus losing their autonomy without necessarily gaining safety. In some respects, the search for autonomy-promoting approaches to maintaining safety can be seen as the nursing equivalent of the hunt for the 'perfect' drug.

## Discussion

This chapter has reviewed the risks inherent in the negotiation of nurse patient interactions during the provision of nursing care. It has identified two competing ethical principles which provide a dichotomous framework for analysing this aspect of care. One principle seeks to maximise beneficence, through decisions which promote the patient's best interests, while the other seeks to maximise patient autonomy. In many cases, beneficence and autonomy promotion will not conflict because no obvious treatment of choice can be identified, patients are presumed to be capable of choosing rationally, and the exercise of autonomy is deemed therapeutic in its own right, as illustrated by the discussion, above, of the Rodin and Langer (1977) study.

However, when nurses or other professionals are confronted with situations where, in their judgements, a patient's decision is clearly not in their best interests, the principles of beneficence and autonomy will conflict, and the professional will be faced with the ethical dilemma discussed in this chapter. The professional's concern will involve the patient's wish to take risks which the professional judges unacceptable, as when a frail elderly person wishes to return home but the professional feels that they are not capable of doing so safely. However, professionals will sometimes encourage clients to take risks which clients find unacceptable, as with some of the adults with learning difficulties discussed in Chapter 9.

The consumerist ethos enshrined in recent government policy has favoured the autonomy side of the argument. The extent to which patients actually feel they have more choice following the reforms, and the extent to which, in various contexts, they want or do not want more choice, can both be questioned. However, the balance of official opinion, and the atmosphere in which nurses have to work, has shifted towards autonomy. The assumption that doctor, or nurse, knows best is greeted with considerably more scepticism than it would have been in 1948, at the birth of the National Health Service. But, at the same time, professionals can be held accountable when society judges that they have 'allowed' patients to take 'unacceptable' risks, as when an elderly, independent person refuses help, and dies alone, in distressing circumstances.

The transition from a paternalistic health-care model to one emphasising patient rights and autonomy poses many difficulties for health-care practitioners who may position themselves at different points to their health-care employers, and even to their colleagues, on the continuum from beneficence to autonomy. Moreover, individual positions on this continuum may ebb and flow as events unfold and circumstances change. This oscillation can be very disconcerting for practitioners, as organisational policies and public expectations can, at times, appear contradictory.

Risk management is an inescapable element in nursing practice, and manifests itself continuously in the daily decisions nurses make. Risk can never be eliminated, as the safety of patients cannot be guaranteed even if they give up all autonomy. On the other hand, blanket autonomy cannot be given to all patients, because their freedom might create unacceptable risks to the wellbeing of others, or they might risk self-harm but lack the capacity to take rational decisions.

The categorisation of nursing models by Leddy and Pepper (1993), presented above, both raises the dilemma of risk versus autonomy in a theoretical form, and provides a framework for developing practice and research. More research is needed into the microprocesses of negotiation and decision-making along the autonomy/beneficence and risk/safety continua. Better understanding of the impact of these processes on both patients and nurses can contribute to the specification of an appropriate infrastructure of support which will enable practitioners to develop confidence in their ability to support patients through these complex decision-making processes.

# 16

# Child protection and the management of risk

## Margaret Moran and Richard W. Barker

## Introduction

Both government and the wider society are determined to ensure that children should, as far as possible, be brought up free from the risk of abuse. The child-protection system is underpinned by a generally held belief that it minimises the risk of abuse. This view, in turn, depends on the assumption, recently questioned (Jackson, Sanders and Thomas, 1995; Corby, 1996; Parton, 1996) that abusive behaviour can be predicted.

The prevalence of child abuse depends on how it is defined (Cleaver and Freeman, 1995). For example, if the definition includes smacking, then a high number of children will be classified as at risk (see below). The cultural theory of risk (Douglas, 1966, 1985) maintains that cultural groups emphasise dangers which affect the core values holding them together. Deliberate harm by parents against their children, particularly sexual abuse, violates the most fundamental bond in our society. It is widely treated as a far more serious danger to children than, for example, the risks associated with traffic and child poverty (Jackson, Sanders and Thomas, 1995).

What, if anything, is considered abusive to children varies considerably between different historical periods and cultures. In the nineteenth century, sparing the rod meant spoiling the child, but physical punishment has been made illegal in some European countries. Poor Nepalese and Thai villagers openly sell their daughters into urban prostitution. Male and female circumcision can each be viewed positively or negatively according to religious beliefs, and opposing beliefs may be held even within the same religious group. Defenders of the female version remain concerned that a failure to circumcise may reduce the marriageability of their daughters, and thus be a cruel act. Since social value systems change continually, and are affected by external influences, disagreements within societies concerning what should count as abuse may be expected.

Until recently, the child-protection system in the UK has tended to focus on intrafamilial abuse, and to ignore other sources, such as risks to children in residential care. At the time of writing, in 1996, the government had highlighted the latter by ordering an inquiry following disclosures that hundreds of children and young people have been sexually abused in Clwyd and Cheshire. The perceived victimisation of these young people has led politicians like Stephen Dorrell to move from labelling them as deviant and criminal to defining them as one of the most vulnerable sections of our community (BBC Radio News, 13 June 1996). This chapter, however, will be concerned solely with intrafamilial abuse.

## The historical and organisational context of child protection

Current debates about risk and child protection must be analysed in their recent historical and organisational context. Four influences on the development of child-protection services in the UK since the 1960s are outlined below.

### THE BATTERED BABY SYNDROME

Kempe *et al*. (1962, p. 24) defined the battered baby syndrome as follows:

> The battered child syndrome is a clinical condition in young children who have received serious physical abuse, and is a frequent cause of common injury or death. Although the findings are quite variable, the syndrome should be considered in any child exhibiting evidence of possible trauma or neglect, or where there is a marked discrepancy between any clinical findings and the historical data as supplied by the parents.

The notion of the battered baby influenced practice on both sides of the Atlantic. Parton (1985) argued that professionals who promoted the baby-battering concept had agendas other than simply discovering a problem and responding to it. The medicalisation of abuse gave the concept additional gravitas, and underpinned calls for a more formal organisational response. As well as preventing harm to children, formal recognition of child abuse could serve to improve professional standing. In the UK, the NSPCC vigorously publicised both the problem and their contribution to its management. This strategy helped to ensure the survival and growth of the NSPCC, an organisation whose future looked precarious at that time.

### THE DEVELOPMENT OF SOCIAL SERVICES DEPARTMENTS

The Seebohm Report (1968) crucially influenced the development of modern social service departments. The Committee's Report recommended the merging of the three small-scale local authority Children's, Welfare and Mental Health Departments into an integrated, generic local authority service for families. From April 1971, social services departments, rapidly to become large-scale bureaucracies, were established. They were more concerned, at the time, with juvenile delinquency than with child abuse, which was considered a potential causal factor in delinquency rather than a problem in its own right. However, social services departments soon came to give child abuse and neglect greater priority than juvenile justice.

## PUBLIC INQUIRIES INTO CHILD-PROTECTION CASES

Over the last 25 years, a series of public inquiries has highlighted the risks to children in families of being abused. The inquiry into the death of Maria Colwell in 1973 sparked central and local government to develop procedures designed to improve inter-agency communication, and so reduce the probability that services would fail to respond effectively when children were at risk. This inquiry marked the beginnings of a trend to hold professionals responsible for not protecting children, rather than simply blaming the abusers. Subsequently, over 30 public inquiries have been held. Some have had a significant impact on professional and public responses to the risk of child abuse and neglect. For example, the inquiry into the death of Jasmine Beckford, in 1985, triggered a tightening-up of procedural guidelines. The inquiry into child sexual abuse in Cleveland (DHSS, 1988) influenced the passing of the 1989 Children Act, currently the main civil legislation concerned with child abuse and neglect.

While valuable lessons have been learnt from such inquiries, they can create the false impression that the risk of abuse can, ultimately, be eliminated. The Beckford inquiry (London Borough of Brent, 1985, p. 288) illustrated the confusion which surrounds thinking about risk, by saying on the same page, 'We do not define high risk mainly because we do not think it is susceptible to definition', and 'The attempt to isolate such [high risk] cases from the majority of child abuse cases must always be made'. The risk of child abuse will never be eradicated completely in societies like the UK. Power over the lives of children rests firmly with parents, and agents of the state may intervene in the private arena of family life only in strictly defined and regulated circumstances.

## THE INCREASING REGULATION OF CHILD-PROTECTION WORK

Since the early 1970s, the procedural regulation of child-protection work has increased massively, with the twin aims of regulating the state's intervention into parent–child relationships, and improving practice. The DHSS publication *The Battered Baby* (1970) gave advice to agencies on the management of cases. A further circular (DHSS, 1974) emphasised the need for the co-ordination of services through the mechanism of case conferences. Following the death of Maria Colwell, local Area Review Committees, consisting of representatives from health, welfare, education and justice agencies, were established (DHSS, 1974), with mainly advisory powers to monitor area child-protection services. In 1976, central government mandated local authority areas to establish confidential at-risk registers, in order to keep track of children deemed to be at risk of further abuse or neglect. Following implementation of the 1989 Children Act, *Working Together under the Children Act* (DOH, 1991, pp. 6–7) confirmed that each local authority area (133 in 1995) should have an Area Child Protection Committee with the tasks of co-ordinating, monitoring and reporting on local child-protection services.

'At-risk' registers, usually held by local social services departments, have been renamed 'child-protection' registers. They record all children in the area about whom there are both child-protection concerns, and interagency plans to respond. At least biannual reviews of such cases have to be undertaken. Children's names are placed on these registers if it is considered that one or more identifiable incidents of abuse have adversely affected the child, and that further incidents are likely; or if future significant harm (a concept drawn from the 1989 Children Act) to the child is expected. Four different categories of registration can be used, all centrally concerned with the 'risk' of abuse or neglect, although the term features explicitly in none of them.

The four categories (DOH, 1991, pp. 48–9 ) are:

**Neglect:** The persistent or severe neglect of a child, or the failure to protect a child from exposure to any kind of danger, including cold or starvation, or extreme failure to carry out important aspects of care, resulting in the significant impairment of the child's heath or development, including non-organic failure to thrive.

**Physical injury:** Actual or likely physical injury to a child, or failure to prevent physical injury (or suffering) to a child, including deliberate poisoning, suffocation and Munchausen's Syndrome by Proxy.

**Sexual abuse:** Actual or likely sexual exploitation of a child or adolescent.

**Emotional abuse:** Actual or likely severe adverse effect on the emotional and behavioural development of a child caused by persistent or severe emotional ill-treatment or rejection.

Counts of children's names on registers do not measure the extent of child abuse, but do give one indicator of official state activity. On 31 March 1994, 34 900 children were recorded on the English registers, a rate of 31.7 per 10 000 of the population under 18. During the previous year, 28 500 children's names had been added and 26 200 children's names removed from the registers (DOH, 1995).

## The child-protection system

Perceptions of abuse depend on the social context. Public opinion can have a substantial effect on both public policy and the detailed working of the child-protection system. For example, in 1987, a public inquiry was instituted in Cleveland, amid widespread concern that children had been forcibly removed from home on the basis of insufficient evidence of sexual abuse. The outcome shaped policy and practice for the future, and influenced the Children Act 1989, which emphasised the need to assess the child in context, and to consider placing children within the family where possible. Child-protection agencies are expected both to eliminate the risk of abuse going undetected, and to avoid disrupting non-abusive families. Similar problems of balancing sensitivity and specificity can be found in all preventive endeavours based on selecting critical cases with imperfect predictive tools, for example in maternal genetic testing (see Chapter 7).

When public and professional opinions do not correspond, the public are likely to see any professional action as unreasonable, and the various stakeholders may lose faith in the efficacy of the system. The degree of public support for the child-protection system will, in turn, depend on the extent of shared understanding of the concept of 'risk'. Lay people and professionals generally agree that drastic preventive action is required in 'heavy end' cases involving severe beating, physical injury, sexual abuse or serious neglect. In 'grey' areas, involving less severe damage and less convincing evidence, the public sometimes deem professionals to be heavy-handed.

Debate between professionals and lay people over the appropriateness of current levels of state intervention rages strongly in this area. Cleaver and Freeman (1995, p. 157) cite recent research from both the UK and the US (e.g. Creighton 1988; Crittenden, 1988) indicating *'an increasing preoccupation with less serious cases'*. Cleaver and Freeman (1995, p. 6) suggest that *'Social workers fear that every case is a Jasmine Beckford tragedy.'* Even if abuse is confirmed, children will usually remain at home, and parents may receive help. However, the difficulty involved in assessing the risk of child abuse is illustrated by the West case. In 1995 Mr West committed suicide in prison, and his wife was found guilty of complicity in the murder of a number of children, including some of her own. Justice and welfare agencies contacted the West children several times, but interpreted what they judged to be minor instances of abuse as indicative of a relatively normal family situation.

The following hypothetical case (see Figure 16.1) will highlight some of the main issues in contention.

---

### The case of Jenny Bond

Six-year-old Jenny Bond is taken to the hospital by her grandmother who has noticed bruising on her legs and weals on her bottom. Jenny is in pain, and whimpered when her Gran was drying her after the bath. When questioned by her Gran, Jenny said that her younger brother, Jack had hit her. But as he is only three this, Gran thought this unlikely.

Jenny lives with her Mum, Joan, aged 31, her Dad, Robert, aged 50, and three brothers. Jenny, the second youngest, is the result of an affair between Joan and her boss at work. Robert forgave Joan, accepting the child as his own, although Gran says that he treats her more harshly than the others, and that she takes care of her more.

Both parents work, Joan as a senior administrator in a law firm, and Robert as owner of a haulage company. They live in a modern house on a large estate. No previous family problems have been recorded. Robert is currently seeing a psychiatrist because he is depressed. He has said that he smacked Jenny to punish her for defiance. Joan thinks that the whole business has got out of hand. Robert, she says, is a very caring father, has accepted Jenny as his own, and really wanted a daughter anyway. She feels that he disciplines the children appropriately, and that they would not have been subjected to so much fuss if her mother had not overreacted.

What issues do you feel are raised by this case, and what is your reaction to what has happened?

---

**Figure 16.1**   The case of Jenny Bond

Consideration of the issues raised by this case, and of the way in which the child-protection system might respond, will help to highlight the points at which public and professional opinion may vary. Twenty years ago, this case would probably not have been brought to the attention of the child-protection system. Although the bruises to the child might have aroused some concern, it was generally believed, at that time, that smacking did little harm, and that parents were entitled to discipline their children. Minor injuries would have been seen as no more than a sign of over-chastisement, rather than abuse.

## THE STAGES OF WORK IN CHILD-PROTECTION CASES

*Working Together under the Children Act 1989* (DOH, 1991) highlights six stages of the child-protection process, each of which would include risk appraisal. The stages are:

1   Problem identification and referral
2   Immediate protection and investigation planning
3   Investigation and the initial assessment
4   The initial child-protection conference, and possible registration
5   Comprehensive assessment and planning
6   Implementation, review, and possible deregistration.

Child-protection agency involvement might cease at any of these stages if the child was judged not to be suffering presently, or at serious risk of future harm. Such decisions must now be taken multi-professionally, in partnership with parents, rather than by a single agency. The notion of 'partnership' is contentious to many practitioners, as it ignores power differences both between professionals and parents, and between parents. Partnership, therefore, can at times be particularly hard to achieve, but research, albeit undertaken before the implementation of the 1989 Children Act, for example by Cleaver and Freeman (1995), suggests that the non-involvement of parents can lead, often unintentionally, to abuses of professional power, or to decisions which, although made with good intentions, prove counterproductive. Professionals face the dilemma that they must treat parents as a potential source of both problems and solutions.

### Problem identification and referral

Behaviour which might be classified as abusive affects many children who are not referred to helping agencies. In our case study, Jenny was taken to a hospital where her injuries were recognised, and seen as indicative of possible abuse. A referral has been made to the child-protection agencies. A designated member of the hospital staff would check the child-protection register, to look for entries which might indicate any previous abuse of Jenny or her siblings. Until recently, hospital accident and emergency staff would not have been trained to recognise abuse, and would not have had a statutory obligation to pursue such a matter further.

## Immediate protection and investigation planning

Once a referral has been made, immediate decisions have to be taken about the current risk to the child. Jenny might be admitted to hospital for a short period (if beds were available) while her injuries were treated, and to safeguard her. If her parents refused consent, and Jenny was felt to be significantly at risk, consideration would have to be given to applying to a magistrate for an Emergency Protection Order (Section 44, Children Act 1989), to enable the local authority to protect her for an initial period of up to eight days. The main agencies involved at this stage might be social and health services, and the police. They would have the difficult task of collaborating, and working in partnership with the parents, while protecting the child from the risk of future harm. Social services would take primary responsibility for the management of the case at this time.

## Investigation and the initial assessment

The preliminary assessment aims to gather information which may lead to a decision not to proceed with an initial child-protection conference, because the professionals involved are satisfied that there is no further significant risk to the child. If they are still concerned about the risk to the child, the information will be used at the child-protection conference in order to decide what further action, if any, should be taken. Many investigations of isolated, less severe incidents do not progress beyond this initial stage, because the professionals agree that further involvement is not needed (Cleaver and Freeman, 1995, p. 63).

However, because of the risk to agencies of making a mistake, they tend to lean towards caution. As in the case of defensive medicine, the optimal balance of risks for the service-provider may not be in the best interest of the child or the family. Agencies are unlikely to be censured for being overprotective in cases like that of Jenny. Parton (1996, p. 101) cites the conclusion of the Audit Commission (1994) *'that much field social work time is used in carrying out inappropriate child protection investigations'*.

The conduct of the initial assessment, a process described by Cleaver and Freeman (1995) as *'the confrontation stage'*, also gives rise to problems. These researchers found that, in a context of suspicion, parents and professionals were unlikely to share their perspectives. Parents felt guilt and shame, tried to conceal what was happening within their community, and attempted to present themselves as favourably as possible. In communities where hostility toward the child-protection process meets with some general approval, parents can receive wider support for being unco-operative towards professionals. Parton (1985) points out that the vast majority of child-abuse referrals come from poor communities, not necessarily because abuse occurs more frequently there, but because agencies police them at a higher level than in more affluent areas.

Previous involvement with professionals, and the experience itself, may influence parents' attitude towards the initial assessment process. Farmer and Owen (1995) found that a greater degree of co-operation between professionals and families at an early stage was associated with a more successful outcome for the child. This study found, as did Cleaver and Freeman (1995), that 70 per cent of parents became more sympathetic to professional concerns as the inquiry unfolded, and came to regard it as having conferred some benefits. Parents may be persuaded, through good professional practice, to accept professional concerns, despite, or perhaps because of, their fears of losing their children, or of criminal prosecution.

At this stage the immediate context of the suspected abuse would be considered. For example, a cigarette burn on a child's hand might indicate deliberate cruelty, or result from an accident. Such ambiguities are difficult to resolve unless a history of injuries can be uncovered. Evidence, for example from the GP, might uncover a previous history of apparent accidents. Questions would then need to be asked about whether the child was being neglected, or subjected to non-accidental injury.

The nature of the abuse would also be considered. In our case example, it is alleged that Jenny has been smacked. Research suggests a wide divergence between professionals and lay definitions of physical abuse. Most parents hit their children, even babies in nappies. A recent British study (Smith et al., 1995, pp. 83–5) concluded that 91 per cent of their sample of children, and 75 per cent of those under the age of one, had been hit, although half of the parents interviewed thought that they should not have been. A majority of the public would probably see the father's behaviour in our case study as excessive, but within the normal range of permissible parental behaviour towards children. Many adults have themselves been beaten by their own parents, and commonly believe that 'It never did us any harm.' Half of the children interviewed thought that their parents should smack them, and intended to smack their own children. Child-protection professionals who do see such behaviour as problematic define normal behaviour and risk factors differently. Risk appraisal, in each case, is embedded in implicit or explicit normative judgements.

Professionals have to decide whether the abuse which, as they see it, has occurred puts the child at risk. A plethora of research suggests that abuse has short- and long-term adverse effects on children. For example, Gibbons, Thorpe and Wilkinson (1990), found that physically abused children were more likely to show behavioural problems at home and at school, had greater difficulty with relationships, and scored lower on certain cognitive tests. However, this study also found that when physical abuse occurred as an isolated event, and was not associated with neglect, sexual abuse or a generally violent family climate, the outlook for the child was relatively good. Such research provides a justification for professional intervention, but has to be treated with caution as a guide to risk factors. The studies rely on correlational data, and may confound identified abuse with other possible risk factors such as socioeconomic deprivation or family stress. They are generally based on known cases, and may confound the damaging effects of the abusive behaviour with adverse consequences of the child-protection process itself, such as stigmatisation, family breakdown, being taken into care. These consequences arise through the processes of reflexive recursion, as discussed in Chapter 2.

As with any other complex social or health category, the concept of abuse provides an 'iconic device' covering a wide range of phenomena. At the extreme, physical violence to children which causes serious injury, and clearly sexual contact between parents and young children, are widely rejected as unacceptable in contemporary Western cultures. However, in 'grey' areas, as in our illustrative case study, the classification of parental behaviour as abusive is contentious. Whether the child is seen as being at risk will depend on whether marginally acceptable/unacceptable parental behaviour is categorised as abusive, and so as launching the child into the damaging trajectory identified in epidemiological research.

So many interacting variables affect child development that the consequences of particular forms of 'abuse' on individual children cannot be predicted with certainty. Research-based risk analysis must therefore fall back on aggregate estimates of future probabilities which do not allow outcomes in individual cases to be forecast. But professionals have to make decisions about individuals, taking into account both the risk that child-protection intervention might cause secondary damage, and the risk to the child, the family and their own standing if an eventually serious case remains undetected.

In the present case, the investigation suggests that the physical abuse is an isolated event, but that it has occurred in a context of long-term family problems.

## The initial child-protection conference and possible registration

The initial child-protection conference is used, primarily, for the exchange of information between professionals and family members, and to decide whether registration will be required. However, practice seems somewhat variable. Giller, Gormely and Williams. (1992) found, in each of four geographical areas, that official guidelines provided for professionals did not discuss risk analysis. Farmer and Owen (1995, p. 159) concluded that risk assessment varied in thoroughness depending on which method was chosen, and that certain patterns of reasoning were used *'over and over again in the run-up to the final decision'*. They give examples of four methods of assessment: summing up all the concerns, cumulatively; comparing present and past situations for the child, to plot a future trajectory; focusing on specific incidents or abusers; and attempting to unravel family dynamics. Farmer and Owen comment on the lack of a shared theoretical framework between professionals, and conclude that the overuse of any one assessment method necessarily precludes discussion which could enhance effective decision-making, especially where complex issues of race, gender, class and disability are involved.

Thoburn, Lewis and Shemmings (1995, p. 133) concluded that, in terms of the *Working Together* guidelines, the conference was probably or definitely not needed in about one-quarter of the cases. As already noted, in an atmosphere of intense media and public concern, professionals seem to be minimising the risk of failing to prevent tragic consequences, thereby accepting the higher risk of the damaging effects of intervention. A case known to the authors illustrates the way in which intervention may, recursively, increase the risk it was designed to prevent. A school reported that a pupil had been severely bruised, and the child confirmed that his father had hit him the previous evening. A visit to the family followed. The father, a large and intimidating man, and the mother both expressed anger with the child for telling the school nurse what had happened. The professionals decided that the investigation had increased the risk to the child, who was temporarily removed on a Place of Safety Order, as it was then known. A child-protection conference was then held.

Recent practice has been influenced by a financially driven constraint, not yet documented, in that convening professionals for informal meetings has become virtually impossible. Agencies, attempting to manage limited resources, will often only agree to attend formal meetings. In consequence, families are inadvertently moved up the risk escalator (see Chapter 2) to a higher intensity of procedure than the severity of the case would have warranted if less formal options could have been selected.

In our illustrative case, the parents describe their marital relationship as poor at the initial child-protection conference, but say they intend to stay together for the sake of the children. The father's depression is linked to business trouble, and debts which threaten the family home. Jenny has said that her dad had never hit her this hard before. She had been asked three times to set the table for her Mum coming home, and had continued watching television. Her dad went 'mental', and hit her with a big wooden spoon he was using to stir the bolognese sauce. She says that he cried afterwards, and apologised, and that he doesn't usually pick on her. All the family agree that Jenny is Dad's favourite. Even Gran accepts that her father does spoil her, and that she went over the top when she saw Jenny's bruises. The parents agree they need counselling, as the father's medication does not seem to be working, and acknowledge they have never really worked through the aftermath of the wife's affair.

The decision to register the child is based on a judgement by parents and professionals that there has been at least one identifiable incident of abuse which has adversely affected the child, and that future significant harm to the child is likely. Practice examples, in the authors' experience, suggest, however, that professionals are using registration as a means of gaining resources for children and families. As with the case conference, organisationally driven attempts to ration and control resource allocation has the unintended consequence of pushing families up the risk escalator.

Jenny would probably not be registered according to standard criteria, given the absence of evidence suggesting a probability of future harm, and indications that the family are actively seeking help. Thoburn, Lewis and Shemmings, (1995, p. 133) noted that 62 per cent of cases resulted in the child being registered, but that, in many other cases, a decision was made to offer help to the family or the child. Some parents welcomed the offer of services, even though the child's name was not placed on the register. In our case, the psychiatrist might offer counselling to the parents. The conference can only make a decision about whether or not the child should be registered, and on the identity of the key worker. (All children who are registered would be allocated a key worker charged with overseeing and co-ordinating the treatment plan.) Otherwise, responsibility for managing the case falls to the individual agencies involved. However, the conference can make recommendations, for example about whether police action should be taken against the abuser. Thoburn, Lewis and Shemmings, (1995) observed that such action was deemed necessary in only 9 per cent of the cases they examined.

Child-protection conferences must make complex, difficult decisions. Farmer and Owen (1995) found that the key agencies participating were health, education, police and social services. But, with the exception of health visitors, the health services were not well represented. Farmer and Owen noted that where senior health workers were involved, they often said very little, (or nothing at all in 10 per cent of the meetings) as their main aim seemed to be to supervise the health visitors. This lack of health-service representation, they felt, has implications for treatment as well as assessment, as health professionals often possess information about other family members, for example the mother, which can help the conference in planning intervention. They also found that participants' degree of influence depended on their status.

Most conferences now include parents, but their contribution varies according to local custom, and may involve full participation, or attendance only at parts of the conference where decisions are not being made. Mothers attend more commonly than fathers. As a result, women become responsible for both the problem and the solution, even where the abuse has been mainly carried out by a father or partner. Both parents and children have great difficulty in participating effectively in such an intimidating context, particularly when the family come from a minority ethnic group, and communication is affected by language difficulties or cultural differences.

## Comprehensive assessment and planning

In a minority of cases, the initial child-protection conference recommends that further assessment should be undertaken before services are provided. Browne and Saqi (1988) identified five different models which professionals have used to explain child maltreatment, and to underpin comprehensive assessment.

**Psychopathic:** Fifty years ago child abuse was thought to be a rare event. In North America, it was seen as the result of organic illness suffered by known perpetrators.

**Social or environmental:** Problems of housing, unemployment and other social issues have been linked to aggressive behaviour.

**Special victim:** Some studies (e.g. Rusch, Hall and Griffen, 1986) have suggested that certain children 'provoke' abuse. For example, premature babies tend to have a high-pitched cry, which mothers may find irritating. Children with learning difficulties, disabilities, health or behavioural problems can put stress on parents and increase the likelihood of abuse.

**Psychosocial:** This model suggests that certain social and psychological factors can make some adults, for example those who have been mistreated themselves, more prone to abuse children.

**Integrated model:** It is now broadly accepted that a combination of all the above factors will play a part in the abuse of children.

If the initial child-protection conference had recommended a comprehensive assessment, it would have adopted an integrated approach, and considered the economic and social circumstances of the family, the mental health history of both parents, their own history of abuse, and the circumstances surrounding the child's behaviour. Questions would be asked of the parents, about whether they thought that their relationship had an impact on what happened to Jenny; of the doctor, to ascertain whether they felt the father's depression had contributed to what happened; of the grandmother, about whether she thought that the way the father was reared had had any impact; and of Jenny, about her behaviour, and its effect at the time of the smacking.

The comprehensive assessment should be used to generate a care plan, the implementation of which is intended to ameliorate the factors judged to have led to the abuse, and to reduce future levels of risk. However, the multifactorial, interactional causation of abuse makes prediction of its recurrence problematic (Jackson, Sanders and Thomas, 1995) and its management difficult.

### Implementation, review and possible deregistration

Children whose names are placed on the child-protection register should become the subject of an interagency plan which is formally reviewed every six months. If the child is judged to be no longer at risk, they would be deregistered. Farmer and Owen (1995, p. 274) found that, after 18 months, 80 per cent of the children had been deregistered. The interventions which professionals and parents at the deregistration conference judged to have been successful included counselling, material help and psychiatric treatment. However, the impact of these interventions on the risk of abuse, and their long-term effects, remain uncertain.

Farmer and Owen (1995) found varied parental reactions to the removal of their child's name from the register. Those who had felt stigmatised by registration, or concerned about the spread of gossip in the community, were relieved. Others regretted the loss of valued social work support.

## Discussion

The child-protection system lacks a well-validated risk-assessment methodology. Previous tools have included, for example, a checklist of predisposing factors such as the extreme youth of the mother, or observation of eye contact between mother and baby. But these instruments have been discredited because of the risk of false negatives and positives. Most young mothers do not abuse their children, while an older mother with the potential to abuse might not be detected. Despite huge investment, the effectiveness of the child-protection system in reducing the risk to children has not been established. As in other preventive industries, those on the payroll have an interest in not questioning its value.

A comparatively simple, although not uncommon, case has been used to illustrate some of the issues involved in child protection. Child sexual abuse, for example, raises more complex issues, in relation to detection, treatment and criminal justice. In such cases, co-operation between family members and professionals may be less likely. The involvement of the criminal-justice system, and the time taken to bring cases to court, will also delay the provision of help to the child.

In only a small number of cases do things go badly wrong, although it does not follow that disaster is avoided in other families **because of** the child-protection system. Its preventive value is simply unknown. The scapegoating of professionals, both for being over-zealous, and for failing to protect children, is associated with the intense publicity given to these cases. Dracup, in Chapter 5, discusses the power of hindsight effects (e.g. seeing the probability of an event leading to disaster as higher if you know that one has actually occurred) and argues that those who conduct official inquiries need to know much more about such psychological processes.

In the absence of sound risk indicators, the central dilemma of sensitivity versus specificity remains. If the scale of investigations is reduced, the number of horrendous cases which are not detected, or detected too late, may increase. If the scale of investigation is increased, then more families will suffer adverse consequences, including stigmatisation, stress and family break-up, from being caught in the child-protection net. Child-protection involves multiagency, multiprofessional activities which raise complex moral, political and clinical questions. It is designed to work, in partnership with families, to protect children and to manage risk. To work effectively, those involved in assessing risk in child-protection cases need not only professional knowledge and expertise, but also public support, and understanding of the risk-management dilemma they face.

# Risk and community care for people with mental illness

# 17

Heather Scott

| |
|---|
| Introduction |
| Schizophrenia and risk |
| Labelling and risk |
| Discussion |

## Introduction

*He thinks he's Jesus. You think he's a killer. They think he's fine.* (SANE, 1989, Poster)

This caption, used in a 1989 poster campaign by the charity SANE (Schizophrenia, A National Emergency), encapsulates widely differing perspectives about the risks associated with 'mental illness'. Few health issues have been more in the public eye in the UK in recent years than the treatment and care of people diagnosed as mentally ill. Their situation has many parallels with those described elsewhere in this book, but differs in two important respects. First the nature of 'mental illness' is contested particularly intensely. Second, specific legislation has been developed, in the UK, as in many other countries, with the aim of controlling the behaviour of people diagnosed as mentally ill in certain circumstances.

Very few people diagnosed as suffering from 'mental illness' pose a significant threat to others (Joseph, 1993). However, the UK media have, in recent years, drawn public attention, often in a sensationalist way, towards a number of tragic cases, most of which involve killings by someone with a history of psychiatric problems. A more detailed and considered picture of these events has been provided by the reports of the independent inquiries which must be held following fatal incidents. Thirty-six such reports were published between 1985 and 1996, with a number still in progress (Sheppard, 1996). The reports contain painstaking accounts of the circumstances leading up to the fatal incident, sometimes traced back over many years, and provide examples of risk appraisal.

As a result of these cases, much professional attention is now directed at improving the assessment and management of risks associated with mental illness. However, risks are viewed selectively, as argued in Chapters 1 and 2. Consideration of the position of people with mental health problems raises a number of challenging ethical and social issues. This chapter examines the dominant preoccupation with the perceived dangerousness of people categorised as having a serious mental illness. The discussion focuses on schizophrenia, the diagnostic label born by most of the individuals who have been the subject of recent public attention in the UK, with illustrations from selected reports of independent inquiries, particularly *The Falling Shadow* (Blom-Cooper, Hally and Murphy, 1995), and the *Report of the Inquiry into the Care and Treatment of Christopher Clunis* (North East Thames and South East Thames Regional Health Authorities, 1994).

The first Report describes the mental health care received by Andrew Robinson until, in September 1993, he murdered Georgina Robinson (no relation), an occupational therapist working at the mental health unit in which he was detained as an inpatient. Andrew, a white male, aged 36 years at the time of the attack, had first been diagnosed as schizophrenic some 15 years previously, following an assault, involving a shotgun, on a young woman with whom he had become infatuated. He was convicted, and ordered to be detained under the 1959 Mental Health Act in Broadmoor, a secure psychiatric hospital. He was released in 1982, and the restriction order was discharged in 1986. Following his conviction for the manslaughter of Georgina Robinson, Andrew Robinson was again detained, under the Mental Health Act 1983, and readmitted to Broadmoor Hospital.

The second Report mentioned above contains an account of contact between health and social services and Christopher Clunis, a young Black man, prior to his murder of Jonathan Zito, a complete stranger, at a London underground station, in December 1993. As a result, Clunis was, like Robinson, detained, under the Mental Health Act 1983, in Rampton Special Hospital.

## Schizophrenia and risk

Schizophrenia is one of the most feared, as well as controversial, of diagnoses. Over the past 40 years, the nature and even the existence of mental disorders such as schizophrenia have been widely debated by psychiatrists, philosophers and sociologists. Although psychiatrists now widely accept that 'schizophrenia is pre-eminently a condition which responds to changes in social circumstances' (Bebbington and Kuipers, 1993, p. 82), biomedical approaches remain dominant in the field of treatment and care. Doubt exists about whether 'schizophrenia' describes a single entity or a number of different phenomena, and many issues remain a source of contention among psychiatrists, patients and their families. These issues include the role of genetic factors in the aetiology of schizophrenia, the relationship between relapse and family interaction, and the value of long-term medication (Rogers, Pilgrim and Lacey, 1993; Solomon, 1994).

Despite such controversies, few would dispute the negative impact that 'schizophrenia' can have on the lives of patients, their families and the wider community. Forty years ago, people experiencing such distress and disability would, almost inevitably, have been detained compulsorily in a psychiatric hospital, often for the remainder of their lives. Today, most patients live outside hospital, and inpatient treatment is limited to brief admissions during acute phases or relapse. However, a significant number of patients, particularly those from ethnic minorities, find currently available services neither appropriate nor acceptable. They tend to have contact with services only at points of crisis, against their will (Bingley, 1995; Moodley, 1995).

Table 17.1 identifies major risks which have been associated with 'schizophrenia', and suggests their probable direction. Although not comprehensive, this list does illustrate the multidimensional range of the negativities associated with schizophrenia. According to epidemiologists, schizophrenia is found in all cultures and societies. Individuals throughout the world have a lifetime chance of 1: 100 of developing the disorder (WHO, 1973). Figures for outcome vary, but transcultural studies have found that patients do significantly better in the developing than in highly industrialised countries (Sartorius, 1989, p. 195). In developed countries, only 15.5 per cent of those experiencing a first acute episode of schizophrenia have no relapse or impairment. About 26 per cent experience multiple episodes and some impairment, and almost 20 per cent suffer severe, continuing disability. The figures for developing countries are 37 per cent, 12.8 per cent and 12 per cent respectively (Sartorius, 1989, p. 201). These differences may result from cul-

**Table 17.1**   Risk and schizophrenia

| Risk type | Risk most likely to whom? |
|---|---|
| Labelling effects | The patient |
| Loss of civil rights | The patient |
| Side effects of medication | The patient |
| Economic exclusion | The patient |
| Homelessness | The patient |
| Exploitation by others | The patient |
| Long-term emotional effects | The patient and relatives |
| Family stress | The patient and relatives |
| Verbal and physical aggression | The patient, relatives and professionals |
| Accountability, litigation and inquiries | Professionals |
| Costs of treatment and care | The public |

tural variations, for example in the social labelling and stigmatisation of deviant individuals.

Within individual countries, certain groups may be more likely to receive the diagnosis of schizophrenia, and to have poorer outcomes. In Britain, young African-Caribbean men experience very high rates of diagnosis of schizophrenia, admission to hospital and treatment through coercive means (Fernando, 1995). Browne (1995) explains the greater use of coercion with this group, through detention in locked wards, high doses of medication, and categorisation as 'offender-patients', in terms of the professional and public stereotying of young African-Caribbean men as violence prone.

## Labelling and risk

The media, in the UK, often discuss deaths associated with mental health problems in a sensationalist and stigmatising manner, with headlines such as 'Freed to kill in the community' (*Daily Express*, 2/07/93) and 'Mistakes let psychopath kill' (*Daily Telegraph*, 30/04/96). However, this heightened public concern about the dangerousness of mentally ill people living in the community is not universally shared in other countries. As well as giving examples of positive media coverage of issues associated with mental illness in Italy, Ramon (1996) points out that the UK appears to be alone in Europe in introducing training courses designed to teach nurses and other workers how to respond to violent behaviour. The present author's own discussions with providers of public mental health services in the United States and Australia suggest that they do not share the UK preoccupation with the risk of the mentally ill becoming violent.

In theory, two possible explanations for this cultural variation can be suggested. First, the incidence of violent assaults by former psychiatric patients might be higher in the UK than in comparable countries. Second, heightened concern might result from cultural selective attention to the risk of mentally ill patients becoming violent, as ideological changes emphasising individual responsibility rather than social rights have increased the 'otherness' of people who do not conform, including those with mental health problems (Marshall and Bottomore, 1990). Estimates of the real incidence of serious violent offences carried out by mentally disordered people vary, but one comprehensive study in Germany (Hafner and Boker, 1982) estimated that only 0.05 per cent (5 per 10 000) of people suffering from schizophrenia committed violent offences.

Media use of words such as 'turned loose' (*Daily Telegraph*, 26/09/95) and 'caged' (*Newcastle Journal*, 30/03/96) associate the idea of the containment of dangerous wild animals with mental illness. As shown in Chapter 4 with respect to HIV-positive people, the media communicate the dangerousness of feared social groups through images, metaphors and symbols rather than through quantitative statistics.

Politicians react to public and media concerns, but decide how strongly to respond, and whether to try to exacerbate or to calm public fears. The Conservative Health Minister pledged, when announcing the proposed

*Patients Charter: Mental Health Services* (DOH, 1996a), that patients would not be sent home if there was the *'slightest risk to carers, relatives or the public'* (Community Care, 11–17/1/1996, p. 1). Such overblown political claims, implying the possibility of total risk removal (Crichton, 1995), devalue the positive aspects of the Charter, particularly assurances about service quality, and fail to recognise that adversity can never be fully predicted or prevented. Thus a small number of sensational cases exert a disproportionate effect on public policy, leading to the prioritisation of security and protection for the public over treatment needs (Joseph, 1993).

The adverse effects of such policies may be felt by patients who are not prone to violent behaviour as well as by those who are, with neither group receiving appropriate treatment and care. Christopher Clunis could not be admitted to hospital in April 1988 when he was psychotic, and in need of assessment and treatment, because no beds were available (North East Thames and South East Thames Regional Health Authorities, 1994). At the same time, it has been estimated that half of all patients in Britain's three secure psychiatric hospitals do not need the high levels of security they provide (Community Care, 29/6–5/7/1995).

## Risk dilemmas and mental illness

### MENTAL ILLNESS AND VIOLENCE

The focus of public and political attention on the tragedies described in the inquiry reports has contributed to a change in social attitudes towards people with mental illnesses. In earlier stages of the shift from institutional to community care, 'risk' was seen in more positive terms, as a necessary element in the enhancement of individual independence, choice and quality of life for patients (Personal Social Services Council, 1977). As for people with learning difficulties, rehabilitation programmes preparing patients to return from psychiatric hospital to the community were devised as sequences of small steps which, when successfully accomplished, would give the individual, their family, and the public, confidence in their ability to live with greater freedom and autonomy. Such positive reinforcement was expected to lead to the increasing integration of patients into the 'community', and, in turn, to reduced levels of patient stress and the consequent risk of relapse. In this virtuous circle, individuals would progress to the point at which they could live with little or no support from mental health services.

The success of this downwards 'risk escalator' (see Chapter 2) has been widely questioned. It depends on the creation of 'therapeutic alliances' between patients, professionals and others involved in their care, and on the provision of appropriate support. The evidence from reports such as that on Christopher Clunis convey a picture, not of calculated and sensible risk-taking with therapeutic aims, but of professional neglect. Individuals experiencing mental health problems, particularly those who do not fit the system, or whom professionals find difficult to work with, often receive a piecemeal service, characterised by a succession of brief contacts which preclude adequate need assessment. All too often, such fragmented intervention results only in the prescription of medication. In the absence of any therapeutic alliance, service-users are likely to discontinue medication, and to be reluctant to seek further help from psychiatric and social services. Lack of appropriate response to their mental health needs may lead to increasing stresses, for example difficulties with benefits and homelessness, which, in turn, exacerbate the initial mental health problems. If their mental health continues to deteriorate, patients' behaviour may become increasingly disturbed, resulting in harm to themselves or others, bringing them to the attention of the police, and making them the target of coercive action. Thus the fears of the public are realised, and stereotypes reinforced. The escalator, in practice, takes patients upwards towards maximal risk-avoiding intervention and constraint on their autonomy.

Such upward spirals continue to occur despite evidence both of the cumulative disabling effects of repeated psychotic episodes (Bhugra and Leff, 1993), and of the effectiveness of intervention systems which identify and respond to 'early warning' signs of relapse (Falloon and Fadden, 1993). 'Risk' now seems synonymous, in the public's mind, with the danger of violence to others, even though the mentally ill are more likely to harm themselves than others. The otherness of the mentally ill is further reinforced when it is combined with the otherness of being racially or ethnically distinct, as with Black people, over-represented under the forensic sections of the Mental Health Act (Browne, 1995).

Mental health legislation has always reflected a shifting balance between the protection of the rights of the mentally ill individual, on the one hand, and of society on the other. In the UK, the Mental Health Act 1983 emphasised the former, and the number of compulsory admissions fell in the years immediately following its implementation. However, this trend has been dramatically reversed, with a growth of 55 per cent in compulsory admissions between 1989–90 and 1994–95 (DOH, 1996b, p. 53). Recently, a series of new measures, designed to increase the level of supervision and control of discharged patients, has shifted the policy balance back towards the protection of society. These measures have included the Care Programme Approach, Supervision Registers and, most recently, the introduction of Supervised Discharge under the Mental Health (Patients in the Community) Act 1995.

Despite public concern, the increased risk of those diagnosed as suffering from schizophrenia becoming seriously violent is small (Boyd, 1996, p.82). According to the recent *Report of the Confidential Inquiry into Homicides and Suicides by Mentally Ill People* (Boyd, 1996), people classified as legally abnormal are responsible for less than one-fifth of the homicide convictions in Britain, although to these must be added those who commit suicide after the killing. People with schizophrenia pose more threat to themselves than to others, being 100 times more likely to kill themselves than another person (Hafner and Boker, 1982). Where psychotic patients have murdered, the killings have often occurred in situations of upset or relationship crisis (Joseph, 1993). In this respect, they do not differ from those carried out by the rest of the population. In around half of violent offences committed by people with schizophrenia, the victim was associated with the delusional system of the offender (Joseph, 1993).

The random killings of strangers, such as the murder of Jonathan Zito by Christopher Clunis occur, contrary to public perception, much less frequently (North East Thames and South East Thames Regional Health Authorities, 1994). However, the perceived threat to public safety posed by former psychiatric patients in the community, and illustrated by the emotive wording of the SANE poster, has provoked moral panic (Cohen, 1980).

## PROFESSIONAL AND LAY PERSPECTIVES

Professional views often stand in sharp contrast to those of both the public and the families of people with schizophrenia. Inquiry reports show that professionals repeatedly minimised the significance of violent incidents. For example, Christopher Clunis committed a series of violent attacks over a four-year period, but only one charge of breach of the peace was brought.

The most valuable information about Andrew Robinson was provided by his parents, but their concerns were frequently ignored, particularly where their views conflicted with those of experts. The inquiry report contrasts the report of a home assessment carried out by a community psychiatric nurse with a letter to the psychiatrist from Andrew's father less than three weeks earlier (Blom-Cooper, Hally and Murphy, 1995, p.98). The former's assessment read:

> Andrew appeared relaxed and was very friendly, imparted information freely, and there was no evidence of any psychotic symptoms ... I was impressed by the way in which Andrew presented himself today and I think that his time in Torquay has been beneficial to him. (Blom-Cooper, Hally and Murphy, 1995, p. 98)

Andrew's father wrote:

> I think I ought to let you know that my wife and I are not at all happy about Andrew, who has become very 'high' recently. This may not be immediately detectable in a short interview, but to us as his parents it is only too clear ... But his basic illness is the real cause – he continues to 'hear voices' (or however one describes it). (Blom-Cooper, Hally and Murphy, 1995, p. 98)

Elsewhere, Andrew's father wrote to the visiting registered nurse:

> I am sure you are aware that, since ceasing to take medication last November, Andrew has become very unwell, and as always when he refuses medication, we know (from 16 years experience!) that it can only end in some disaster. We feel as though we are sitting waiting for a time-bomb to go off! (Blom-Cooper, Hally and Murphy, 1995, p. 144).

Official reports contain numerous examples of desperate but unanswered appeals from parents and other close relatives, friends and voluntary workers. Such appeals produced no response, or ones that complainants found grossly inadequate in relation to the intensity of the concerns they had expressed. Professionals and family carers appear, sometimes, to have different priorities with respect to risk management.

Both maximising and minimising concern about the risk of mentally ill people being violent towards others may have damaging consequences.

Maximising risk concern increases public fear, leading to greater stigmatisation and avoidance of the mentally ill. As a result, patients may experience increased stress which, in turn, increases the risk of relapse into psychosis, and thus brings about a self-fulfilling prophecy, as argued above. Defensive practice by professionals may lead to periods of detention which are longer, and in more secure conditions, than would otherwise have been judged necessary.

Minimisation may have positive advantages for the individual, reducing the damaging consequences of labelling, limiting the iatrogenic effects of medication and institutional care, and increasing autonomy. However, if an optimum balance between autonomy and need for the support and supervision necessary to maintain recovery is not achieved, these strategies may increase the risk of patient violence both to others and to themselves. In forming judgements about the optimum balance, mental health professionals need to consider the following two critical issues. First, the therapeutic validity of a risk-minimisation strategy for a patient depends on the assumption that individuals will respond positively to environments which maximise their autonomy (see Table 2.3, Chapter 2). But relatives often believe, rightly or wrongly, that the patient's illness prevents them from benefiting from a normalising strategy. Second, professionals may base their decisions on knowledge of the low **population** incidence of violence. But, as pointed out in Chapter 2, such general information does not allow the behaviour of **individuals** to be accurately predicted (Gigerenzer, 1991).

One consequence of 'care in the community' has been a shift of responsibility for care of people with mental health problems (as well as other groups of service-users) from trained professionals to untrained family members and volunteers. Solomon (1994) estimates that between 30 per cent and 90 per cent of discharged patients return to their families. Families are major providers of care, but the voice of those closest to the person with schizophrenia often remains unheard (Creer and Wing, 1974). The inquiry reports on Andrew Robinson and Christopher Clunis, discussed above, indicate that even people who have severely disordered ideas can often conceal their problems from professionals during a brief contact. Because of the time they spend with the individual, relatives and other carers may well have the fullest and most accurate knowledge of a patient's changing mental state. But, paradoxically, because of their low status, as non-experts, in the health and social care system, lay people may find that their views are ignored or discounted by professionals, particularly where assessments conflict or professionals are required to ration scarce resources. However, those personally involved with a patient, for example close relatives, may feel that they, not professional gatekeepers, would be most affected if anything went wrong.

## COMMUNICATION AND CONFIDENTIALITY

Problems of information transmission play an important part in failures of care. Here, professionals face another dilemma, as they have to balance concern for confidentiality and informed consent against the requirement to base risk assessment on adequate information. Ethical considerations about confidentiality can sometimes be used to legitimise neglect.

Mental health professionals clearly found Christopher Clunis difficult to work with, and *'the more disturbed [he] became, the less effective care he received'* (North East Thames and South East Thames Regional Health Authorities, 1994, p.37). People with relevant information, including his sister, were not consulted. By regarding him as homeless, a succession of professionals, particularly social workers, were able to treat him as a short-term 'case', and thereby justify not seeking further information about his previous circumstances and history of contact with mental health services. On occasion, professionals used client consent and confidentiality as reasons for not seeking further information. Similarly, a doctor and community psychiatric nurse did not disclose Christopher Clunis' history of violence to residential staff caring for him on the grounds of confidentiality (North East Thames and South East Thames Regional Health Authorities, 1994, p.48).

The report on Andrew Robinson also complained that *'information that was available failed to register, while information that was not readily at hand was not sought'* (Blom-Cooper, Hally and Murphy, 1995, p.139). The risk which Andrew presented was underplayed, not least by the repeated minimising of his 'index offence', involving a shotgun, for which he had been committed to Broadmoor (Blom-Cooper, Hally and Murphy, 1995, p.139).

For mental health professionals, caution in disclosing information about patients may indicate respect for their privacy and autonomy. However, the examples demonstrate the possible consequences of unwillingness or failure to share information with others involved in providing care and support. Moreover, there is some evidence that families of people with serious mental illness are given less information than relatives in coronary care units and trauma centres. Such a *'lack of critical information can elevate a health crisis to a catastrophic disaster'* (McElroy and McElroy, 1994, p. 243).

## MEDICATION AND RISK

The maintenance of neuroleptic medication, which can produce side effects ranging from unpleasant sensations to Parkinsonism and permanent neurological damage (tardive dyskinesia), produces further dilemmas. While in Broadmoor, Andrew Robinson was constantly troubled by the side effects of prescribed medication, and was subsequently noted to be suffering from akathisia and drug-related movement disorder (Blom-Cooper, Hally and Murphy, 1995). Similarly, Christopher Clunis complained of the side effects of medication, and sought to see a psychiatrist about his symptoms on two occasions, in 1989. On the first occasion, no action was taken. On the second, he refused to accept the prescribed depot injection unless he was given an appointment to see a psychiatrist. An appointment was made, but with a six-week waiting time and, in the event, the psychiatrist did not see him for 13 weeks (North East Thames and South East Thames Regional Health Authority, 1994). This lack of prompt response suggests both a minimisation of Christopher Clunis' difficulties (perhaps in comparison with other demands on resources available at that time) and a possible reluctance to engage with service-users perceived as 'difficult' or unco-operative.

A psychiatrist who believes that maintenance of medication is required to prevent a patient relapsing into a psychotic state may discount their complaints about side effects. The psychiatrist may prioritise reducing the risk of relapse, while the patient balances this risk against a current quality of life which may be damaged by unpleasant physical and mental sensations caused by the pharmaceutical regime. Patients may also resent being offered only medication in response to wider problems of money, accommodation or loneliness (Rogers, Pilgrim and Lacey, 1993). Too often, medication becomes a battleground between psychiatrist and the patient. family carers frequently become alarmed at the deterioration they perceive in their relative's mental state when medication is not taken, but they and their relative often seek help in meeting a range of other needs, for accommodation, work, and social support.

## RELAPSE AND RECOVERY

Clinicians and service-users may hold sharply divergent views about the priority which should be given to avoiding relapse. Clinicians may share the view of McElroy and McElroy (1994, p. 252) that relapses involve *'unpleasant, frightening experiences that are to be avoided because evidence exists that some patients never regain their previous level of functioning'*. Patients, however, have to balance future uncertainties against present need, for example to escape from an unstimulating environment, or to avoid drug side effects. As Kersker (1994, p. 334) argues: *'Risks may lead temporarily to relapse and re-hospitalisation, but a static environment is deadly to recovery.'*

## Discussion

The inquiry reports considered in this chapter give examples of good practice generating positive results, even with patients reluctant to engage with services, and able to conceal disturbed thoughts and feelings. In the case of Andrew Robinson, a period of successful care was achieved by means of a Guardianship Order (under Section 7 of the Mental Health Act 1983) combined with a detailed care contract, and well co-ordinated multidisciplinary teamwork (Blom-Cooper, Hally and Murphy, 1995, pp.136–7). Research provides more general evidence of the effectiveness of well-planned systematic approaches to treatment and care. The Maudsley Outreach Support and Treatment Team (MOST) has reported that 90 per cent of service users (70 per cent of whom were Black) were successfully engaged. Significantly, no violent incidents or suicides occurred (Moodley, 1995, p. 132).

However, in the absence of appropriate and acceptable services, or of any services at all, compulsory admission and prison become the only available options. Patients like Christopher Clunis, perceived as unco-operative, may well have asked for help at some point, but have received a minimal response or not been followed up. Individuals who do not fit the system or who *'collide with services'* (Moodley, 1995, p. 121) are most likely to lose out in such circumstances. A lack of any social services mental health provision in Oxfordshire before 1990 was acknowledged at the inquiry following the murder of Jonathan Newby by John Rous (Davies, 1995). Specific service and policies may be poorly co-ordinated, particularly in the disjointed internal 'market' created by the NHS and Community Care Act 1990. But the inquiry reports demonstrate that people coping with severe difficulties and chaotic lives need cohesive care.

The reports (Sheppard, 1996) document individual tragedies for victims, perpetrators and their families. They contain many recommendations aimed at preventing similar situations in the future. However, with the exception of *The Falling Shadow* (Blom-Cooper, Hally and Murphy, 1995), they do not provide recommendations at the level of the structure or organisation of services: a surprising omission, given the evidence, in many of the reports, of the fragmentation of services and poor communication. The reports do, however, draw attention to the lack of resources available for those with serious mental health problems. Professionals are faced with the overwhelming task of allocating scarce services, time and beds to meet the urgent and competing needs of people in acute distress. Unable to offer the stability, consistency and relationships that many service-users need, they are obliged to ration resources by limiting intervention to a series of piecemeal short-term responses to complex, often long-term, needs. In this no-win situation, they, like the child-protection workers, discussed in Chapter 16, frequently resort to defensive practice.

Government policy, in the UK, supports a case-management approach. Thornicroft (1993, p. 420) describes case management as *'a unifying concept which promises to represent a patient group where there has been neglect, to integrate services where there has been fragmentation, and to offer care shaped by the needs of the patients rather than of service providers'*. The risk of the mentally ill becoming violent, so alarming to the public, the media and politicians, could be dramatically reduced if resources could be found to fund better services. The WHO has estimated (Sartorius, 1989, p. 324) that *'approximately 50 per cent of all mental, neurological and psychosocial problems could be prevented if there existed the political will to do so and if concerted action by all concerned could be brought about'*. To date, this political will appears to be lacking. Segregating those classified as dangerous appears to be the *de facto* treatment of choice, although it is not necessarily cheaper, over the long term, than offering decent mental health services to all in need.

# 18

# Reconceptualising risk in health-promotion practice

## Susan Milner

## Introduction

This chapter begins by briefly discussing the definition of risk within the practice of health promotion. The reductionist, epidemiological framework within which risk is usually conceptualised in health promotion is then critically reviewed. Expansion of the discourse relating to risk in health promotion is then explored, and it is argued that the predominant medical paradigm acts as a conceptual and theoretical constraint on the development of health-promotion practice. A paradigm shift is required to facilitate the development of a new approach, based on a holistic approach to health and healing. Such an approach acknowledges health as a state of balance between environmental and social influences, and recognises both the interdependence of mind and body and natural healing processes.

## Health and health promotion

Health promotion, as a field of study and practice, attempts to improve the health status of individuals and communities. It is, therefore, an umbrella term covering activities ranging from individually focused health education to changes in public policy, and legal and fiscal measures. Professional and lay people undertake such activities in a broad range of settings, using a variety of approaches. There have been many attempts to define what health promotion actually 'is' or sets out 'to do'.

> [Health promotion incorporates] diverse, but complementary, methods or approaches, including communication, education, legislation, fiscal measures, organizational change, community development and spontaneous local activities against health hazards. It offers new challenges to existing professional groups, commerce and corporate bodies, cultural norms and the inertia of health institutions ... it reiterates the 'Health for All' components of intersectoral action and advocacy for health, stressing the need to go beyond health care and equity in access to a healthy life. (Kickbusch, 1986, pp. 437–8)

This definition emphasises efforts to change both behaviour and social structures, and so reflects a shift away from 'health education' as the only health-promotion method in use.

Analysis of the professional practice of health promotion requires prior consideration of the nature of health and its determinants. These conceptual issues have been well rehearsed elsewhere (WHO, 1948, 1984; Dubos and Pines, 1965; Seedhouse, 1986; Aggleton, 1990). 'Health' emerges as a complex phenomenon differentially defined and experienced by individuals and communities.

Patterns of ill health in industrialised societies have changed since the middle of the nineteenth century. Infectious diseases have been replaced, as the main killer conditions, by chronic degenerative diseases such as heart disease and cancer. This shift is often referred to as the 'epidemiological transition' (Wilkinson, 1996) and is associated with an important change in professional health-promotion practice. The untreatability of these diseases has led to increased scrutiny of the causes of ill-health, but not to a serious search for the determinants of health (Antonovsky, 1984). However 'health' is defined, it is linked to an individual's life experience through complex causal pathways.

## Determinants of ill-health: The 'web of causation'

Epidemiology involves the study of ill-health in populations rather than in individuals, and provides the main theoretical driving force for the professional practice of health promotion in the developed world. As pointed out in Chapter 2, risk analysis which attributes population parameters to individuals operates through a heuristic device which may distort as well as illuminate. Contemporary epidemiologists acknowledge that an individual's risk of contracting specific diseases depends on many interacting and interdependant variables: the 'web of causation' (MacMahon, Pugh and Ipsen, 1960; Susser, 1985; Krieger, 1994). This web depends, for its empirical survival, on statistical techniques of multivariate analysis. The underlying model of pathogenesis assumes that improvements to the public's health depend on experts' ability to identify 'risk factors', and to predict the results of breaking supposed chains of causality or, at least, selected strands of the causal web. Thus, the epidemiologist's view of public health depends on statistical notions of risk, rather than individuals' personal experience of their own health. Current professional health-promotion practice is based around these supposed risk factors.

However, Krieger (1994) argues that the widespread adoption of this form of causal reasoning and risk analysis may be misplaced. She believes that too much emphasis has been placed on issues of epidemiological methods, and on questions about the validity of causal inferences involved in the web of causation, while too little consideration has been given to what she terms 'epidemiological theory' i.e. explanations of the changing patterns of health and ill-health in different societies. The societal dynamics of health (the why) are ignored in favour of the modelling of complex relationships between supposed risk factors (the what).

This trend may reflect the professionalisation, in the 1950s and 1960s, of a growing medical breed, the epidemiologists, who inherited a research philosophy and agenda from the world of acute infectious disease, which they then attempted to apply to the emerging reality of chronic degenerative diseases. Most research was based on individually oriented theories of disease causation, with population risk treated as the sum of individual risks resulting from lifestyle and genetic factors. Single agent-germ theories of disease were replaced with more complex models of 'host, agent and environment'. Advocates of social medicine focused attention on 'social determinants' of health, and epidemiologists responded with new study designs and statistical methods, including the *'approximation of prospectively determined relative risks with odds ratios derived from case-control studies'* (Krieger, 1994, p. 890). These clumsy epidemiological formulae attempt to mechanistically reduce the many elusive and interacting variables which impinge on health status to the mathematical, population-based, equations of risk assessment. The types of risk factors usually included in this web of causation are summarised in Table 18.1.

The importance attributed to different types of risk factor in health promotion has shifted over the past 30 years. The weightings attached to risk factors determine how (and by whom) health promotion is undertaken. Traditionally, and still predominantly, efforts to improve health have concentrated on disease prevention through narrowly defined forms of health education which focus on individuals and their behaviour. Certain behaviours are classified as bad for health, for example smoking, drinking too much alcohol, not taking exercise, not making proper use of health services. This approach to health promotion is based on the notion of individual choice. It assumes that people can, and should, protect their health by following the health promoter's expert, epidemiologically based advice, and has been criticised as 'victim-blaming' (Ryan, 1976).

This simplistic model of health maintenance does not take into account the determinants of a person's health status other than individual lifestyle choices. Notions of risk in health promotion began to expand in the late 1970s to include the social and economic determinants of health (Tudor Hart,

Table 18.1   An epidemiological perspective on the web of causation

| Individual risks | Environmental/social risks |
| --- | --- |
| Inherited disease susceptibility | Pollution |
| Physiological variations | Housing |
| Biological threats (e.g. infection) | Education |
| Preconceptual or *in utero* exposure to risk factors | Income |
| Lifestyle risk factors | Employment |
| | Access to transport |
| | Ethnicity |
| | Social class |
| | Area of residence |
| | Access to services |

1971; Townsend and Davidson, 1982). Populations living in areas of multiple deprivation experience higher morbidity and mortality rates than the rest of the population. These health inequalities have not been reduced by the introduction of the NHS, or by the efforts of health promoters over the decades, and may be increasing (Whitehead, 1987; Townsend, Phillimore and Beattie, 1988; Phillimore, Beattie and Townsend, 1994; Wilkinson, 1996).

Since the mid-1980s there has been a further shift in risk-factor assessment, to include an array of environmental factors thought to impact on health. Godlee and Walker (1991, p. 1124) argue that the unhealthy habits of *'an energy hungry and throwaway society'*, rather than the behaviour of individuals, have the most serious detrimental impact on health. After many years of lobbying from pressure groups, environmental sources of health risks, for example threats to the safety of the air, water and food supply, have started to attract more mainstream attention. In consequence, the need to consider health issues alongside industrial, agricultural and transport policy, and to combat the vested interests of powerful, international commercial organisations (Hancock, 1993), have been highlighted.

The politics and practice of health promotion have, to date, predominantly focused on the above types of risk factor, as they are the ones that have been identified and studied. Within the risk categories just discussed, individual lifestyle variables have been given the most attention because their control requires little action from the political system. But are these the right risk factors? Are they only ones that matter? How do all these risk factors interact at the level of the individual? Do other unidentified and unstudied aspects of human experience have an impact on health?

As epidemiology extends its empire, everything becomes 'risky': being a man or a woman; poverty or opulence; employment or unemployment;

being old or young; living in a town or the countryside. The risk-factor approach to health promotion assigns huge numbers of individuals to the halfway-house status of being 'at risk'. These individuals have no clinical pathology, no symptoms, have usually made no approaches to the medical services, but come under the medical gaze, and are subjected to proactive, and often unwelcome, attempts to reduce their supposed risk status. If life is so risky, how can risk be avoided? But risk is not a neutral term. It is socially constructed and ideologically loaded (Lupton, 1993; Skolbekken, 1995). It can be used to blame the individual for their own ill-health. Instead of 'lives' people now have 'lifestyles'. Private health has become public property. Illnesses, such as heart disease, and conditions which put individuals into categories marked as high risk, for example obesity, are increasingly seen as a sign of misbehaviour. Some lifestyle features, for example smoking or having multiple sexual partners, are officially challenged, while others, such as mountain-climbing or regular car-driving, are considered acceptable even though they carry at least as much health risk (Fitzgerald, 1994).

A health promotion agenda directed against selected disapproved behaviours was reinforced by the publication of the first national health strategy for England, *The Health of the Nation* (DOH, 1992). As a result of this strategy, most professional health-promotion resources are now being concentrated on disease prevention in the following areas:

- Coronary heart disease and stroke
- Cancers
- Mental illness
- HIV/AIDS and sexual health
- Accidents

and associated risk related to:

- Smoking
- Diet and nutrition
- Blood pressure
- Injecting drug use
- Alcohol consumption
- Sun-bathing
- Sexual practices

Attempts to reduce exposure to these 'risk factors' involve the promotion of individual behaviour change through health education and/or social engineering tactics such as fiscal or legal measures. A proliferation of vertical health-promotion programmes, focusing on either an ill-health problem, such as CHD, or a risk factor, for example exercise, has resulted. Health-promotion practice thus mirrors medical practice by compartmentalising human experience.

Preventing diseases or injuries before they occur seems to make good sense, in theory at least. Health-promotion professionals agree less about what needs to be done at a practical level to bring about these desired improvements in public health, or even about what these improvements should be. These difficulties are well illustrated in the government's *Health of the Nation* strategy which focused professional health-promotion efforts on individually oriented lifestyle-change issues, and excluded other determinants of health.

## Iatrogenesis

Health-promotion professional practice aims to improve public health in a variety of ways (Downie, Fyfe and Tannahill, 1990; Tones and Tilford 1994). Most interventions are designed to prevent disease, through encouraging immunisation, mass screening, control of occupational health and safety hazards, and educating the public about health and lifestyle issues (Stone, 1986).

In all these areas, however, attempts to promote health can be counterproductive, as argued in Chapter 1. Vaccinations carry a 'small' risk to individuals, for example the risk of brain damage to children receiving the whooping-cough vaccine. Immunisation is no longer seen as an unmitigated benefit to the community, and some parents do not accept that they should run the private and individual risk of brain damage to their child in order to protect the whole community for the public good. After years of campaigning to persuade parents to position their babies face-down to sleep, this advice has now been shown to be incorrect, and may have contributed to the incidence of cot deaths (Ogden, 1993).

The promotion of high-factor screens for sunbathers may simply encourage users to stay in the sun for longer (McGregor and Young, 1996). Screening programmes, whether for high-risk groups or for the general population, are also fraught with problems such as test inaccuracies (see Chapter 7), increased anxiety, overtreatment, and uncertainty over the impact of early diagnosis on prognosis (Oliver, 1992; Clarke, 1995a; Raffle, Alden and Mackenzie, 1995). Such activities should not simply be accepted at face value as self-evidently beneficial, but should be subjected to constant scrutiny and critical review.

## A new science of health

Disenchantment with mainstream medical practice is growing, as is the number of people seeking advice and treatment from other types of healer. At the same time, research is progressively undermining the paradigm on which the practice of modern medicine is based (Capra, 1975, 1982; Chopra, 1989; Zohar, 1991; Zohar and Marshall, 1994).

The return, in terms of improved health, of many medical practices cannot be readily identified. Modern medicine is often credited with improving the health of the population through its victory over the 'germ'. However, closer examination of the past epidemiology of the major infectious diseases reveals that they were already declining before the introduction of immunisation and antibiotics, as a result of wider social improvements, such as clean water, and better sanitation, housing and nutrition (Powles 1973; McKeown, 1979).

The *Oxford Textbook of Medicine* (Horrobin, 1988, p. 2.1) argued that:

*Medicine has acquired the attitude of pure science where things are done with no clear practical end in terms of benefit to the patient. With perhaps two exceptions, peptic ulcer and renal failure, there is no common disease in which it is possible to demonstrate convincingly that those receiving treatment in 1985 are much better off than those receiving the best treatment in 1960. In other common conditions there is nothing that medicine has done which has dramatically improved either the survival or the comfort of patients.*

Medical practice has had little effect on the nation's health at a population level. It has been estimated that only about 5 per cent of deaths in the UK can be prevented through 'good' medical practice (Martini *et al.*, 1977). Western biomedicine has had little impact on overall death rates from cancers and heart disease, our biggest killers (Jacobson, Smith and Whitehead, 1991). Martini *et al.'s* study (1977) found, for every indicator assessed, that socioeconomic status predicted morbidity and mortality rates better than the provision of local medical services. MacKenbach, Bouvier-Colle and Jougla (1990) drew the same conclusion, even though they confined their analysis to a group of conditions, accounting for about 10 per cent of all deaths, which medical experts identified as most preventable through good treatment.

Although medicine, to date, has had less impact, at the population level, than socioeconomic factors, some forms of treatment do improve the quality and/or quantity of life for individuals, for example hip replacements, cataract removal, appendicectomy. To illustrate this point by analogy Wilkinson (1996, p. 66) suggests that an army medical corps may provide a highly effective and beneficial service to those on the battlefield, without influencing the number of casualties in a battle.

Limited improvement in the treatment of many diseases has been matched by a lack of progress in preventing major health problems such as cancer, diabetes, heart disease and mental illness. Weir and Whittaker (1996) argue that the failure to effect improvements across such a broad spectrum of activities should call into question the explanatory power of the underlying theoretical paradigm. Unanswered questions include:

- Why do some people with 'unhealthy' lifestyles stay well?
- Why do some people with 'healthy' lifestyles become ill?
- Why do poorer people have worse health status?
- Why do some people diagnosed as terminally ill recover completely?
- How is the placebo effect to be explained?
- Why do people who retire often die quickly?
- Why does the death of a spouse lead to increased morbidity and mortality for the survivor?
- Can people literally lose heart?
- Why are the above questions largely ignored within mainstream medical practice?

## What's wrong with the current paradigm?

Capra (1982) has argued that medical practice still operates within the mechanistic paradigm about life which developed from the ideas of René

Descartes (1596–1650) and Isaac Newton (1642–1727). Bunton and MacDonald (1992, p. 231) define a paradigm as:

*A wider concept than theory. It constitutes the agreed upon way of looking at and interpreting the world, or a particular field of study, and predicts the course of further investigations and study. A theoretical paradigm refers to the context within which a theory exists.*

Kuhn (1962) argued that scientific thinking does not evolve smoothly, but progresses through periodic revolutions, as an existing paradigm is increasingly challenged by new thinking, and eventually becomes redundant, replaced by a new way of looking at the world.

The mechanistic and reductionist paradigm which still prevails in medicine emerged from attempts in the sixteenth and seventeenth century to break free from the perceived dogma and superstition of the day. Galileo argued that science should restrict its investigations only to objective properties which could be measured. An understanding of the universe in inanimate and mechanical terms began to replace the notion of an organic and living entity (Capra, 1982), a text written by God.

Descartes thought of the material universe as a machine which worked according to mechanical laws. To be studied, the universe had, first, to be reduced to its component parts, which could then be investigated in a simpler, more manageable form. Descartes believed that the reduction of complex systems into simpler component parts could be used in the study of the body, but not the mind, which was the province of God!

## THE MIND–BODY PROBLEM

What is the mind? What happens when we think? Can thought be reduced to a physical activity, involving no more than the stimulation of a collection of nerve endings? Do human beings possess non-physical souls? In everyday life, we draw common-sense, taken-for-granted, distinctions between the mental and the physical, for example between emotions and bodies, or between thinking and acting. But how do the 'physical' and the 'mental' relate together? Philosophers refer to this issue as the 'mind–body problem'. A number of philosophical schools of thought would answer the above questions quite differently (White, 1989).

Those who see the mind and body as separate entities are called mind–body dualists. Those who regard the mind and body as essentially the same, i.e. all flesh and blood with no separate mind substance, are known as physicalists.

René Descartes raised the mind-body problem in its modern form when he postulated **the Cartesian division**, the separation of mind from body. Descartes believed that the body and mind were separate entities with different properties. Mental processes, such as thinking, could not be reduced to physical ones, such as brain cells firing. Struggling to explain their connection, for example when thoughts are translated into action, he suggested that mind and body interacted via the pineal gland. Mind–body dualism underpins the belief, in many religions, that individuals possess 'a soul' which can endure after their death.

The plausibility of mind–body dualism stems from the difficulty involved in explaining the complexities of consciousness in terms of purely physical processes. The main criticism of dualism is that it does not explain how the mind and body interact. Several other philosophical positions have attempted to describe dualism without interaction. **Psychophysical parallelism** maintains that the mind and body run separately, but in parallel, with no causal link. The harmony of this arrangement, they argued, has been pre-arranged by God! **Occasionalism** claims that mind and body are linked, through God's continual intervention. **Epiphenomenalism**, another dualist position, maintains that physical bodily events can cause mental events, but that mental events cannot cause either physical or further mental events. On this view, which seems implicit in much medical practice, mind becomes an irrelevance, and free will an illusion.

Other philosophical approaches reject the dualist starting point of the above positions. **Physicalism**, or materialism, holds that only the physical exists, and that all mental events can be explained in terms of physical ones, usually events in the brain. Several subvarieties of physicalism have been developed. One of the main ones, **Type-identity theory**, asserts that mental events are identical to physical ones. A particular thought equates with a specific state of the brain. Whenever this specific brain state occurs, it results in the same thought.

**Behaviourism** offers a different perspective on the mind–body problem from that provided by dualists and physicalists. Behaviourists, both philosophers and psychologists, argue that accounts of 'mental states' represent no more than shorthand descriptions of our behaviour or intended behaviour. **Methodological behaviourism** maintain that only observable behaviour can be studied scientifically, and that attempts to study the mind through the private world of introspection should be abandoned. **Logical behaviourists** believe that our mental language does not refer to private non-physical entities, but is logically related to observable behaviour.

In the second half of this century there have been heated debates about the relationship between mind and brain. Many aspects of human experience belong to the realm of mind that we usually refer to as consciousness. Such feelings include pleasure, pain, choosing, having a sense of meaning, belonging, loving and spirituality. Despite a huge increase in our knowledge of the brain and how it appears to function physiologically, we still have difficulties in accounting for consciousness and the interactions between mind and body.

## THE BODY AND NOT THE MIND

The assumption of component parts of the body with an independent existence has informed the practice of modern medicine to date. The notion of the body as a machine has been supported by continual 'scientific' discovery, for example of the circulatory system, of the cell, the germ. Classical germ theory recognised that infection required an interplay between factors relating to the 'Germ + Environment + Host'. However, the host is often seen as the passive unfortunate victim of the infection, and the body as a hierarchy of systems, as shown below.

Body
Systems
Organs
Tissues
Cells
DNA

Psychiatrists have attempted to apply a similar framework to the study of the mind, reduced to the brain. Mental illness is explained in terms of biochemical imbalances, to be corrected through pharmaceutical or surgical intervention.

Antonovsky (1984) criticised the pathogenic paradigm which underpins epidemiology and most current health-promotion practice. This paradigm is based on the assumption that the normal human state is one of homeostasis and order (see also Chapter 15). When this order is disrupted, by microbiological, physical, chemical or psychosocial factors (stressors), various neuropsychological, immunological and endocrinological regulatory mechanisms come into play. If the homeostatic mechanisms are overwhelmed by stressors, dis-ease occurs. Treatment is then required to reinforce, enhance or replace the regulatory mechanisms and restore the individual to a state of homeostasis or health.

Antonovsky argues that, within this pathogenic paradigm, people are simply classified as either healthy or diseased. Professional interest, both preventive and curative, focuses on particular pathogens or resultant diseases. Professionals think vertically about the specific cause(s) of specific diseases instead of looking for horizontal connections, such as common stressors or generalised human capacities for dealing with them. The paradigm presupposes the 'badness' of stress. But a certain amount of exposure to 'stressors' benefits health. For example, childhood infections help to build up immunity, and emotional arousal can enhance performance.

The pathogenic paradigm focuses attention on 'the case' for treatment, and the 'high-risk group' for prevention. Deviant cases, relative to this paradigm, those who remain disease-free despite high exposure to stressors, or those who succumb for no apparent reason, receive less attention. Few questions are asked about smokers who don't get lung cancer, or 'high-risk' individuals who don't develop coronary problems. Thus, the 'symptoms of wellness' are largely ignored in this paradigm.

Antonovsky proposes a 'salutogenic', or 'health development', paradigm. He argues that the natural human state involves constant disorder and lack of homeostasis. Salutogenesis is the active process of managing that state of flux in order to prevent the body becoming overwhelmed and succumbing to disease. Thus, health is actively created and sustained despite the natural tendency towards disease and death, as Illich (1977) argued with respect to the iatrogenic effects of modern medicine. Health, not disease, is the mystery which should be studied. Such studies would not be constrained within vertical programmes looking at specific diseases and their supposed risk factors. Instead, horizontal links, for example common protective coping mechanisms which cut across the pathogenic process, should be explored. Inquiry would focus on the whole population, rather than on subgroups identified as being 'at risk' for specific conditions.

Health-promotion practitioners have developed a growing interest in the part played by psychosocial factors in determining an individual's health status. Often these psychosocial variables are reduced to the idea of 'stress'. Psychosocial factors, for example bereavement, loss of employment, lack of control and support, lack of a confiding relationship and depression have been shown to predict the occurrence of cancer and heart disease more powerfully than more widely quoted risk factors such as smoking, diet and hypertension (Eyer, 1980; Morris, Cook, and Shaper, 1994; Baker, Israel and Schurman, 1996; North et al., 1996). Programmes that have attempted to address some of these variables seriously have prolonged the lives of cancer patients and started to clear atheroma from diseased arteries (Capra, 1982; Chopra, 1989; Weir, 1991; Weir and Whittaker, 1996). But how are such psychosocial responses mediated? How does a thought or feeling become translated into a physical manifestation?

## MIND–BODY MEDICINE

Many practitioners of alternative therapies do not accept the conceptual separation of mind and body, or the mechanistic/reductionist model of ill-health. A rejection of the Cartesian division opens up new possibilities for both medical practice and health-promotion. Mental techniques can be used to influence the physiological and immunological basis of health and illness. This approach is commonly found in Eastern medicine, and its value has been demonstrated through the use of biofeedback techniques in Western medical practice (Capra, 1982; Bass and Wade, 1984; Chopra, 1989; Frasure-Smith, Lesperance and Talajic, 1993).

Ayurveda, a system of medicine peculiar to India, has been described as the knowledge of how to live. The term originates from two Sanskrit words: *ayus*, meaning life, and *vid*, meaning knowledge. Ayuverda is a holistic system, dealing with the body, mind and spirit. Western practitioners have tended to dismiss it as a collection of superstitions, but it is now attracting more attention as a valid therapy (Weir and Whittaker, 1996). In Ayurvedic medicine, the patient is expected to take an active (rather than passive/compliant) part in their own cure. Treatment involves meditation, diet, massage, herbal therapies, fasting, purification and aromatherapy. These therapies aim to promote the self-healing potential of the body. Breathing, meditation and a range of bodywork therapies are used to attempt to release energy and emotional blocks. Many Eastern therapies, and Western alternative therapies, are simply nonsensical under the predominant biomedical model. There is an increasing demand, much of it from within the medical profession itself, for a general paradigm shift which would allow for the development of an expanded model of mind, and a greater understanding of the role of consciousness in human health and healing (Capra, 1982; Chopra, 1989; Weir, 1991; Weir and Whittaker 1996).

# Some problems of explanation in current health promotion

The reductionist medical paradigm describes the heart as a pump, and is concerned with the flow of blood through the arteries. If they become blocked, angina and heart attacks can occur. Health promoters, within this paradigm, have the task of preventing arteries from clogging up by persuading people not to undertake certain types of behaviour, such as smoking, eating fatty foods. When prevention fails, clinicians can attempt to clear-out or bypass problem areas through surgical interventions which alleviate symptoms but do not affect the underlying disease process. However, Rose (1985) has pointed out that the modern epidemic of heart disease remains largely unexplained. Behavioural factors account for little of the social class gradient in heart disease, and even individuals in the lowest category for behavioural risk factors are still more likely to die prematurely from heart disease from than any other cause.

Only a minority of CHD patients have a history of the classical risk factors (Graboys, 1984). Patients with the most blocked-up arteries may not experience the most chest pain (Freeman and Nixon, 1985a). Anxiety and over-breathing may be responsible for such divergences. The hyperventilation experienced in emotional distress or exhaustion can lead to changes in blood chemistry and constriction of the coronary arteries (Bass and Wade, 1984; Freeman and Nixon, 1985b).

In post-heart-attack patients, social isolation and stress have been identified as the major predictors of recurrent illness (Frasure-Smith, Lesperance and Talajic, 1993). Drawing on the work of clinicians treating patients with cancer and heart disease, Weir and Whittaker (1996) identify 'meaning and enthusiasm' as the central components of health and wellbeing. Peace of mind, a loving family and a supportive community have all been recognised as protectors and promoters of health (Wilkinson, 1996; Denollet et al., 1996).

Such findings call into question the mechanistic models of heart disease. A heart attack may not result from an easily explained mechanical blockage, but from a dynamic combination of factors associated with life demands, coping and social support, which bring about prolonged periods of emotional exhaustion. In this paradigm, CHD is seen as arising from a chain of psychobiological events (Capra, 1982; Chopra, 1989).

Similarly, research into inequalities in health across social groups provides support for the close interaction between mind and body in the development and maintenance of health. Wilkinson (1996, p. 54) argues that these inequalities do not simply result from physical differences, but are affected by 'psychosocial pathways'. Societies rich enough to meet the population's basic need for food and shelter have gone through the 'epidemiological transition', discussed above. Within this group, the more egalitarian, rather than the richest, societies enjoy the best health (Wilkinson, 1996 p. 75). Wilkinson concludes that 'feeling in control', having social support and 'social cohesion' are the key health-promoting factors which account for health inequalities in social groups in developed countries.

If the health-promotion profession takes this psychosocial dimension in the aetiology of ill-health seriously, it needs to rethink the current notion of 'risk', and the sorts of intervention to which it gives rise. Individuals are asked to change their behaviour (with all the incumbent difficulties entailed) on the strength of possible future benefit. An avoidance of adversity cannot be guaranteed. Conversely, those who continue with an 'unhealthy' lifestyle may suffer no ill-effects. These contradictions can be best explained when a holistic paradigm of health and healing is applied.

'Holism' can be understood at two levels. The first level involves acceptance that all parts of the body interact, and that the functioning of one element should not be considered in isolation. For example, the new science of psychoneuroimmunology recognises the integration of the neurological, endocrinological and immunological functions of the body.

The second level of 'holism' incorporates the traditional shamanistic view of human beings as integral parts of an ordered system of nature, continually interacting with that larger system. This view fits entirely with the modern systems view of the world. Explanations of illness in a new paradigm would look beyond the biological mechanisms of the disease process, and would seek the root causes of illness in social relationships, environmental influences and psychological patterns (Capra, 1982). This philosophy is at the core of Hippocratic medicine, the historical progenitor of modern Western medicine. Unfortunately the emphases in the Hippocratic Corpus on health as a state of balance, environmental influences, the interdependence of mind and body and the inherent healing power of nature were lost with the acceptance of the Cartesian Division, and the rise of reductionism in medical practice. The 'new' paradigm would be better described as the rediscovery of an old one. The nature of such a paradigm, and its use to explain the many contradictions currently encountered in health-promotion, are well-documented in Capra's classic *The Turning Point* (1982) and Chopra's *Quantum Healing* (1989). Both argue for a new understanding of consciousness which combines recent scientific thinking with traditional holistic views of health and healing.

## Health development and mind–body health promotion

Acceptance of mind-body interaction means that 'mental health', often defined in terms of feelings of 'wellbeing', becomes central to a new way of thinking about health promotion. Wellbeing seems protective against ill-health at a general rather than specific disease level, and provides a horizontal link between otherwise disparate and unconnected vertical disease-prevention programmes. But problems of definition remain. The term 'wellbeing' has been criticised as a vague woolly notion, not suited to the requirements for reproducible and so-called objective observations (Seedhouse, 1995). However, this type of criticism, framed by the old, reductionist paradigm, may simply not be relevant to health-promotion practice informed by a new one. Placing wellbeing, a subjective and highly variable phenomenon, at the centre of the health-promotion stage will require abandonment of the 'undelimited' approach to expertise, as argued in Chapter 1, since each individual, ultimately, defines their own wellbeing.

In the early 1980s, the professional practice of health-promotion did attempt to take on board some aspects of personal growth and development, recognising them as vital components of health. Self-realisation and self-actualisation entered into the vocabulary used by the small band of health-promotion specialists. However, changes in the NHS over the past ten years, culminating in the publication of *The Health of the Nation* strategy (DOH, 1992), have led to a much greater number of professionals, both within and outside the NHS, becoming involved in health-promotion activities. These activities have been narrowly defined and prescribed by the government, on the basis of the epidemiological model of disease causation. Health-promotion practice which appears to stray beyond these narrow boundaries has been discouraged.

How would professional health-promotion practice differ if informed by a more holistic understanding of health and healing? A new paradigm for health-promotion must engage more seriously with health determinants identified in recent research. These determinants include (Rijke, quoted in Lafaille and Fulder, 1993, p. 80):

- Autonomy
- The will to live
- Vitality
- Experience of meaning and purpose in life
- High quality of relationships
- Creative expression of meaning
- Body awareness
- Consciousness of inner development
- Individuality
- Belonging

Anything which prevents people achieving these 'foundations for health' constitutes a 'risk' to health. Such thinking provides a new conceptual risk framework for the professional practice of health-promotion. Capra (1982, p. 364) argues that a new system of holistic health care, in which health development is paramount, must entail *'restoring and maintaining the dynamic balance of individuals, families and other social groups'*. Achieving this aim requires recognition of the individuality of wellbeing, and of the interdependence between personal health and social and ecological structures.

The same vehicles for promoting health can be used: namely, individual health education, social engineering measures and healthy public policy formulation. The same channels of communication can be used, including parents, teachers, health and other professionals, volunteers and informed lay people. But the mind-set of those involved in health-promotion would need to change to accommodate newly defined objectives relating to such variables as personal autonomy, high-quality relationships and having meaning and purpose in life, rather than those relating to lifestyle issues. For example, health-education curriculum work in schools would be refocused to concentrate on personal growth and development, rather than on behavioural aspects such as food choices and drug-taking. Public policy could be formulated to take into account the need for individuals to feel a sense of control and participation in decision-making. Health-promotion in the workplace could shift its focus away from limited lifestyle-related issues, and address, in a meaningful way, the organisational roots of health problems in the workforce. Some aspects of current health-promotion practice do fit in with this new approach. Other areas of activity, currently at the margin, would occupy a central position in health-promotion based on the new paradigm, for example, bereavement and relationship counselling.

The demand for a new approach to health and healing will continue to increase. New approaches will emerge outside of mainstream professional health-promotion practice. If we fail to take account of the newly articulated determinants of health, and continue to confine professional health-promotion practice within a reductionist *Health of the Nation* framework, we are surely doomed to fail in our attempts to improve public health.

# References

**Aboussouan, L.S., Odonovan, P.B., Moodie, D.S., Gragg, L.A. and Stoller, J.K.** (1993) Hypoplastic trachea in Down's syndrome. *American Review of Respiratory Disease,* **147,** 72–5.

**Abrams, D., Abraham, C., Spears, R. and Marks, D.** (1990) AIDS invulnerability: Relationships, sexual behaviour and attitudes among 16–19 year olds. In Aggleton, P., Davies, P. and Hart, G. (eds) *Aids: Individual, Cultural and Policy Dimensions.* Basingstoke: Falmer Press.

**Adams, J.** (1995) *Risk.* London: UCL Press.

**Aggleton, P.** (1990) *Health.* London: Routledge.

**Ahmad, W.I.U.** (1989) Policies, pills and political will: A critique of policies to improve the health status of ethnic minorities. *Lancet,* **i,** 148–50.

**Ahmad, W.I.U.** (1992) The maligned healer: The 'Hakim' and Western medicine. *New Community,* **18,** 521–36.

**Ahmad, W.I.U.** (1993) *'Race' and Health in Contemporary Britain.* Buckingham: Open University Press.

**Alaszewski, A.** (1986) *Institutional Care and the Mentally Handicapped.* London: Croom Helm.

**Alderman, C.** (1988) Blood pressure measurement. *Nursing Standard,* **44,** 22–3.

**Aldridge, M.** (1996) Dragged to market: Being a professional in the postmodern world. *British Journal of Social Work,* **26,** 177–94.

**Ales, K.L., Druzin, M.L. and Santini, D.L.** (1990) Impact of advanced maternal age on the outcome of pregnancy. *Surgery, Gynaecology and Obstetrics,* **171,** 209–16.

**Allaby, M.A.** (1995) Effectiveness of family planning services for teenagers. *British Medical Journal,* **31,** 1641–3.

**Altman, D.** (1988) *AIDS and the New Puritanism.* London: Pluto Press.

**Alzheimer's Disease Society** (1993) *Deprivation and Dementia.* London: Alzheimer's Disease Society.

**Anders, T.** (1994) *The Evolution of Evil.* Chicago: Open Court.

**Andersen, T.** (1987) The reflecting team: Dialogue and meta-dialogue in clinical work. *Family Process,* **26,** 415–27.

**Anderson, J.M., Elfert, H. and Lai, M.** (1989) Ideology in the clinical context: Chronic illness, ethnicity and the discourse on normalisation. *Sociology of Health and Illness,* **11,** 253–78.

**Anderson, R. and Bury, M.** (eds) (1988) *Living with Chronic Illness: The Experience of Patients and their Families.* London: Unwin Hyman.

**Annandale, E.** (1995) *Working on the Front Line: Risk Culture and Clinical Decision-making in the New NHS.* Paper presented at the ESRC Risk in Organisational Settings Conference, London.

**Anneren, G., Gustafsson, J., Sara, V.R. and Tuvemo, T.** (1993) Normalized growth velocity in children with Down's syndrome during growth hormone therapy. *Journal of Intellectual Disability Research,* **37,** 381–7.

**Anneren, G., Magnusson, C.G.M., Lilja, G. and Nordvall, S.L.** (1992) Abnormal serum IGG subclass pattern in children with Down's syndrome. *Archives of Disease in Childhood,* **67,** 628–31.

**Antonovsky, A.** (1984) The sense of coherence as a determinant of health. In Matarazzo, J.D. (ed.) *Behavioural Health: An Overview.* Chichester: John Wiley.

**Anwar, M.** (1986) Young Asians between two cultures. In Coombe, V. and Little, A. (eds) *Race and Social Work: A Guide to Training.* London: Tavistock.

**Anzueto, A., Andrade, F.H., Maxwell, L.C., Levine, S.M., Lawrence, R.A., Gibbons, W.J. and Jenkinson, S.G.** (1992) Resistive breathing activates the cluathione redox cycle and impairs performance of rat diaphragm. *Journal of Applied Physiology,* 72, 529–34.

**Arber, S.** (1991) Class, paid employment and family roles: Making sense of structural disadvantage, gender and health status. *Social Science and Medicine,* 32, 425–36.

**Arber, S. and Evandrou, M.** (eds) (1993) *Ageing, Independence and the Life Course.* London: Jessica Kingsley.

**Arkes, H.R., Faust, D., Guilmette, T.J. and Hart, K.** (1988) Eliminating the hindsight bias. *Journal of Applied Psychology,* 73, 305–7.

**Arkes, H.R., Wortmann, R.L., Saville, P.D. and Harkness, A.R.** (1981) Hindsight bias among physicians weighing the likelihood of diagnosis. *Journal of Applied Psychology,* 66, 252–4.

**Armstrong, D.** (1987a) Theoretical tensions in biopsychosocial medicine. *Social Science and Medicine,* 25, 1213–18.

**Armstrong, N.** (1987b) Coping with diabetes mellitus: A full time job. *Nursing Clinics of North America,* 22, 559–68.

**Armstrong, P.** (1996) *Beating the Biological Clock.* London: Hodder Headline.

**Audit Commission** (1992) *Community Care: Managing the Cascade of Change.* London: HMSO.

**Audit Commission** (1994) *Seen But Not Heard.* London: HMSO.

**Avis, N.E., Hyg, M.S., Smith, K.W. and McKinlay, J.B.** (1989) Accuracy of perceptions of heart attack risk: What influences perceptions and can they be changed? *American Journal of Public Health,* 12, 1608–11.

**Babb, P.** (1993) Teenage conceptions and fertility in England and Wales 1971–91. *Population Trends,* 74, 12–17.

**Bailey, R.** (1996) Prenatal testing and the prevention of impairment: A woman's right to choose? In Morris, J. (ed.) *Encounters with Strangers: Feminism and Disability.* London: The Women's Press.

**Baker, A.A.** (1976) Slow euthanasia or – she will be better off in hospital. *British Medical Journal,* 2, 571–2.

**Baker, E., Israel, B. and Schurman, S.** (1996) Role of control and support in occupational stress: An integrated model. *Social Science and Medicine,* 43, 1145–59.

**Baldwin, D.** (1983) *All About Children. An Introduction to Child Development.* Oxford: Oxford University Press.

**Barchas, J., DaCosta, F. and Spector, S.** (1967) Acute pharmacology of melatonin. *Nature,* 214, 919–20.

**Baron, J.** (1994) *Thinking and Deciding.* Cambridge: Cambridge University Press.

**Bass, C. and Wade, C.** (1984) Chest pain with normal coronary arteries: A comparative study of psychiatric and social morbidity. *Psychological Medicine,* 14, 51–61.

**Baumgarten, E.** (1980) The concept of competence in medical ethics. *Journal of Medical Ethics,* 6, 180–4.

**Beauchamp, T.L. and Childress, J.F.** (1994) *Principles of Biomedical Ethics,* 4th edn. Oxford: Oxford University Press.

**Bebbington, P. and Kuipers, L.** (1993) Social causation of schizophrenia. In Bhugra, D. and Leff, J. (eds) *Principles of Social Psychiatry.* Oxford: Blackwell Scientific Publications.

**Beck, A.M. and Meyers, N.M.** (1996) Health enhancement and companion animal ownership. *Annual Review of Public Health,* 17, 247–57.

Beck, U. (1992) *Risk Society: Towards a New Modernity.* London: Sage.

Beck, U. (1996) Risk society and the provident state. In Lash, S., Szerszynski, B. and Wynne, B. (eds) *Risk, Environment and Modernity: Towards a New Ecology.* London: Sage.

Becker, G. and Nachtigall, R.D. (1992) Eager for medicalisation: The social production of infertility as a disease. *Sociology of Health and Illness,* **14,** 156–471.

Beck-Gernsheim, E. (1996) Life as a planning project. In Lash, S., Szerszynski, B. and Wynne, B. (eds) *Risk, Environment and Modernity: Towards a New Ecology.* London: Sage.

Bell, J.A., Pearn, J.H. and Firman, D. (1989) Childhood deaths in Down's syndrome: Survival curves and causes of death from a total population study in Queensland, Australia, 1976 to 1985. *Journal of Medical Genetics,* **26,** 764–8.

Bellini, J. (1986) *High Tech Holocaust.* Newton Abbot: David & Charles.

Benefits Agency (1996) *Benefits Information Guide.* Benefits Agency. An Executive Arm of the Department of Social Security. London: HMSO.

Benner, P. (1984) *From Novice to Expert.* Menlo Park, California: Addsion Wesley.

Bennet, G.C.J. and Ebrahim, S. (1995) *The Essentials of Health Care in Old Age,* 2nd edn. London: Edward Arnold.

Benzeval, M., Judge, K. and Smaje, C. (1995) Beyond class, 'race' and ethnicity: Deprivation and health in Britain. *Health Service Research,* **50,** 237–52.

Beral, V. (1979) Reproductive mortality. *British Medical Journal,* **11,** 632–4.

Berkowitz, G.S., Skovron, M.L., Lapinski, R.H. and Berkowitz, R.L. (1990) Delayed childbearing and the outcome of pregnancy. *New England Journal of Medicine,* **322,** 659–64.

Bernstein, P.L. (1996) *Against the Gods: The Remarkable Story of Risk.* New York: John Wiley.

Bhaduri, R. (1992) Self-determination: Lessons to be learnt from social work practice in India: A comment. *British Journal of Social Work,* **23,** 187–91.

Bhatt, A. and Dickinson, R. (1992), An analysis of health education materials for minority communities by cultural and linguistic group. *Health Education Journal,* **51/2,** 72–7.

Bhopal, R.S. (1986) The interrelationship of folk, traditional and Western medicine within an Asian Community in Britain. *Social Science and Medicine,* **22,** 99–105.

Bhugra, D. and Leff, J. (eds) (1993) *Principles of Social Psychiatry.* Oxford: Blackwell Scientific Publications.

Bingley, W. (1995) Law and guidelines. In Fernando, S. (ed.) *Mental Health in a Multi-ethnic Society: A Multi-disciplinary Handbook.* London: Routledge.

Black, D. (1986) Schoolgirl mothers (Editorial). *British Medical Journal,* **293,** 1047.

Black, R.B. (1979) The effects of diagnostic uncertainty and available options on perceptions of risk. *Birth Defects: Original Articles Series,* **15,** 341–54.

Blair, A. (1993) Social class and the contextualisation of illness experience. In Radley, A. (ed.) *World of Illness.* London: Routledge.

Blank, R.H. (1992) *Mother and Fetus: Changing Notions of Maternal Responsibility.* London: Greenwood Press.

Blaxter, M. (1983) The causes of disease. Women talking. *Social Science and Medicine,* **17,** 59–69.

Blaxter, M. (1990) *The Health and Lifestyle Survey.* London: Routledge.

Block, R. (1980) *Factors Related to Maternal Overprotection of the Mentally Retarded.* Unpublished dissertation, United States International University.

Blockley, D.I. (1980) *The Nature of Structural Design and Safety.* Chichester: Ellis Horwood.

**Blom-Cooper, L., Hally, H. and Murphy, E.** (1995) *The Falling Shadow: One Patient's Mental Health Care, 1978–1993.* London: Duckworth.

**Bloom, J.** (1982) Social support, accommodation to stress and adjustment in breast cancer. *Social Science and Medicine,* **16**, 1328–38.

**Bloor, M.** (1995) A user's guide to contrasting theories of HIV-related risk behaviour. In Gabe, G. (ed.) *Medicine, Health and Risk: Sociological Approaches.* Oxford: Blackwell.

**Blum, M.** (1979) Is the elderly primipara really at high risk? *Journal of Perinatal Medicine,* **7**, 108–12.

**BMA** (1994) *Confidentiality and People under 16.* London: British Medical Association.

**Bond, J. and Bond, S.** (1986) *Sociology and Health Care: An Introduction for Nurses and Other Health Professionals.* Edinburgh: Churchill Livingstone.

**Boore, J.R.P., Champion, R. and Ferguson, M.C.** (1987) *Nursing the Physically Ill Adult.* Edinburgh: Churchill Livingstone.

**Booth, T. , Simmons, K. and Booth, W.** (1989) Transition shock and the relocation of people from mental handicap hospitals and hostels. *Social Policy and Administration,* **23**, 211–18.

**Bosch, H.K.** (1994) Independent living services and programs: Integration into the community. In C.A. Michaels, (ed.) *Transition Strategies for Persons with Learning Disabilities.* San Diego, CA: Singular Publishing Co.

**Bound, J.P., Francis, B.J. and Harvey, P.W.** (1995) Down's syndrome: Prevalence and ionizing radiation in an area of North-west England 1957–91. *Journal of Epidemiology and Community Health,* **49**, 164–70.

**Bourne, G.** (1995) *Pregnancy,* 4th edn. London: Cassell Publications.

**Bowden, D.** (1995) A priority in the health service. *Managing Risk,* April, **1**.

**Bowers, B.J.** (1987) Intergenerational caregiving: Adult caregivers and their ageing parents. *Advanced Nursing Science,* **9**, 20–31.

**Bowler, I.** (1993) 'They're not the same as us'; Midwives' stereotypes of South Asian descent maternity patients. *Sociology of Health and Illness,* **15**, 157–77.

**Bowling, A., Jacobson, B. and Southgate, L.** (1993) Health service priorities: Explorations in consultation of the public and health professionals on priority setting in an inner London health district. *Social Science and Medicine,* **7**, 851–7.

**Boyd, W.** (Chair) (1996) *Report of the Confidential Inquiry into Homicides and Suicides by Mentally Ill People.* London: Royal College of Psychiatrists.

**Bradbury, J.A.** (1989) The policy implications of differing concepts of risk. *Science Technology and Human Value,* **14**, 380–99.

**Brandford, D. and Collacott, R.A.** (1994) Comparison of community and institutional prescription of antiepileptic drugs for individuals with learning disabilities. *Journal of Intellectual Disability Research,* **38**, 561–6.

**Branholm, I.B. and Degerman, E.A.** (1992) Life satisfaction and activity preferences in parents of Down's syndrome children. *Scandinavian Journal of Social Medicine,* **20**, 37–44.

**Brazier, M.** (1992) *Medicine, Patients and the Law.* Harmondsworth: Penguin Books.

**Brearley, P.** (1979) Understanding risk. *Social Work Today,* **10**, 28.

**Brearley, P.** (1982) *Risk and Ageing.* London: Routledge & Kegan Paul.

**Brook Advisory Centres** (Extracts) (1994) Teenage pregnancy: Key facts. *MIDIRS, Midwifery Digest,* **4**, 292–3.

**Brook Press Release** (1995) 40% increase in under-16s visiting Brook Clinics. *Family Planning Today,* Third Quarter, **3**.

**Brookfield, S.** (1990) Using critical incidents to explore learners' assumptions. In

Mezirow, J. and Associates (eds) *Fostering Critical Reflection in Adulthood.* California: Josey Bass.

Brooking, J.J. (1989) A survey of current practices and opinions concerning patient and family participation in hospital care. In Wilson-Barnett, J. and Robinson, S. (eds) *Directions in Nursing Research.* London: Scutari Press.

Browne, D. (1995) Sectioning: The Black experience. In Fernando, S. (ed.) *Mental Health in a Multi-ethnic Society: A Multi-disciplinary Handbook.* London: Routledge.

Browne, K. and Saqi, S. (1988) Approaches to screening for child abuse and neglect. In Browne, K., Davies, C. and Stratton, P. (eds) *Early Prediction and Prevention of Child Abuse.* Chichester: John Wiley.

Brugge, K.L., Grove, G.L., Clopton, P., Grove, M.J. and Piacquadio, D.J. (1993) Evidence for accelerated skin wrinkling among developmentally delayed individuals with Down's syndrome. *Mechanisms of Ageing and Development,* **70,** 213–25.

Brunner, L.S. and Suddarth, D.S. (1992) *The Textbook of Adult Nursing.* London: Chapman & Hall.

Buchwald, H. (1992) Cholesterol inhibition, cancer and chemotherapy. *Lancet,* **339,** 1154–6.

Bulmer, M. (1980) Why don't sociologists make more use of official statistics? *Sociology,* **14,** 505–23.

Bunton, R. and MacDonald, G. (eds) (1992) *Health Promotion: Disciplines and Diversity.* London: Routledge.

Bunton, R., Nettleton, S. and Burrows, R. (1995) *The Sociology of Health Promotion. Critical Analysis of Consumption, Lifestyle and Risk.* London: Routledge.

Burckhardt, C.S. (1987) Coping with chronic illness. *Nursing Clinics of North America,* **22,** 543–50.

Burgess, D. (1996) *An Evaluation of the Ability of Senior Student Nurses to Identify Ergonomic and Other Risks to Carers Arising from Moving and Handling Patients and Loads.* Unpublished MSc Thesis, Msc Health Sciences, University of Northumbria.

Burghes, L. (1995) *Single Lone Mothers: Problems, Prospects and Policies.* London: Family Policies Studies Centre.

Burke, A. and Virmani, R. (1994) Exercise as a factor in sudden cardiac arrest. *Cardiovascular Pathology,* **3,** 99–104.

Burroughs, J. and Hoffbrand, B. (1990) A critical look at nursing observations. *Postgraduate Medical Journal,* **66,** 370–2.

Bury, J.K. (1985) Teenage pregnancy. *British Journal of Obstetrics and Gynaecology,* **92,** 1081–3.

Butcher, L.A. (1994) Family focused perspective of chronic illness. *Rehabilitation Nursing,* **19,** 70–4.

Butterworth, T. and Faugier, J. (1992) *Clinical Supervision and Mentorship in Nursing.* London: Chapman & Hall.

Bygren, L.O., Konlaan, B.B. and Johansson, S.E. (1996) Attendance at cultural events, reading books or periodicals and making music or singing in a choir as determinants of survival: Swedish interview survey of living conditions. *British Medical Journal,* **313,** 1577–80.

Capra, F. (1975) *The Tao of Physics.* London: Wildwood House.

Capra, F. (1982) *The Turning Point.* New York: Wildwood House.

Carr-Hill, R.A. (1989) Assumptions of the QALY Procedure. *Social Science and Medicine,* **29,** 469–77.

Carroll, L. (1988) *Alice's Adventures in Wonderland.* First published 1865. Reprinted in *The Complete Works of Lewis Carroll.* Harmondsworth: Penguin.

Carson, D. (1996) Risking legal repercussions. In Kemshall, H. and Pritchard, J. (eds) *Good Practice in Risk Assessment and Risk Management.* London: Jessica Kingsley.

**Cashmore, E.** (ed.) (1988) *Dictionary of Race and Ethnic Relations.* London: Routledge.

**Castel, R.** (1991) From dangerousness to risk. In Burchell, G., Gordon, C. and Miller, P. (eds) *The Foucault Effect.* London: Harvester Wheatsheaf.

**Casti, J.L.** (1992) *Searching for Certainty: What Science Can Know about the Future.* London: Scribners.

**Cattermole, M., Jahoda, A. and Markova, I.** (1990) Quality of life for people with learning difficulties moving into community homes. *Disability, Handicap and Society,* 5, 137–52.

**Chang, A.K., Barrett-Connor, E. and Edelstein, S.** (1995) Low plasma cholesterol predicts an increased risk of lung cancer in elderly women. *Preventative Medicine,* 24, 557–62.

**Chaplin, E.** (1994) *Sociology and Visual Representation.* London: Routledge.

**Chapman, G.E.** (1983) Ritual and rational action in hospitals. *Journal of Advanced Nursing,* 8, 13–20.

**Chapman, S.** (1992) Dogma disputed: Potential endemic heterosexual transmission of human immunodeficiency virus in Australia. *Australian Journal of Public Health,* 10, 128–41.

**Chapman, S and Lupton, D.** (1994) *The Fight for Public Health: Principles and Practice of Media Advocacy.* London: BMJ Publishing Group.

**Charmaz, K.** (1983) Loss of self: A fundamental form of suffering in the chronically ill. *Sociology of Health and Illness,* 5, 168–95.

**Chopra, D.** (1989) *Quantum Healing. Exploring the Frontiers of Mind/Body Medicine.* New York: Bantam Books.

**Christensen-Szalanski, J.J.J. and Bushyhead, J.B.** (1981) Physicians' use of probabilistic information in a real clinical setting. *Journal of Experimental Psychology: Human Perception and Performance,* 7, 928–35.

**Christensen-Szalanski, J.J.J. and Willham, C.F.** (1991) The hindsight bias: A meta-analysis. *Organizational Behavior and Human Decision Processes,* 48, 147–68.

**Cicourel, A.V.** (1973) *Cognitive Sociology.* Harmondsworth: Penguin.

**Clancy, J. and McVicar, A.J.** (1995) *Physiology and Anatomy: A Homeostatic Approach.* London: Edward Arnold.

**Clarke, A.** (1995a) Population screening for genetic susceptibility to disease. *British Medical Journal,* 311, 35–8.

**Clarke, C.L.** (1995b) Care of elderly people suffering from dementia and their co-resident informal carers. In Heyman, B. (ed.) *Researching User Perspectives on Community Health Care.* London: Chapman & Hall.

**Clarke, C.L. and Keady, J.** (1996) Researching dementia care and family caregiving: Extending ethical responsibilities. *Health Care in Later Life,* 1, 85–95.

**Clarke, C.L. and Watson, D.** (1991) Informal carers of the dementing elderly: A study of relationships. *Nursing Practice,* 4, 17–21.

**Clarke, C.L., Heyman, R., Pearson, P. and Watson, D.W.** (1993) Formal carers: Attitudes to working with the dementing elderly and their informal carers. *Health and Social Care,* 1, 227–38.

**Cleaver, H. and Freeman, P.** (1995) *Parental Perspectives in Cases of Child Abuse. Studies in Child Protection.* London: HMSO.

**Clift, S. and Stears, D.** (1991) AIDS education in secondary schools. *Education and Health,* 9, 1–4.

**Clough, R.** (1978) No one could call me a fussy man. *Social Work Today,* 9, 15.

**Coates, V.E. and Boore, J.R.P.** (1995) Self-management of chronic illness: Implications for nursing. *International Journal of Nursing Studies,* 32, 628–40.

Cohen, L.J. (1979) On the psychology of prediction: Whose is the fallacy? *Cognition,* 7, 385–407.

Cohen, M.H. (1993) The unknown and the unknowable: Managing sustained uncertainty. *Western Journal of Nursing Research,* 15, 77–96.

Cohen, S. (1980) *Folk Devils and Moral Panics.* Oxford: Oxford University Press.

Collacott, R.A., Cooper, S.A. and Ismail, I.A. (1994) Multiinfarct dementia in Down's syndrome. *Journal of Intellectual Disability Research,* 38, 203–8.

Colvin, C.R. and Block, J. (1994) Do positive illusions foster mental health? An examination of the Taylor and Brown formulation. *Psychological Bulletin,* 116, 3–20.

Commission for Racial Equality (1992) *Race Relations Code of Practice in Primary Health Care Services.* London: Commission for Racial Equality.

Conceicao, S., Ward, M.K. and Kerr, D.N.S. (1976) Defects in sphygmomanometers: An important source of error in blood pressure recording. *British Medical Journal,* 1, 886–8.

Connor, S. and Kingman, S. (1988) *The Search for the Virus: The Scientific Discovery of AIDS and the Quest for a Cure.* Harmondsworth, Penguin Books.

Cook, F.L., Skogan, W.G., Cook, T.D. and Antunes, G.E. (1978) Criminal victimisation of the elderly: The physical and economic consequences. *The Gerontologist,* 18, 338–49.

Cook, G. (1994) *An Examination of Risk-Taking Practices in Rehabilitative Care for Elderly Patients: A Nursing Dilemma.* Unpublished dissertation, University of Keele.

Cooper, M.G. (ed.) (1985) *Risk. Man-made Hazards to Man,* Oxford: Clarendon Press.

Cooper, S.A. and Collacott, R.A. (1994) Clinical features and diagnostic criteria of depression in Down's syndrome. *British Journal of Psychiatry,* 165, 399–403.

Cooper, S.A. and Collacott, R.A. (1995) The effect of age on language in people with Down's syndrome. *Journal of Intellectual Disability Research,* 39, 197–200.

Cooper, W.G. (1993) Roles of evolution, quantum mechanics and point mutations in origins of cancer. *Cancer Chemistry Biophysics,* 13, 147–70.

Corby, B. (1996) Risk assessment in child protection work. In Kempshall, H. and Pritchard, J. (eds) *Good Practice in Risk Assessment and Risk Management.* London: Jessica Kingsley.

Corrao, G., Lepore, A.R., Torchio, P., Valenti, M., Galatola, G., Damcis, A., Arico, S. and Diorio, F. (1994) The effect of drinking coffee and smoking cigarettes on the risk of cirrhosis associated with alcohol consumption: A case control study. *European Journal of Epidemiology,* 10, 657–64.

Counsel and Care (1993) *The Right to Take Risks.* London: Counsel and Care.

Covello, V.T. and Mumpower, J. (1985) Risk analysis and risk management: An historical perspective. *Risk Analysis,* 5, 103–20.

Covington, D. (1995) *Salvation on Sand Mountain: Snake Handling and Redemption in Southern Appalachia.* Reading, MA: Addison-Wesley.

Cowley, L. (1996) *Information Needs of Women Receiving Adjuvant Chemotherapy for Breast Cancer: Perceptions of Treatment Impact upon Lifestyle.* Unpublished MSc Thesis, MSc Health Sciences, University of Northumbria.

Coyne, A.M. (1986) *Schoolgirl Mothers,* Research Report No. 2. London: Health Education Council.

Crandall, B.F., Lebherz, T.B. and Tabsh, K. (1986) Maternal age and amniocentesis: Should this be lowered to 30 years? *Prenatal Diagnosis,* 6, 237–42.

Crawford, R. (1977) You are dangerous to your health: The ideology and politics of victim blaming. *International Journal of Health Services,* 4, 663–80.

Creer, C. and Wing, J. (1974) *Schizophrenia at Home.* Surbiton, Surrey: National Schizophrenia Fellowship.

**Creighton, S.J.** (1988) The incidence of child abuse and neglect. In Browne, K. Davies, C. and Stratton, P. (eds) *Early Prediction and Prevention of Child Abuse.* Chichester: John Wiley.

**Crichton, J.** (ed.) (1995) *Psychiatric Patient Violence: Risk and Response.* London: Duckworth.

**Criqui, M.H.** (1996) Alcohol and coronary heart disease: Consistent relationship and public health implications. *Clinica Chimica Acta,* **246**, 51–7.

**Crittenden, P.** (1988) Family and dyadic patterns of functioning in maltreating families. In Browne, K., Davies, C. and Stratton, P. (eds) *Early Prediction and Prevention of Child Abuse.* Chichester: John Wiley.

**Cubbon, J.** (1991) The principle of QALY maximization as the basis for allocating health care resources. *Journal of Medical Ethics,* **17**, 181–4.

**Cuckle, H.S., Wald, N.J. and Thompson, S.G.** (1987) Estimating a woman's risk of having a pregnancy associated with Down's syndrome using her age and serum alpha-fetoprotein level. *British Journal of Obstetrics and Gynaecology,* **94**, 387–402.

**Cunningham, A.J.** (1996) *Healing Change: A Qualitative Study of Psychological Self-healing Efforts in Patients with Metastatic Cancer.* Paper presented at the Qualitative Health Research Conference, Bournemouth.

**Davidson, N. and Rakusen, J.** (1982) *Out of Our Hands.* London: Pan Books.

**Davies, B.** (1988) Auditory disorders in Down's syndrome. *Scandinavian Audiology,* S30, 65–8.

**Davies, N.** (Chair) (1995) *Report of the Inquiry into the Circumstances Leading to the Death of Jonathan Newby.* Oxford: Oxfordshire Health Authority.

**Davis, F.** (1991) Identity ambivalence in clothing: The dialectic of the erotic and the chaste. In Maines, D.R. (ed.) *Social Organisation and Social Process: Essays in Honor of Anselm Strauss.* New York: Aldine De Gruyter.

**Davison, C., Davey Smith, G. and Frankel, S.** (1991) Lay epidemiology and the prevention paradox: The implications of candidacy for health education. *Sociology of Health and Illness,* **13**, 1–19.

**Davison, C., Frankel, S. and Davey Smith, G.** (1992) The limits of lifestyle: Re-assessing 'Fatalism' in the popular culture of illness prevention, *Social Science and Medicine,* **6**, 675–85.

**Davison, N. and Reed, J.** (1995) One foot on the escalator: Elderly people in sheltered accommodation. In Heyman, B. *Researching User Perspectives on Community Health Care.* London: Chapman & Hall.

**Dawes, R.M., Mirels, H.L., Gold E. and Donahue E.** (1993) Equating inverse probabilities in implicit personality judgments. *Psychological Science,* **4**, 396–400.

**Day, M.** (1996) Do you really need that aspirin? *New Scientist,* **2033**, 10.

**De Beauvoir, S.** (1960) *The Second Sex.* London: Jonathan Cape.

**Delahaye, F., Bruckert, E., Thomas, D., Emmerch, J. and Richard, J.L.** (1992) Serum cholesterol levels and cancer: Is there a causal relationship? *Archives des Maladies du Coeur et des Vaisseaux,* **85**, 37–45.

**Denollet, J., Sys, S.V., Stroobant, N., Ronbouts, H., Gillebert, T.C. and Brutseart, D.L.** (1996) Personality as independent predictor of long-term mortality in patients with coronary heart disease. *Lancet,* **i**, 417–21.

**Devenny, D.A. and Silverman, W.P.** (1990) Speech dysfluency and manual specialization in Down's syndrome. *Journal of Mental Deficiency Research,* **34**, 253–60.

**DHSS** (1970) *The Battered Baby.* London: HMSO.

**DHSS** (1971) *Better Services for the Mentally Handicapped.* London: HMSO.

**DHSS** (1974) *Memorandum on Non-Accidental Injury to Children.* London. HMSO.

**DHSS** (1976) *Personal and Staff Training: Proposals on Aspects of the Briggs Report on Nursing.* London: HMSO.

**DHSS** (1980) *Mental Handicap: Progress, Problems and Priorities*. London: HMSO.

**DHSS** (1988) *Report of the Inquiry into Child Abuse in Cleveland, 1987 (Butler-Sloss)*. London: HMSO.

**Diachuk, M.G.** (1994) When a child has a birth defect. In Field, P.A. and Marck, P.B. (eds) *Uncertain Motherhood*. Thousand Oaks, CA: Sage.

**DiGuilio, V.S.** (1957) The elderly primipara. *Obstetrics and Gynaecology*, **10**, 525–8.

**Dillner, L.** (1991) Unplanned pregnancies. *British Medical Journal*, **303**, 604.

**Dinani, S. and Carpenter, S.** (1990) Down's syndrome and thyroid disorder. *Journal of Mental Deficiency Research*, **34**, 187–93.

**Dodds, R.** (1997) *The Stress of Tests in Pregnancy*. London: The National Childbirth Trust.

**DOH** (1989) *Caring for People*. London: HMSO.

**DOH** (1990) *The NHS and Community Care Act*. London: HMSO.

**DOH** (1991) *Working Together under the Children Act 1989: A Guide to Arrangements for Inter-Agency Co-operation for the Protection of Children from Abuse*. London: HMSO.

**DOH** (1992) *The Health of the Nation: A Strategy for Health in England*. London: HMSO.

**DOH** (1993) *Changing Childbirth, Part 1: Report of the Expert Maternity Group*, Chair: Baroness Cumberledge. London: HMSO.

**DOH** (1995) *Children and Young Persons on Child Protection Registers, Year ending 31 March 1994*. London: HMSO.

**DOH** (1996a) *The Patients Charter: Mental Health Services: Draft Consultation Edition*. London: Department of Health.

**DOH** (1996b) *Health and Social Services Statistics for England*. London: HMSO.

**DOH/British Diabetics Association** (1995) *St Vincent Joint Task Force for Diabetes: The Report*. London: DOH/BDA.

**Donnenfeld, A.E.** (1995) The risk figure of 1/270. *Journal of Medical Science*, **2**, 1–2.

**Donovan, J.** (1984) Ethnicity and Health. *Social Science and Medicine*, **19**, 663–70.

**Donovan, J.** (1986) *We Don't Buy Sickness, It Just Comes*. Aldershot: Gower.

**Douglas, M.** (1966) *Purity and Danger: Conceptions of Pollution and Taboo*. London: Routledge & Kegan Paul.

**Douglas, M.** (1985) *Risk Acceptability According to the Social Sciences*. New York: Russell Sage Foundation.

**Douglas, M.** (1990) Risk as a forensic resource. *Daedalus*, **119**, 1–16.

**Douglas, M.** (1994) *Risk and Blame: Essays in Cultural Theory*. London: Routledge.

**Downie, R.S., Fyfe, C. and Tannahill, A.** (1990) *Health Promotion: Models and Values*. Oxford: Oxford University Press.

**Doyal, L.** (1979) *The Political Economy of Health*. London: Pluto Press.

**Dracup, C.** (1995) Hypothesis testing: What it really is. *Psychologist*, **8**, 359–62.

**Draper, P.** (1987) Not a job for juniors. *Nursing Times*, **83**, 58–62.

**Dreuilhe, E.** (1987) *Mortal Embrace: Living with AIDS*. London: Faber & Faber.

**Dubos, R. and Pines, M.** (1965) *Health and Disease*. (Nederland) NV: Time Life International.

**Duchon, M.A. and Muise, K.L.** (1993) Pregnancy after age 35. *The Female Patient*, **18**, 69–72.

**Eddy, D.M.** (1982) Probabilistic reasoning in clinical medicine: Problems and opportunities. In Kahneman, D., Slovic, P. and Tversky, A. (eds) *Judgment under Uncertainty: Heuristics and Biases*. Cambridge: Cambridge University Press.

**Edelstein, J. and Linn, M.W.** (1985) The influence of the family on control of diabetes. *Social Science and Medicine*, **21**, 541–4.

**Edgerton, R.B.** (1975) Issues relating to quality of life among mentally retarded persons. In Begab, M.J. and Richardson, S.A. (eds) *The Mentally Retarded and Society: A Social Science Perspective.* Baltimore: University Park Press.

**Edgerton, R.B.** (1988) Aging in the community: A matter of choice. *American Journal on Mental Retardation,* **92,** 331–5.

**Edgerton, R.B., Bollinger, M. and Herr, B.** (1984) The cloak of competence: After two decades. *American Journal of Mental Deficiency,* **88,** 345–51.

**Edstrom, K.** (1972) *Early Complications and Late Sequelae of Induced Abortion. A Review of the Literature.* Working Paper for Consultation on Abortion Care. Geneva: WHO.

**Eisenstadt, S.N.** (1956) *From Generation to Generation.* New York: The Free Press.

**Eisinger, J.** (1991) Early consumer protection legislation: A 17th century law prohibiting lead adulteration of wines. *Interdisciplinary Science Review,* **16,** 61–8.

**Elford, J., Phillips, A., Thompson, A.G. and Sharper, A.G.** (1990) Migration and geographic variations in blood pressure in Britain. *British Medical Journal,* **300,** 291–5.

**Englehardt, H.T.** (1986) *The Foundations of Bioethics.* New York: Oxford English Press.

**Epstein, S.** (1995) The construction of lay expertise: AIDS activism and the forging of credibility in the reform of clinical trials. *Science, Technology and Human Values,* **20,** 408–37.

**Erev, I. and Cohen, B.L.** (1990) Verbal versus numerical probabilities: Efficiency, biases, and the preference paradox. *Organizational Behavior and Human Decision Processes,* **45,** 1–18.

**Eyer, J.** (1980) Social causes of coronary heart disease. *Psychotherapy and Psychosomatics,* **34,** 75–87.

**Falloon, I. and Fadden, G.** (1993) *Integrated Mental Health Care: A Comprehensive Community-based Approach.* Cambridge: Cambridge University Press.

**Family Planning Association** (1994) *Children Who Have Children. A Report.* London: FPA Press Department.

**Family Planning Association** (1996) *Contraceptive Choices.* London: FPA.

**Family Planning Association and Contraceptive Education Service** (1995) New confidentiality guidelines. *Family Planning Today,* Fourth Quarter, **2.**

**Fanon, F.** (1978) Medicine and colonialism. In Ehrenreich, J. (ed.) *The Cultural Crisis of Modern Medicine.* London: Monthly Review Press.

**Farmer, E. and Owen, M.** (1995) *Child Protection Practice: Private Risks and Public Remedies: A Study of Decision-making, Intervention and Outcome in Child Protection Work.* London: HMSO.

**Fawcett, J.** (1989) *Analysis and Evaluation of Conceptual Models of Nursing.* Philadelphia: F.A. Davis.

**Feher, M., Harris-St John, K. and Lant, A.** (1992) Blood pressure measurement by junior hospital doctors: A gap in medical education? *Health Trends,* **24,** 59–61.

**Fernando, S.** (ed.) (1995) *Mental Health in a Multi-ethnic Society: A Multi-Disciplinary Handbook.* London: Routledge.

**Ferrara, D.** (1979) Attitudes of parents of mentally retarded children towards normalisation activities. *American Journal of Mental Deficiency,* **84,** 145–51.

**Field, P.A., Marck, P. B., Anderson, G. and McGeary, K.** (1994) Introduction. In Field, P.A. and Marck, P.B. (eds) *Uncertain Motherhood.* Thousand Oaks, CA: Sage.

**Fielding, G. and Evered, C.** (1980) The influence of patients' speech upon doctors: The diagnostic interview. In St Clair, R. and Giles, H. (eds) *Social and Psychological Contexts of Language.* Hillside, NJ: Erlbaum.

**Firth, W.J.** (1991) Chaos – predicting the unpredictable. *British Medical Journal,* **303,** 1565–8.

Fischhoff, B. (1975) Hindsight < > foresight: The effect of outcome knowledge on judgment under uncertainty. *Journal of Experimental Psychology: Human Perception and Performance*, **1**, 288–99.

Fischhoff, B. (1977) Perceived informativeness of facts. *Journal of Experimental Psychology: Human Perception and Performance*, **3**, 349–58.

Fischhoff, B., Watson, S.R. and Hope, C. (1984) Defining risk. *Policy Sciences*, **17**, 123–39.

Fitzgerald, F.T. (1994) The tyranny of health. *New England Journal of Medicine*, **331**, 196–8.

Forde, D.R. (1993) Perceived crime, fear of crime and walking alone at night. *Psychological Reports*, **73**, 403–7.

Foucault, M. (1973) *The Birth of the Clinic*, trans. A. Sheridan. New York: Vintage.

Francome, C., Savage, W., Churchill, H. and Lewison, H. (1993) *Caesarian Birth in Britain: A Book for Health Professionals and Parents*. London: Middlesex University Press.

Frasure-Smith, N., Lesperance, F. and Talajic, M. (1993) Depression following myocardial infarction. Impact on 6-month survival. *Journal of the American Medical Association*, **270**, 18–19.

Freeman, L.J. and Nixon, P. (1985a) Dynamic causes of angina pectoris. *The American Heart Journal*, **110**, 1087–92.

Freeman, L.J. and Nixon, P. (1985b) Chest pain and hyperventilation syndrome: Some aetiological considerations. *Postgraduate Medical Journal*, **61**, 957–61.

Freeman, R. (1992) The idea of prevention: A critical review. In Scott, S., Williams, G., Platt S. and Thomas, H. (eds) *Private Risks and Public Dangers. Studies in Sociology, No. 43*. Aldershot: Avebury.

Friedan, B. (1977) *The Feminine Mystique*. New York: Dell.

Fuller, R.C. and Meyers, R.R. (1941) Natural history of a social problem. *American Sociologcal Review*, **6**, 321–8.

Furnham, A. (1994) Explaining health and illness: Lay perspectives on current and future health, the causes of illness and the nature of recovery. *Social Science and Medicine*, **39**, 715–25.

Gabe, J. (1995) Health medicine and risk: The need for a sociological approach. In Gabe, J. (ed.) *Medicine, Health and Risk: Sociological Approaches*. Oxford: Blackwell.

Gardner, G. (1991) Unplanned pregnancies. *British Medical Journal*, **303**, 992.

Gartrad, A.R. (1994) Attitudes and beliefs of Muslim mothers towards pregnancy and infancy. *Archives of Disease in Childhood*, **71**, 170–4.

Gellner, E. (1992) *Postmodernism, Reason and Religion*. London: Routledge.

Gerhardt, U. (1989) *Ideas about Illness: An Intellectual and Political History of Medical Sociology*. London: Macmillan.

Gibbons, J., Thorpe, S. and Wilkinson, P. (1990) *Family Support and Prevention: Studies in Local Areas*. National Institute for Social Work, London: HMSO.

Giddens, A. (1991) *Modernity and Self-Indentity: Self and Politics in the Late Modern Age*. Cambridge: Polity Press.

Gigerenzer, G. (1991) How to make cognitive illusions disappear: Beyond 'heuristics and biases'. In Stroebe, W. and Hewstone, M. (eds) *European Review of Social Psychology, Volume 2*. London: John Wiley.

Gigerenzer, G. (1996) On narrow norms and vague heuristics: A reply to Kahneman and Tversky (1996). *Psychological Review*, **10**, 592–6.

Gigerenzer, G., Swijtnik, Z., Porter, T., Daston, L., Beatty, J. and Krüger, L. (1990) *The Empire of Chance: How Probability Changed Science and Everyday Life*. Cambridge: Cambridge University Press.

Giller, H., Gormely, C. and Williams, P. (1992) *The Effectiveness of Child Protection Procedures: An Evaluation of Child Protection Procedures in Four ACPC Areas*. Cheshire

Social Information Systems.

**Gillick, V.** (1986) *Dear Mrs Gillick. The Public Respond.* Hampshire: Marshalls.

**Gillman, M., Heyman, B. and Swain, J.** (1997) Life history or 'case' history: The objectification of people with learning difficulties through the tyranny of professional discourses. *Disability and Society,* in press.

**Gillon, R.** (1985) Autonomy and consent. In Lockwood, M. (ed.) *Moral Dilemmas in Modern Medicine.* Oxford: Oxford University Press.

**Glaser, B. and Strauss, A.** (1967) *The Discovery of Grounded Theory.* Chicago: Aldine.

**Gleser, G.C. and Ihilevich, D.** (1969) An objective instrument for measuring defence mechanisms. *Journal of Consulting and Clinical Psychology,* **33**, 51–60.

**Gochman, D.S.** (ed.) (1988) *Health Behavior: Emerging Reasearch Perspectives.* New York: Plenum.

**Godlee, F. and Walker, A.** (1991) Importance of a healthy environment. *British Medical Journal,* **303**, 1124–6.

**Goffman, E.** (1968) *Asylums: Essays on the Social Situation of Mental Patients and Other Inmates.* Harmondsworth: Pelican Books.

**Goodwin, S. and Managan, P.** (1985) Do older people come from outer space? *Nursing Times,* **81**, 45–6.

**Gould, S.** (1980) *The Panda's Thumb.* Harmondsworth: Penguin Books.

**Graboys, T.B.** (1984) Stress and the aching heart. *New England Journal of Medicine,* **311**, 594–5.

**Graham, H.** (1984) *Women, Health and the Family.* Brighton, Sussex: Harvester Press.

**Graham, H.** (1987) Women's smoking and family health. *Social Science and Medicine,* **25**, 47–56.

**Grande, G.E., Todd, C.J. and Barclay, S.I.G.** (1995) *Symptom Control Skills and Symptom Communication in Palliative Care.* Paper presented at the European Public Health Association Meeting, Budapest.

**Gray, M.** (1979) Forcing old people to leave their homes. *Community Care,* 8 March, 19–20.

**Green, J.** (1994) Women's experiences of prenatal screening and diagnosis. In Abramsky, L. and Chapple, J. (eds) *Prenatal Diagnosis: The Human Side.* London: Chapman & Hall.

**Green, J.M., Dennis, J. and Bennets, L.A.** (1989) Attention disorder in a group of young Down's syndrome children. *Journal of Mental Deficiency Research,* **33**, 105–22.

**Greenhalgh, T.** (1993) In praise of RITA. *British Medical Journal,* **307**, 1012.

**Gribben, M.** (1992) *Seeking Out the Wounded Child.* London: Barnardo's.

**Griffin, C.** (1993) *Representations of Youth: The Study of Youth and Adolescence in Britain and America.* Cambridge: Polity Press.

**Grimley, D.M., Prochaska, J.O., Velicer, W.F. and Prochaska, G.E.** (1995) Contraceptive and condom use, adoption and maintenance: A stage paradigm approach. *Health Education Quarterly,* **22**, 20–35.

**Grinyer, A.** (1995) Risk, the real world and naïve sociology: Perceptions of risk from occupational injury in the health service. In Gabe, J. (ed.) *Medicine, Health and Risk: Sociological Approaches.* Oxford: Blackwell.

**Gubrium, J.F.** (1987) Structuring and destructuring the course of illness: The Alzheimer's disease experience. *Sociology of Health and Illness,* **9**, 1–24.

**Guidotti, R.** (1986) Appropriate perinatal technology. In Phaff, J.M.L. (ed.) *Perinatal Health Services in Europe: Searching for Better Childbirth.* London: Croom Helm.

**Hacking, I.** (1975) *The Emergence of Probability: A Philosophical Study of Early Ideas about Probability, Induction and Statistical Inference.* Cambridge: Cambridge University Press.

Hacking, I. (1990) *The Taming of Chance.* Cambridge: Cambridge University Press.

Hafner, H. and Boker, W. (1982) *Crimes of Violence by Mentally Abnormal Offenders: A Psychiatric and Epidemiological Study in the Federal German Republic.* Cambridge: Cambridge University Press.

Hall, L.A. (1992) Forbidden by government, despised by men: Masturbation, medical warnings, moral panic and manhood in Great Britain, 1850–1890. *Journal of the History of Sexuality,* **2**, 365–87.

Hall, S. (1992) The West and the rest: Discourse and power. In Hall, S. and Geiben, B. (eds) *Formations of Modernity.* Cambridge: Polity Press.

Hammond, M. (1990) Is nursing a semi-profession? *Canadian Nurse,* **86**, 20–3.

Hancock, T. (1993) Health, human development and the community ecosystem: Three ecological models. *Health Promotion International,* **8**, 41–7.

Handwerker, L. (1994) Medical risk: Implicating poor pregnant women. *Social Science & Medicine,* **38**, 665–75.

Handyside, E.C. (1995) The needs of people with HIV, their informal carers and service providers. In Heyman, B. (ed) *Researching User Perspectives on Community Health Care.* London: Chapman & Hall.

Hansen, J.P. (1986) Older maternal age and pregnancy outcome: A review of the literature. *Obstetrical and Gynaecological Survey,* **41**, 726–42.

Hansson, S.O. (1989) Dimensions of risk. *Risk Analysis,* **9**, 107–12.

Hansson, S.O. (1993) The false promise of risk analysis. *Ratio* (New Series), **6**, 16–26.

Harker, L. and Thorpe, K. (1992) The last egg in the basket? Elderly primiparity: A review of findings. *Birth,* **19**, 23–30.

Hartmann, B.W., Kirchengast, S., Albrecht, A., Metka, M. and Huber, J.C. (1995) Hysterectomy increases the symptomology of postmenopausal syndrome. *Gynecological Endocrinology,* **9**, 247–52.

Hasselkus, B.R. (1988) Meaning in family caregiving: Perspectives on caregiver/professional relationships. *The Gerontologist,* **28**, 686–91.

Hayes, M.V. (1992) On the epistemology of risk: Language, logic and social science. *Social Science & Medicine,* **35**, 401–7.

Hayes, R.B., Sackett, D.L., Taylor, D.W., Gibson, E. and Johnson, A.L. (1978) Increased absenteeism from work after detection and labelling of hypertensive patients. *New England Journal of Medicine,* **299**, 741–4.

Health Advisory Service (1995) *People who are Homeless: Mental Health Services.* London: HMSO.

Health Education Authority (1992) *The Facts About HIV and AIDS.* London: Health Education Authority.

Healthcare Service Commissioner (1994) *Annual Report for 1993–94.* London: HMSO.

Heller, R.F., Saltzstein, H.D. and Caspe, W.B. (1992) Heuristics in medical and non-medical decision-making. *The Quarterly Journal of Experimental Psychology,* **44A**, 211–35.

Helman, C. (1989) *Culture, Health and Illness.* Bristol: Wright.

Henry, J.P. (1982) The relation of social to biological disease processes. *Social Science & Medicine,* **16**, 369–80.

Herzlich, C. (1979) *Health and Illness.* London: Academic Press.

Heslon, R., Mitchell, V. and Moane, G. (1984) Personality and patterns of adherence and nonadherence to the social clock. *Journal of Personality and Social Psychology,* **46**, 1079–96.

Hestnes, A., Sand, T. and Fostad, K. (1991) Ocular findings in Down's syndrome. *Journal of Mental Deficiency Research,* **35**, 194–203.

**Heyman, B.** (1995a) (ed.) *Researching User Perspectives on Community Health Care.* London: Chapman & Hall.

**Heyman, B.** (1995b) Patients' views of GPs. In Heyman, B. (ed.) *Researching User Perspectives on Community Health Care.* London: Chapman & Hall.

**Heyman, B. and Huckle, S.** (1993a) Normal life in a hazardous world: How adults with moderate learning difficulties and their carers cope with risks and dangers. *Disability, Handicap and Society,* **8**, 143–60.

**Heyman, B. and Huckle, S.** (1993b) Not worth the risk? Attitudes of adults with learning difficulties and their informal and formal carers to the hazards of everyday life. *Social Science and Medicine,* **12**, 1557–64.

**Heyman, B. and Huckle, S.** (1995a) How adults with learning difficulties and their carers see 'the community'. In Heyman, B. (ed.) *Researching User Perspectives on Community Health Care.* London: Chapman & Hall.

**Heyman, B. and Huckle, S.** (1995b) Talking to people with learning difficulties. In Reed, J. and Procter, S. (eds) *Practitioner Research in Health Care.* London: Chapman & Hall.

**Heyman, B. and Huckle, S.** (1995c) Sexuality as a perceived hazard in the lives of adults with learning difficulties. *Disability and Society,* **10**, 139–55.

**Heyman, B., Swain, J., Gillman, M., Handyside, E.C. and Newman, W.** (1997) Alone in the crowd: How adults with learning difficulties cope with social network problems. *Social Science and Medicine,* **44**, 41–53.

**Hill, D.J., Maher, D.J., Wood, C.E., Lolatgis, N., Lawrence, A., Dowling, B. and Lawrence M.** (1994) The complications of laparoscopic hysterectomy. *Journal of the American Association of Gynecologic Laparascopists,* **1**, 159–62.

**Hill, M.N. and Grim, C.M.** (1991) How to take a precise blood pressure. *American Journal of Nursing,* **91**, 38–42.

**Hillman, M., Adams, J. and Whitelegg, J.** (1990) *One False Move: A Study of Children's Independent Mobility.* London: Policy Studies Institute.

**Hinchliff, S.M., Norman, S.E. and Schober, J.E.** (eds) (1993) *Nursing Practice and Health Care,* 2nd edn. London: Edward Arnold.

**HMSO** (1908) *Report of the Royal Commission on the Care and Control of the Feeble Minded.* London: HMSO.

**HMSO** (1969) *Report of the Committee of Enquiry Into The Allegations of Ill-Treatment of Patients and Other Irregularities At The Ely Hospital, Cardiff.* London: HMSO.

**HMSO** (1978) *Report of the Committee of Enquiry into Normansfield Hospital.* London: HMSO.

**HMSO** (1979) *Report of the Committee of Enquiry into Mental Handicap Nursing and Care,* Chairman Peggy Jay, Vol. 1. London: HMSO.

**HMSO** (1989) *Community Care: Services for People with a Mental Handicap and People with a Mental Illness.* London: HMSO.

**HMSO** (1990) *Caring For People. Community Care in the Next Decade and Beyond.* London: HMSO.

**Høeg, P.** (1994) *Miss Smilla's Feeling for Snow.* London: Flamingo.

**Holden, J.** (1990) Models, muddles and medicine. *International Journal of Nursing Studies,* **27**, 223–34.

**Hollander, D. and Breen, J.L.** (1990) Pregnancy in the older gravida: How old is old? *Obstetric Gynaecology Survey,* **45**, 106–12.

**Holman, C.D.J.** (1996) Ought low alcohol intake to be promoted for health reasons? *Journal of the Royal Society of Medicine,* **89**, 123–9.

**Hood, C. and Jones, K.C.** (eds) (1996) *Accident and Design.* London: UCL Press.

**Hood, C.C., Jones, D.K.C., Pigeon, N.F., Turner, B.A. and Gibson, R.** (1992) Risk management. In The Royal Society *Risk: Analysis, Perception and Management. Report of a Royal Society Study Group.*

**Horner, T.M., Guyer, M.J. and Kalter, N.M.** (1993) Clinical expertise and the assessment of child sexual abuse. *Journal of the American Academy of Child Adolescent Psychiatry,* **32,** 925–31.

**Horrobin, D.F.** (1988) *Oxford Textbook of Medicine.* Oxford: Oxford University Press.

**Hough, M. and Mayhew, P.** (1983) *British Crime Survey: First Report.* London: HMSO.

**Howlett, B.C., Ahmad, W.I.U. and Murray, R.** (1992) An exploration of White, Asian and Afro-Caribbean peoples' concepts of health and illness causation. *New Community,* **18,** 281–92.

**Hudson, F. and Ineichen, B.** (1991) *Taking It Lying Down: Sexuality and Teenage Motherhood.* Hong Kong: Macmillan Education.

**Husted, G.L. and Husted, J.H.** (1991) *Ethical Decsion-making in Nursing.* St Louis: Mosby Year Book.

**Iliffe, S., See Thai, S., Hanes, A., Gallivan, S., Goldenberg, E., Boor, A. and Morgan, P.** (1992) Are elderly people living alone an at-risk group? *British Medical Journal,* **305,** 1001–4.

**Illich, I.** (1977) *Limits to Medicine.* Harmondsworth: Pelican Books.

**Illsley, R. and Taylor, R.** (1974) *Sociological Aspects of Teenage Pregnancy.* Occasional Paper No. 1. MRC Unit, Aberdeen: University of Aberdeen.

**Ineichen, B. and Hudson, F.** (1994) *Teenage Pregnancy.* National Children's Bureau, March. Reprinted in *MIDIRS Midwifery Digest* March 1995, **5,** 1, 39–41.

**International Medical Advisor Panel** (1994) IMAP statement on emergency contraception. *International Planned Parenthood Federation Medical Bulletin,* **28,** 1–2.

**Jackson, S., Sanders, R. and Thomas, N.** (1995) *Setting Priorities in Child Protection: Perception of Risk and Agency Strategy.* Paper presented at the ESRC Risk in Organisational Settings Conference, London.

**Jacobson, B., Smith, A. and Whitehead, M.** (eds) (1991) *The Nation's Health: A Strategy for the 1990s.* London: King Edward Fund for London.

**James, G.D., Yee, L.S. and Pickering, T.G.** (1990) Winter–summer differences in the effect of emotion, posture and place of measurement on blood pressure. *Social Science and Medicine,* **31,** 1213–17.

**Jeffrey, R.** (1979) Normal rubbish: Deviant patients in casualty departments. *Sociology of Health and Illness,* **1,** 98–107.

**Jenkins, R.** (1986) Social anthropological models of inter-ethnic relations. In Rex, J. and Mason, D. (eds) *Theories of Race and Ethnic Relations.* Cambridge: Cambridge University Press.

**Jerrome, D.** (1992) *Good Company: An Anthropological Study of Old People in Groups.* Edinburgh: Edinburgh University Press.

**Jewell, D.** (1987) Taking blood pressure. *Update,* **35,** 934–41.

**Johnson, A.G.** (1989) *Human Arrangements: An Introduction to Sociology.* Florida: Harcourt Brace Jovanovich.

**Johnston, M.** (1986) Preoperative emotional states and postoperative recovery. *Advances in Psychosomatic Medicine,* **15,** 1–22.

**Jolly, A.** (1991) Taking blood pressure. *Nursing Times,* **87,** 40–3.

**Jones, M.** (1996) *Choosing Older Motherhood.* London: Vermilion.

**Jones, C. and Bassell, S.** (1987) *So Good So Far? A Study of Quality of Life of Residents Discharged from Llanfrecha Grange.* Pontypod: Gwent Health Authority.

**Jones, S.K., Jones, K.T. and Frisch, D.** (1995) Biases of probability assessment: A comparison of frequency and single-case judgments. *Organizational Behavior and Human Decision Processes,* **61,** 109–22.

**Joseph, P.** (1993) Social factors in forensic psychiatry. In Bhugra, D. and Leff, J. (eds) *Principles of Social Psychiatry.* Oxford: Blackwell Scientific Publications.

**Josephs, D.H.** (1993) Risk: A concept worthy of attention. *Nursing Forum,* **28,** 12–16.

**Kahneman, D. and Tversky, A.** (1972) Subjective probability: A judgment of representativeness. *Cognitive Psychology,* **3,** 430–54.

**Kahneman, D. and Tversky, A.** (1973) On the psychology of prediction. *Psychological Review* **80,** 237–51.

**Kahneman, D. and Tversky, A.** (1979) Prospect theory: An analysis of decision under risk. *Econometrika,* **47,** 263–91.

**Kahneman, D. and Tversky, A.** (1996) On the reality of cognitive illusions. *Psychological Review,* **103,** 582–91.

**Kaplan, R.M.** (1995) *The Power Behind Your Eyes: Improving Your Eyesight with Integrated Vision Therapy.* Rochester, Vermont: Healing Art Press.

**Kay, B.** (1996) Qualifying existence. *Nursing Times,* **18,** 31–2.

**Keady, J. and Nolan, M.** (1994) Younger onset dementia: Developing a longitudinal model as the basis for a research agenda and as a guide to interventions with sufferers and carers. *Journal of Advanced Nursing,* **19,** 659–69.

**Kee, F., Gaffney, B. and McDonald, P.** (1995) *Treatment or Prevention? The Patient's Perspective.* Paper presented at the European Public Health Association Meeting, Budapest.

**Kelly, M.P. and May, D.** (1982) 'Good' and 'bad' patients: A review of the literature and theoretical critique. *Journal of Advanced Nursing,* **7,** 147–56.

**Kemp, F., Foster, C. and McKinlay, S.** (1993) Blood pressure measurement technique of clinical staff. *Journal of Human Hypertension,* **7,** 95–102.

**Kempe, C., Silverman, F., Steele, B., Droegemueller, W. and Silver, H.** (1962) The battered child syndrome. *Journal of the American Medical Association,* **181,** 17–24.

**Kemshall, H. and Pritchard, J.** (eds) (1996) *Good Practice in Risk Assessment and Risk Management.* London: Jessica Kingsley.

**Kennard, A., Goodburn, S., Golightly, S. and Piggott, M.** (1995) Serum screening for Down's syndrome. *Midwives,* **108,** 207–10.

**Kennedy, B.J., Tellegen, A., Kennedy, S. and Havernick, N.** (1976) Psychological responses of patients cured of advanced cancer. *Cancer,* **38,** 2184–91.

**Kersker, S.** (1994) The consumer perspective on family involvement. In Lefley, H. and Wasow, M. (eds) *Helping Families Cope with Mental Illness.* Chur, Switzerland: Harwood Academic Publishers.

**Key, M.** (1989) The practice of assessing elders. In Stevenson, O. (ed.) *Age and Vulnerability: A Guide to Better Care.* Age Concern Handbooks. London: Edward Arnold.

**Kickbusch, I.** (1986) Issues in health promotion. *Health Promotion,* **1,** 437–42.

**Kilgour, D. and Speedie, G.** (1985) Taking the pressure off. *Nursing Mirror,* **160,** 39–40.

**King, I.M.** (1981) *A Theory for Nursing: Systems, Concepts, Process.* New York: John Wiley.

**Kingsley, S. and Douglas, R.** (1991) Developing service strategies: The transition to community care. In McNaught, A. (ed.) *Managing Community Health Services,* London: Chapman & Hall.

**Kinney, W.R. Jr and Uecker, W.** (1982) Mitigating the consequences of anchoring in auditor judgments. *The Accounting Review,* **LVII,** 55–67.

**Kitson, A.L.** (1987) A comparative analysis of lay-caring and professional (nursing) caring relationships. *International Journal of Nursing Studies,* **24,** 155–65.

**Kitwood, T. and Bredin, K.** (1992) Towards a theory of dementia care: Personhood and well-being. *Ageing and Society,* **12,** 269–87.

**Kohner, N.** (1994) *Clinical Supervision in Practice.* London: Kings Fund Centre.

**Kolb, D.** (1984) *Experiential Learning.* London: Prentice Hall.

**Konje, J.C., Palmer, A., Watson, A., Hay, D.M. and Imrie, A.** (1992) Early teenage pregnancies in Hull. *British Journal of Obstetrics and Gynaecology,* **99,** 969–73.

**Krakoff, L.R.** (1994) *Management of the Hypertensive Patient.* New York: Churchill Livingstone.

**Krause, I.** (1989) Sinking heart: A Punjabi communication of distress. *Social Science & Medicine,* **29,** 563–75.

**Kreger, B.E., Anderson, K.M., Schatzkin, A. and Splansky, G.L.** (1992) Serum cholesterol level, body mass index, and the risk of colon cancer: The Framingham study. *Cancer,* **70,** 1038–43.

**Krieger, N.** (1994) Epidemiology and the web of causation: Has anyone seen the spider? *Social Science and Medicine,* **39,** 887–903.

**Kringlen, E.** (1994) Is the concept of schizophrenia useful from an aetiological point of view? A selective review of findings and paradoxes. *Acta Psychiatrica Scandinavia Supplement,* **384,** 17–25.

**Kroker, A. and Kroker, M.** (1988) Panic sex in America. In Kroker, A. and Kroker, M. (eds) *Body Invaders: Sexuality and the Postmodern Condition.* London: Macmillan Education.

**Kuhn, T.** (1962) *The Structure of Scientific Revolutions.* Chicago: University of Chicago Press.

**Lafaille, R. and Fulder, S.** (eds) (1993) *Towards a New Science of Health.* London: Routledge.

**Lakoff, G. and Johnson, M.** (1981) *Metaphors We Live By.* Chicago: University of Chicago Press.

**Lane, K.** (1995) The medical model of the body as a site of risk: A case study of childbirth. In Gabe, G. (ed.) *Medicine, Health and Risk: Sociological Approaches.* Oxford: Blackwell.

**Langford, J.** (1992) Over 35 and at risk? *New Generation,* **11,** 4–5.

**Lash, S., Szerszynski, B. and Wynne, B.** (eds) (1996) *Risk, Environment and Modernity: Towards a New Ecology.* London: Sage.

**Law, M.G., Rosenberg, P.S., McDonald, A. and Kaldor, J.M.** (1996) Age-specific HIV incidence among homosexually active men in Australia. *Medical Journal of Australia,* **164,** 715–18.

**Lawler, J.** (1991) *Behind the Screens: Nursing, Somology, and the Problem with the Body.* Edinburgh: Churchill Livingstone.

**Lazarides, L.** (1996) Editorial. *Nutritional Therapy Today,* **6,** 1–2.

**Lazarus, R.S.** (1992) Coping with the stress of illness. In Kaplan, A. (ed.) *Health Promotion and Chronic Illness: Discovering a New Quality of Health.* Geneva: WHO Regional Publications, European Series, **44,** 11–32.

**Lazarus, R.S. and Folkman, S.** (1984) Coping and adaptation. In Gentry, W.D. (ed.) *The Handbook of Behavioural Medicine.* New York: Guilford.

**Leary, M.R.** (1982) Hindsight distortion and the 1980 presidential election. *Personality and Social Psychology Bulletin,* **8,** 257–63.

**Leddy, S. and Pepper, J.M.** (1993) *Conceptual Bases of Professional Nursing.* Philadelphia: J.B. Lippincott.

**Lee, P.N.** (1994) Smoking and Alzheimer's disease: A review of the epidemolgic evidence. *Neuroepidemiology,* **13,** 131–44.

**Lefcourt, H.M.** (1992) Durability and impact of the locus of control construct. *Psychological Bulletin,* **112,** 411–14.

**Lehner, P.E., Laskey, K.B. and Dubois, D.** (1996) An introduction to issues in higher order uncertainty. *IEEE Transactions on Systems, Man and Cybernetics – Part A: Systems and Humans,* **26,** 289–92.

**Leininger, M.M.** (1985) Nature, rationale and importance of research methods in nursing. In Leininger, M.M. (ed.) *Qualitative Research Methods in Nursing.* Philadelphia: W.B. Saunders.

**Lewis, L.W. and Timby, B.K.** (1993) *Fundamental Skills and Concepts in Patient Care.* London: Chapman & Hall.

**Li, S. and Adams, A.S.** (1995) Is there something more important behind framing? *Organizational Behavior and Human Decision Processes,* **62,** 216–19.

**Lloyd, B.** (1995) Guidelines to reduce risk and improve the quality and cost-effectiveness of care. *Managing Risk,* April, 5.

**Lo, S.V., Kaul, S. and Kaul, R.** (1994) Teenage pregnancy: Contraceptive use and non-use. *British Journal of Family Planning,* **20,** 79–83.

**Lomax, A.** (1921) *The Experiences of an Asylum Doctor.* London: Allan & Unwin.

**London Borough of Brent** (1985) *A Child in Trust: The Report of the Panel of Inquiry into the Circumstances Surrounding the Death of Jasmine Beckford.* Wembley, Middlesex: London Borough of Brent.

**Lopez, P.M., Stoner, D. and Gilmour, H.** (1995) Epidemiology of Down's syndrome in a Scottish city. *Paediatric and Perinatal Epidemiology,* **9,** 331–40.

**Lorber, J.** (1975) Good patients and problem patients: Conformity and deviance in a general hospital. *Journal of Health and Social Behaviour,* **16,** 213–25.

**Lundh, L.G.** (1987) Placebo, belief and health: A cognitive-emotional model. *Scandinavian Journal of Psychology,* **28,** 128–43.

**Luoto, R., Kaprio, J., Reunanen, A. and Rutanen, E.M.** (1995) Cardiovascular morbidity in relation to ovarian function after hysterectomy. *Obstetrics and Gynecology,* **85,** 515–22.

**Lupton, D.** (1993) Risk as moral danger: The social and political functions of risk discourse in public health. *International Journal of Health Services,* **23,** 425–35.

**Lupton, D.** (1994a) *Medicine as Culture: Illness, Disease and the Body in Western Societies.* London: Sage.

**Lupton, D.** (1994b) *Moral Threats and Dangerous Desires: AIDS in the News Media.* London: Taylor & Francis.

**MacDonald, G. and Smith, C.** (1990) Complacency, risk perception and the problem of HIV education. *AIDS Care,* **2,** 63–8.

**Macintyre, S.** (1977) Old age as social problem. In Dingwall, R., Heath, C., Reid, M. and Stacey, M. (eds) *Health Care and Health Knowledge.* London: Croom Helm.

**MacKay, C.** (1994) Violence to health care professionals: A health and safety perspective. In Wykes, T. (ed.) *Violence and Health Care Professionals.* London: Chapman & Hall.

**MacKenbach, J.P., Bouvier-Colle, M.H. and Jougla, E.** (1990) 'Avoidable' mortality and health services: A review of aggregate data studies. *Journal of Epidemiology and Community Health,* **44,** 106–11.

**MacKinnon, M.** (1993) *Providing Diabetes Care in General Practice: A Practical Guide for the Primary Health Care Team.* London: Class Publishing.

**MacLachlan, R.A., Fidler, K.E., Yeh, H., Hodgetts, P.G., Pharand, G. and Chau, M.** (1993) Cervical spine abnormalities in institutionalized adults with Down's syndrome. *Journal of Intellectual Disability Research,* **37,** 277–85.

**MacMahon, B., Pugh, T.F. and Ipsen, J.** (1960) *Epidemiologic Methods.* Boston, USA: Little Brown.

**Males, M.A.** (1995) Adult involvement in teenage childbearing and STD. *Lancet,* **346,** 64–5.

**Manderson, L.** (1987) Hot–cold food and medical theories: Overview and introduction. *Social Science & Medicine*, **25**, 329–30.

**Mansfield, P.K.** (1986a) Like a boxer over the hill? Assessing the prejudice against mid-life childbearing. *Health/PAC Bulletin*, **16**, 15–21.

**Mansfield, P.K.** (1986b) Re-evaluating the medical risks of late childbearing. *Women and Health*, **11**, 37–60.

**Mansfield, P.K.** (1986c) *Pregnancy for Older Women: Assessing the Medical Risks.* New York: Praeger Publications.

**Mansfield, P.K.** (1988) Midlife childbearing: Strategies for informed decision-making. *Psychology of Women Quarterly*, **12**, 445–60.

**Marino, B.** (1993) Congenital heart disease in patients with Down's syndrome: Anatomic and genetic aspects. *Biomedicine and Pharmacotherapy*, **47**, 197–200.

**Marks, D.F. and Clarkson, J.K.** (1972) An explanation of conservatism in the book-bag-and-pokerchips situation. *Acta Psychologica*, **36**, 145–60.

**Marks, D.F. and Clarkson, J.K.** (1973) Conservatism as non-Bayesian performance: A reply to De Swart. *Acta Psychologica*, **37**, 55–63.

**Marmot, M. and Elliot, P.** (1992) *Coronary Heart Disease Epidemiology: From Aetiology to Public Health.* Oxford: Oxford Medical Publications.

**Marshall, M.** (1990) Proud to be old. In McEwen, E. (ed.) *Age: The Unrecognised Discrimination.* London: Age Concern England.

**Marshall, T. and Bottomore, T.** (1990) *Citizenship and Social Class.* London: Pluto Press.

**Martin, E.** (1994) *Flexible Bodies: Tracking Immunity in American Culture from the Days of Polio to the Age of AIDS.* Boston: Beacon Press.

**Martin, P.** (1997) *The Sickening Mind: Brain, Behaviour, Immunity and Disease.* London: HarperCollins.

**Martin, J. and White, A.** (1985) *Infant Feeding: OPCS Infant Feeding Survey.* London: HMSO.

**Martin, L.R., Friedman, H.S., Tucker, J.S., Schwartz, J.E., Criqui, M.H. and Wingard, D.L.** (1995) An archival prospective study of mental health and longevity. *Health Psychology*, **14**, 381–7.

**Martini, C.J., Allan, G.H., Davison, J. and Backett, E.M.** (1977) Health indexes sensitive to medical care intervention. *International Journal of Health Services*, **7**, 293–309.

**Mason, D.** (1990) A rose by any other name … ?: Categorisation, identity, and social science. *New Community*, **17**, 123–33.

**Mason, J.M.** (1994) Cost per QALY league tables: Their role in pharmacoeconomic analysis. *Pharmacoeconomics*, **5**, 472–81.

**Mawby, R.I.** (1988) Age, vulnerability and the impact of crime. In Maguire, M. and Pointing, J. (eds) *Victims of Crime: A New Deal?* Milton Keynes: Open University Press.

**Maxfield, M.** (1987) *Explaining Fear of Crime: Evidence from the 1984 British Crime Survey.* London: HMSO.

**Mazzoni, D.S., Ackley, R.S. and Nash, D.J.** (1994) Abnormal pinna type and hearing loss correlations in Down syndrome. *Journal of Intellectual Disability Research*, **38**, 549–60.

**McElroy, E. and McElroy, P.** (1994) Family concerns about confidentiality and the seriously mentally ill: Ethical implications. In Lefley, H. and Wasow, M. (eds) *Helping Families Cope with Mental Illness.* Chur, Switzerland: Harwood Academic Publishers.

**McGeary, K.** (1994) The influence of guarding on the developing mother–unborn child relationship. In Field, P.A. and Marck, P.B. (eds) *Uncertain Motherhood: Negotiating the Risks of the Childbearing Years.* Thousand Oaks, CA: Sage.

**McGee, R. and Stanton, W.R.** (1993) A longitudinal study of reasons for smoking in adolescence. *Addiction*, **88**, 265–71.

**McGregor, J.M. and Young, A.R.** (1996) Sunscreens, suntans and skin cancer. *British Medical Journal,* **312,** 1621–2.

**McGrother, C.W. and Marshall, B.** (1990) Recent trends in incidence, morbidity and survival in Down's syndrome. *Journal of Mental Deficiency Research,* **34,** 49–57.

**McKee, C.** (1991) Breaking the mold: A humanistic approach to nursing practice. In McMahon, R. and Pearson, A. (eds) *Nursing as Therapy.* London: Chapman & Hall.

**McKenna, F.P., Warburton, D.M. and Winwood, M.** (1993) Exploring the limits of optimism: The case of smokers' decision making. *British Journal of Psychology,* **84,** 389–94.

**McKeown, T.** (1979) *The Role of Medicine: Dream, Mirage or Nemesis.* Oxford: Blackwell.

**McKie, L., Al-Bashir, M., Anagnostopoulou, T., Csepe, P., El-Asafahani, A., Fonseca, H., Funiak, S., Javetz, R. and Samsuridjal, S.** (1993) Defining and assessing risky behaviours. *Journal of Advanced Nursing,* **18,** 1911–16.

**McVicker, R.W., Shanks, O.E.P. and McClelland, R.J.** (1994) Prevalence and associated features of epilepsy in adults with Down's syndrome. *British Journal of Psychiatry,* **164,** 528–32.

**Medicines Control Agency** (1995) *Medicines Act Leaflet: A Guide to What is a Medicinal Product.* London: Medicines Control Agency.

**Mellanby, A., Phelps, F. and Tripp, J.H.** (1993) Teenagers, sex and risk taking. *British Medical Journal,* **307,** 25.

**Menzies, I.E.P.** (1970) *The Functioning of Social Systems as a Defence Against Anxiety.* London: Tavistock.

**Mestel, R.** (1995) The lengths some men will go to. *New Scientist,* **1976,** 9.

**Meyer, T.J. and Mark, M.M.** (1995) Effects of psychosocial interventions with adult cancer patients: A meta-analysis of randomised experiments. *Health Psychology,* **14,** 101–8.

**Michaels, C.A.** (ed.) (1994) *Transition Strategies for Persons with Learning Disabilities.* San Diego, CA: Singular Publishing.

**Middleton, D. and Curnock, D.** (1995) *Talk of Uncertainty: Doubt as an Organisational Resource for Co-ordinating Multi-Disciplinary Activity in Neonatal Intensive Care.* Paper presented at the ESRC Risk in Organisational Settings Conference, London.

**Mikkelsen, M., Hallberg, A., Poulsen, H., Frantzen, M., Hansen, J. and Peterson, M.B.** (1995) The epidemiologic study of Down's syndrome in Denmark, including family studies of chromosomes and DNA markers. *Developmental Brain Dysfunction,* **8,** 4–12.

**Miles, R.** (1984) Marxism versus the sociology of race relations. *Ethnic and Racial Studies,* **7,** 217–37.

**Mili, F., Lynch, C.F., Khoury, M.J., Flanders, W.D. and Edmonds, L.D.** (1993) Risk of childhood cancer for infants with birth-defects 2. A Record linkage study, Iowa, 989. *American Journal of Epidemiology,* **137,** 639–44.

**Milner, M., Barry Kinsella, C., Unwin, A. and Harrison, R.F.** (1992) The impact of maternal age on pregnancy and its outcome. *International Journal of Gynaecology and Obstetrics,* **38,** 281–6.

**Ministry of Health** (1965) *Improving the Effectiveness of the Hospital Service for the Mentally Subnormal.* London: HMSO.

**Minois, G.** (1987) *History of Old Age.* Chicago: The University of Chicago Press.

**Mitchell, T.R. and Kalb, L.S.** (1981) Effects of outcome knowledge and outcome valence on supervisors' evaluations. *Journal of Applied Psychology,* **66,** 604–12.

**Modeer, T., Barr, M. and Dahllof, G.** (1990) Periodontal disease in children with Down's syndrome. *Scandinavian Journal of Dental Research,* **98,** 228–34.

Moore, S. and Rosenthal, D. (1993) *Sexuality in Adolescence.* London: Routledge.

Moodley, P. (1995) Reaching out. In Fernando, S. (ed.) *Mental Health in a Multi-ethnic Society: A Multi-disciplinary Handbook.* London: Routledge.

Morris, J.K., Cook, D.G. and Shaper, A.G. (1994) Loss of employment and mortality. *British Medical Journal,* **308**, 1135–9.

Morris, P. (1969) *Put Away: A Sociological Study of Institutions for the Mentally Retarded.* London: Routledge & Kegan Paul.

Motluk, A. (1997) Losers get an attack of nerves. *New Scientist,* **2067**, 15.

Mueller, M.R. (1995) Significant symbols, symbolic boundaries and quilts in the time of AIDS. *Research in the Sociology of Health Care,* **12**, 3–23.

Murphy, R.J.L. (1979) Removing the marks from examination scripts before re-marking them: Does it make any difference? *British Journal of Educational Psychology,* **49**, 73–8.

Namnoum, A.B., Gehlbach, D.L., Hickman, T.N., Rock, J.A. and Goodman, S.B. (1995) The incidence of symptom recurrence after hysterectomy for endometriosis. *Fertility and Sterility,* **64**, 898–902.

Nash, J. (1979) *We Eat the Mines and the Mines Eat Us: Dependency and Exploitation in Bolivian Tin Mines.* New York: Columbia University Press.

National Health Service Executive (1996) *Promoting Clinical Effectiveness: A Framework for Action in and through the NHS.* London: Department of Health.

Nespoli, L., Burgio, G.R., Ugazio, A.G. and Maccario, R. (1993) Immunological features of Down's syndrome – a review. *Journal of Intellectual Disability Research,* **37**, 543–51.

Nettleton, S. (1995) *The Sociology of Health and Illness.* Cambridge: Polity Press.

Neugarten, B.L. (1979) Time, age and the life cycle. *American Journal of Psychiatry,* **136**, 887–94.

Neugarten, B.L., Moore, J.W. and Lowe, J.C. (1965) Age norms, age constraints, and adult socialisation. *American Journal of Sociology,* **70**, 710–17.

Newby, N.M. (1996) Chronic illness and the family life-cycle. *Journal of Advanced Nursing,* **23**, 786–91.

Niven, N. (1989) *Health Psychology: An Introduction for Nurses and Other Health Professionals.* Edinburgh: Churchill Livingstone.

Norman, A. (1980) *Rights and Risk,* 2nd edn. London: Centre for Policy on Ageing.

Norman, A. (1987) *Aspects of Ageism.* London: Centre for Policy on Ageing.

North, F.M., Syme, S.L., Feeney, A., Shipley, M. and Marmot, M. (1996) Psychosocial work environment and sickness absence among British civil servants: The Whitehall II Study. *American Journal of Public Health,* **86**, 332–40.

North East Thames and South East Thames Regional Health Authorities (1994) *Report of the Inquiry into the Care and Treatment of Christopher Clunis.* London: HMSO.

Northcraft, G.B. and Neale, M.A. (1987) Experts, amateurs, and real estate: An anchoring-and-adjustment perspective on property pricing decisions. *Organizational Behavior and Human Decision Processes,* **39**, 84–97.

Northern Region Genetics Service (1995) *Maternal Serum Screening in the Northern Region: Information for Health Professionals.* Newcastle upon Tyne: Northern Region Genetics Service.

Novakovic, B., Fears, T.R., Wexler, L.H., McClure, L.L., Wilson, D.L., McCalla, J.L. and Tucker, M.A. (1996) The experience of cancer in children and adolescents. *Cancer Nursing,* **19**, 54–9.

Oakley, A. (1993) *Essays on Women, Medicine and Health.* Edinburgh: Edinburgh University Press.

Obrdlik, A.J. (1942) Gallows humour: A sociological phenomenon. *American Journal of Sociology,* **47**, 709–16.

**O'Brien, E. and O'Malley, K.** (1981) *Essentials of Blood Pressure Management.* Edinburgh: Churchill Livingstone.

**Office for National Statistics** (1996) *Monitor: Population and Health.* 24 September, London: The Government Statistical Services.

**Ofman, U.S.** (1995) Sexual quality of life in men with prostate cancer. *Cancer,* **75**, 1949–53.

**Ogden, J.** (1993) Getting it wrong. *Nursing Times,* **89**, 18.

**Oliver, M.F.** (1992) Doubts about preventing coronary heart disease. *The British Medical Journal,* **304**, 393–4.

**OPCS** (1992) *Population Trends.* London: Office of Population Censuses and Surveys.

**OPCS** (1993a) *Congenital Malformation Statistics Notifications: A Statistical Review of Notifications of Congenital Malformations Received as Part of the England and Wales Monitoring System, 1991.* London: HMSO.

**OPCS** (1993b) *Population Trends.* London: Office of Population Censuses and Surveys.

**Orem, D.** (1980) *Nursing: Concepts of Practice.* New York: McGraw Hill.

**Pain, R.H.** (1994) Elderly women and fear of violent crime: The least likely victims? *British Journal of Criminology,* **35**, 584–98.

**Paley, J.** (1996) Intuition and expertise: Comments on the Benner debate. *Journal of Advanced Nursing,* **23**, 665–71.

**Parkinson, M.** (1990) Taking risks. *Nursing the Elderly.* February, **8**.

**Parse, R.R.** (1981) *Man – Living – Health: A Theory of Nursing.* New York: John Wiley.

**Parton, N.** (1985) *The Politics of Child Abuse.* Basingstoke: Macmillan.

**Parton, N.** (1996) Social work, risk and the 'blaming system'. In Parton, N. (ed.) *Social Theory, Social Change and Social Work.* London: Routledge.

**Pascall, G.** (1986) *Social Policy: A Feminist Analysis.* London: Tavistock.

**Paterson, B.** (1994) A phenomenological study of the decision making experience of individuals with long-standing diabetes. *Canadian Journal of Diabetes Care,* **18**, 10–19.

**Pattie, A.H. and Gilleard, C.J.** (1979) *Manual for the Clifton Assessment Procedures for the Elderly (CAPE).* Sevenoaks, England: Hodder & Stoughton Educational.

**Pellegrino, E. and Thomasma, D.** (1988) *For the Patient's Good: The Restoration of Beneficence in Health Care.* New York: Oxford University Press.

**Pennington, D.C., Rutter, D.R., McKenna, K. and Morley, I.E.** (1980) Estimating the outcome of a pregnancy test: Women's judgements in foresight and hindsight. *British Journal of Social and Clinical Psychology,* **19**, 317–24.

**Perske, R.** (1972) The dignity of risk and the mentally retarded. *Mental Retardation,* **10**, 24–7.

**Personal Social Services Council** (1977) *Residential Care Reviewed.* London: Personal Social Services Council.

**Peters, T.** (1987) *Thriving on Chaos.* London: Harper & Row.

**Petrie, J.C., O'Brien, E.T., Littler, W.A. and De Swiet, M.** (1986) Recommendations on blood pressure measurement. *British Medical Journal,* **292**, 611–15.

**Petrou, S. and Renton, A.** (1993) The QALY: A guide for the public health physician. *Public Health,* **107**, 327–36.

**Phillimore, P., Beattie, A. and Townsend, P.** (1994) The widening gap: Inequality of health in Northern England, 1989–1991. *British Medical Journal,* **308**, 1125–8.

**Phillips, L.D. and Edwards. W.** (1966) Conservatism in a simple probability inference task. *Journal of Experimental Psychology,* **72**, 346–54.

**Phoenix, A.** (1991) *Young Mothers?* Cambridge: Polity Press.

**Piaget, J.** (1932) *The Moral Judgement of the Child.* New York: Harcourt Brace & World.

**Piaget, J. and Inhelder, B.** (1958) *The Growth of Logical Thinking from Childhood to Adolescence.* London: Routledge.

**Pine, D.S., Cohen, P. and Brook, J.** (1996) Emotional problems during youth as predictors of stature during early adulthood: Results from a prospective epidemiologic study. *Pediatrics,* **97**, 856–63.

**Pitz, G.P.** (1968) Information seeking when available information is limited. *Journal of Experimental Psychology,* **76**, 25–34.

**Platt, L.** (1995) *Young Women and Sex: Reproductive Ideologies.* Norwich: Social Work Monographs, No. 131.

**Points, T.C.** (1957) The elderly primipara. *Obstetrics and Gynaecology,* **9**, 348–54.

**Porter, R.** (1986) Plague and panic. *New Society,* 12 December, 11–13.

**Potter, P.A. and Perry, A.G.** (1995) *Basic Nursing: Theory and Practice.* St Louis: Mosby.

**Powles, J.** (1973) On the limitations of modern medicine. *Science, Medicine and Man,* **1**, 1–30.

**Poyner, B. and Hughes, N.A.** (1978) *Classification of Fatal Home Accidents.* London: The Tavistock Institute of Human Relations.

**Prasher, V.P.** (1995) Overweight and obesity amongst Down's syndrome adults. *Journal of Intellectual Disability Research,* **39**, 437–41.

**Pratt, C., Schmall, V. and Wright, S.** (1987) Ethical concerns of family caregivers to dementia patients. *The Gerontologist,* **27**, 632–8.

**Prendergast, S. and Prout, A.** (1990) Learning about birth: Parenthood and sex education in English secondary schools. In Garcia, J., Kilpatrick, R. and Richards, M. (eds) *The Politics of Maternity Care.* Oxford: Clarendon Press.

**Pueschel, S.M., Bernier, J.C. and Pezzullo, J.C.** (1991) Behavioral observations in children with Down's syndrome. *Journal of Mental Deficiency Research,* **35**, 502–11.

**Puri, B.K. and Singh, I.** (1995) Season of birth in Down's syndrome. *British Journal of Clinical Practice,* **49**, 129–30.

**Quadrango, J.** (1982) *Aging in Early Industrial Society.* New York: Academic Press.

**Qureshi, B.** (1989) *Transcultural Medicine.* Dordrecht: Kluwer Academic.

**Rabinow, P.** (1984) *The Foucault Reader.* Harmondsworth: Penguin Books.

**Radcliffe-Brown, A.R.** (1965) *Structure and Function in Primitive Society.* First published 1940. New York: The Free Press.

**Raffle, A.E., Alden, B. and Mackenzie, E.F.D.** (1995) Detection rates for abnormal cervical smears: What are we screening for? *Lancet,* **345**, 1469–73.

**Ramon, S.** (1996) *Mental Health in Europe: Ends, Beginnings and Rediscoveries.* Basingstoke: Macmillan/MIND.

**Rankin, J.M.** (1996) *Ethnicity and Health Beliefs.* Unpublished report, University of Newcastle upon Tyne.

**Rapp, R.** (1988a) The power of positive diagnosis: Medical and maternal discourses on aminocentesis. In Michaelson, K.L. (ed.) *Childbirth in America: Anthropological Perspectives.* MA, USA: Bergin & Harvey.

**Rapp, R.** (1988b) Chromosomes and communication: The discourse of genetic counselling. *Medical Anthropology Quarterly,* **2**, 143–57.

**Rapp, R.** (1993) Amniocentesis in sociocultural perspective. *Journal of Genetic Counselling,* **2**, 183–96.

**Raz, N., Torres, I.J., Briggs, S.D., Spencer, W.D., Thorton, A.E., Loken, W.J., Gunning, F.M., Mcquain, J.D., Driesen, N.R. and Acker, J.D.** (1995) Selective neuroanatomical abnormalities in Down's syndrome and their cognitive correlates – evidence from MRI morphometry. *Neurology,* **45**, 356–66.

**Reed, J. and Payton, V.R.** (1996) *Working to Create Continuity: Older People Managing* *the Move into the Care Home Setting.* Report No. 76, University of Newcastle upon Tyne, Centre for Health Services Research.

**Reed, M. and Harvey, D.L.** (1994) The new science and the old: Complexity and realism in the social sciences. *Journal for the Theory of Social Behaviour,* **22,** 355–80.

**Reif, L.** (1973) Managing a life with chronic illness. *American Journal of Nursing,* **73,** 261–4.

**Renn, O., Burns, W.J., Kasperson, J.X. and Kasperson, R.E.** (1992) The social amplification of risk: Theroretical foundations and empirical applications. *Journal of Social Issues,* **4,** 137–60.

**Rescher, N.** (1983) *Risk: A Philosophical Introduction,* Washington DC: University Press of America.

**Richardson, D.** (1987) *Women and the AIDS Crisis.* London: Pandora.

**Richardson, S.A.** (1989) Letting go: A mother's view. *Disability, Handicap and Society,* **4,** 81–92.

**Richardson, S.A. and Ritchie, J.** (1989) *Letting Go.* Milton Keynes: Open University Press.

**Riggs, J.E.** (1996) The protective influence of cigarette smoking on Alzheimer's and Parkinson's diseases: Quagmire or opportunity for neuroepidemiology? *Neurological Clinics,* **14,** 353.

**Rijke, R.** (1993) Health in medical science: From determinism towards autonomy. In Lafaille, R. and Fulder, S. (eds) *Towards a New Science of Health.* London: Routledge.

**Rittel, H.W.J. and Weber, M.M.** (1974) *Dilemmas in a General Theory of Planning.* New York: Petrocelli.

**Roberts, H., Smith, S. and Bryce, C.** (1993) Prevention is better … . *Sociology of Health and Illness,* **15,** 447–63.

**Robinson, C.A.** (1993) Managing life with a chronic illness: The story of normalisation. *Qualitative Health Research,* **3,** 6–28.

**Rodin, J. and Langer, E.J.** (1977) Long-term effects of a control-relevant intervention with the institutionalised aged. *Journal of Personality and Social Psychology,* **35,** 897–902.

**Roeden, J.M. and Zitman, F.G.** (1995) Aging in adults with Down's syndrome in institutionally based and community based residences. *Journal of Intellectual Disability Research,* **39,** 399–407.

**Rogers, M.E.** (1970) *An Introduction to the Theoretical Basis of Nursing.* Philadelphia: F.A. Davis.

**Rogers, W.S.** (1991) *Explaining Health and Illness.* Hemel Hempstead: Harvester Wheatsheaf.

**Rogers A., Pilgrim, D. and Lacey, R.** (1993) *Experiencing Psychiatry: Users' Views of Services.* Basingstoke: Macmillan/MIND.

**Rokeach, M. and Ball-Rokeach, S.J.** (1989) Stability and change in American value priorities. *American Psychologist,* **47,** 397–411.

**Rooff, M.** (1957) *Voluntary Societies and Social Policy.* London: Routledge & Kegan Paul.

**Rook, S., Catalano, R. and Dooley, D.** (1989) The timing of major life events: Effects of departing from the social clock. *American Journal of Community Psychology,* **17,** 233–59.

**Roper, N., Logan, W.W. and Tierney, A.J.** (1980) *The Elements of Nursing.* Edinburgh: Churchill Livingstone.

**Rose, G.** (1985) Strategy of prevention: lessons from cardiovascular disease. *International Journal of Epidemiology,* **14,** 32–8.

**Rose, K.S.B.** (1994) A review of Down's syndrome studies and ionising radiation. *Journal of the British Nuclear Energy Society,* **33,** 145–51.

**Rosenstock, I.M.** (1985) Understanding and enhancing patient compliance with diabetic regimens. *Diabetes Care,* **8,** 610–16.

**Ross, J.W.** (1989) An ethics of compassion, a language of division: Working out the AIDS metaphors. In Corless, I.B. and Pittman-Lindeman, M. (eds) *AIDS: Principles, Practices and Politics.* New York: Hemisphere.

**Rothman, B.K.** (1988) The decision to have or not to have amniocentesis for prenatal diagnosis. In Michaelson, K.L. (ed.) *Childbirth in America: Anthropological Perspectives.* MA, USA: Bergin & Harvey.

**Rotter, J.B.** (1990) Internal versus external control of reinforcement: A case history of a variable. *American Psychologist,* **45,** 489–93.

**Roy, C.** (1980) The Roy adaptation model. In Riehl, J.P. and Roy, C. (eds) *Conceptual Models for Nursing Practice.* Norwalk: Appelton, Century Crofts.

**Roy, S.**(1996) Risk management. *Nursing Standard,* **10,** 51–4.

**Royle, J.A. and Walsh, M.** (1992) *Watson's Medical-Surgical Nursing and Related Physiology.* London: Baillière Tindall.

**Ruchelli, E., Uri, A., Duncan, L., Dimmick, J., Huff, D. and Witzleben, C.** (1990) Severe infantile subacute and chronic liver disease in Down's syndrome. *Laboratory Investigation,* **62,** 7.

**Rundle, R.** (1992) Parsons revisited: A reappraisal of the community nurse role. In Jolley, M. and Brykczynska, G. (eds) *Nursing Care: The Challenge to Change.* London: Edward Arnold.

**Rusch, R.G., Hall, J.C. and Griffen, H.C.** (1986) Abuse provoking characteristics of institutionalized mentally retarded individuals. *American Journal of Mental Deficiency,* **90,** 618–24.

**Ruskin, C.** (1987) *The Quilt: Stories from the NAMES Project.* New York, Pocket Books.

**Russell, J.K.** (1988) Early teenage pregnancy. *Maternal and Child Health,* **13,** 43–6.

**Rutter, M. and Smith, D.J.** (1995) *Psychosocial Disorders in Young People.* London: John Wiley.

**Ryan, T.** (1993) Therapeutic risk taking in mental health nursing. *Nursing Standard,* **7,** 29–31.

**Ryan, W.** (1976) *Blaming the Victim.* New York: Vintage Books.

**Ryan, J. and Thomas, F.** (1987) *The Politics of Mental Handicap.* London: Free Association.

**Sackett, D.L. and Haynes, R.B.** (1995) On the need for evidence-based medicine. *Evidence-Based Medicine,* **1,** 5–6.

**Said, E.** (1978) *Orientalism: Western Concepts of the Orient.* Harmondsworth: Penguin Books.

**Samuels, A.** (1993) The legal liability of the nurse: The lawyer's view. *Medical Science Law,* **33,** 305–9.

**Santow, G.** (1995) Education and hysterectomy. *Australian and New Zealand Journal of Obstetrics and Gynaecology,* **35,** 60–9.

**Sapolsky, H.M.** (1990) The politics of risk. *Daedalus,* **119,** 83–96.

**Sarafino, E.P.** (1990) *Health Psychology: Biopsychosocial Interactions.* New York: John Wiley.

**Sartorius, N.** (1989) Course and outcome in schizophrenia: A preliminary communication. In Cooper, B. and Helgason, T. (eds) *Epidemiology and the Prevention of Mental Disorders.* London: Routledge.

**Scanlon, C. and Sanders, T.** (1995) *Essentials of Anatomy and Physiology.* Philadelphia: F.A. Davis.

**Schiller, N.G., Crystal, S. and Lewellen, D.** (1994) Risky business: The cultural construction of AIDS risk groups. *Social Science and Medicine,* **38,** 1337–46.

**Schloo, B.L., Vawter, G.F. and Reid, L.M.** (1991) Down's syndrome: Patterns of disturbed lung growth. *Human Patholgy,* **22,** 919–23.

**Schneider, W., Gruber, H., Gold, A. and Opwis, K.** (1993) Chess expertise and memory for chess problems in children and adults. *Journal of Experimental Child Psychology,* **56,** 328–49.

**Schon, D.A.** (1983) *The Reflective Practitioner.* London: Temple Smith.

**Schon, D.A.** (1987) *Educating the Reflective Practitioner.* California: Jossey Bass.

**Schrag, C.** (1992) *The Resources of Rationality: A Response to the Postmodern Challenge.* Bloomington, Indianapolis: Indiana University Press.

**Schulz, R.** (1976) Effects of control and predictability on the psychological well-being of the institutionalized aged. *Journal of Personality and Social Psychology,* **33,** 563–73.

**Schuman, A.N. and Marteau, T.M.** (1993) Obstetricians' and midwives' contrasting perceptions of pregnancy. *Journal of Reproductive and Infant Psychology,* **11,** 115–18.

**Scott, J.** (1994) *What Young People Want from Family Planning Services.* Ipswich: Suffolk Health Authority.

**Scull, A.T.** (1979) *Museums of Madness: The Social Organisation of Insanity in Nineteenth-Century England.* Harmondsworth: Allen Lane.

**Searle, J.R.** (1995) *The Construction of Social Reality.* Harmondsworth: Allen Lane.

**Seebohm Report** (1968) *Report of the Committee on Local Authorities and Allied Personal Social Services.* London: HMSO.

**Seedhouse, D.** (1986) *Health: The Foundations for Achievement.* Chichester: John Wiley.

**Seedhouse, D.** (1995) 'Well-being': Health promotion's red herring. *Health Promotion International,* **10,** 61–7.

**Shaw, E.D. and Beals, R.K.** (1992) The hip joint in Down's syndrome: A study of its structure and associated disease. *Clinical Orthopaedics and Related Research,* **278,** 101–7.

**Sheldon, T.A. and Parker, H.** (1992) Race and ethnicity in health research. *Journal of Public Health Medicine,* **14,** 104–10.

**Sheppard, D.** (1996) *Learning the Lessons,* 2nd edn. London: The Zito Trust.

**Shiloh, S. and Saxe, L.** (1989) Perceptions of risk in genetic counselling. *Psychology and Health,* **3,** 45–61.

**Silverman, D.** (1987) *Communication and Medical Practice: Social Relations in the Clinic.* London: Sage.

**Silverton, L.** (1993) *The Art and Science of Midwifery.* Wiltshire: Prentice Hall.

**Singer, E., Garfinkel, R., Cohen, S.M. and Srole, L.** (1976) Mortality and mental health: Evidence from the Midtown Manhattan restudy. *Science & Medicine,* **10,** 517–25.

**Skeat, W.W.** (1972) *The Complete Works of Chaucer.* Edited from Numerous Manuscripts by W.W. Skeat: Volume IV, *The Canterbury Tales.* Oxford: Clarendon Press.

**Skolbekken, J.** (1995) The risk epidemic in medical journals. *Social Science & Medicine,* **40,** 291–305.

**Slovic, P.** (1987) Perceptions of risk. *Science,* **236,** 280–5.

**Slovic, P., Fischhoff, B. and Lichtenstein, S.** (1982) Facts versus fears: Understanding perceived risk. In Kahneman, D., Slovic, P. and Tversky, A. (eds) *Judgment under Uncertainty: Heuristics and Biases.* New York: Cambridge University Press.

**Smaje, C.** (1996) The ethnic patterning of health: New directions for theory and research. *Sociology of Health and Illness,* **18,** 139–71.

**Smigel, K.** (1996) Beta carotene fails to prevent cancer in two major studies: CARET intervention stopped. *Journal of the National Cancer Institute,* **88,** 144.

**Smith, P.** (1992) *The Emotional Labour of Nursing.* London: Macmillan.

**Smith, T.** (1993) Influence of socioeconomic factors on attaining targets for reducing teenage pregnancies. *British Medical Journal,* **306,** 1232–5.

**Smith, A. and Russell, J.** (1991) Using critical learning incidents in nurse education. *Nurse Education Today,* **11,** 284–91.

**Smith, A. and Russell, J.** (1993) Critical incident technique. In Reed, J. and Procter, S. (eds) *Nurse Education: A Reflective Approach.* London: Edward Arnold.

**Smith, G., Cantley, C. and Ritman, V.** (1983) Day care made simple. *Health and Social Services Journal,* **93,** 692–3.

**Smith, M., Bee, P., Heverin, A. and Nobes, G.** (1995) *Parental Control within the Family: The Nature and Extent of Parental Violence to Children.* London: HMSO.

**Soininen, H., Partanen, J., Jousmaki, V., Helkala, E.L., Vanhanen, M., Majuri, S., Kaski, M., Hartikainen, P. and Riekkinen, P.** (1993) Age-related cognitive decline and electroencephalogram slowing in Down's syndrome as a model of Alzheimer's disease. *Neuroscience,* **53,** 57–63.

**Solomon, P.** (1994) Families' views of service delivery: An empirical assessment. In Lefley, H. and Wasow, M. (eds) *Helping Families Cope with Mental Illness.* Chur, Switzerland: Harwood Academic Publishers.

**Sontag, S.** (1984) *Illness as Metaphor.* Harmondsworth: Penguin Books.

**Sontag, S.** (1989) *Illness as Metaphor/AIDS and its Metaphors.* New York: Anchor Books.

**Sorensen, K.C. and Luckmann, J.** (1986) *Basic Nursing: A Psychophysiological Approach,* 2nd edn. Philadelphia: W.B. Saunders.

**Spanos, N.P., Stenstrom, R.J. and Johnston, J.C.** (1988) Hynosis, placebo and suggestion in the treatment of warts. *Psychosomatic Medicine,* **50,** 245–60.

**Spiegel, D., Bloom, J., Kraemer, H.C. and Gottheil, E.** (1989) Effect of psychosocial treatment on survival of patients with metastatic breast cancer. *Lancet,* **ii,** 888–91.

**Stacey, M.** (1988) *The Sociology of Health and Healing.* London: Unwin Hyman.

**Stahlberg, D., Eller, F., Maass, A. and Frey, D.** (1995) We knew it all along: Hindsight bias in groups. *Organizational Behavior and Human Decision Processes,* **63,** 46–58.

**Stainton, M.C.** (1992) Mismatched caring in high-risk perinatal situations. *Clinical Nursing Research,* **1,** 35–49.

**Stetz, K., Lewis, F. and Primomo, J.** (1986) Family coping strategies and chronic illness in the mother. *Family Relations,* **35,** 515–22.

**Stevenson, C.** (1995) *Negotiating a Therapeutic Context in Family Therapy.* Newcastle upon Tyne: Unpublished PhD thesis, University of Northumbria.

**Stevenson, C. and Cooper, N.** (1997) Qualitative and quantitative research. *The Psychologist,* **10,** 159–60.

**Stewart, I.** (1995) Toss a lucky coin and win every time? *New Scientist,* **147,** 46–7.

**Stockwell, F.** (1972) The unpopular patient. *Royal College of Nursing Research Project Series 1, No. 2.* London: Royal College of Nursing.

**Stone, D.A.** (1986) The resistible rise of preventive medicine. *Journal of Health Politics, Policy and Law,* **11,** 671–96.

**Stone, J.** (1995) *Mobility for Special Needs.* London: Cassell.

**Stoppard, T.** (1968) *Rosencrantz and Guildenstern are Dead.* London: Faber & Faber.

**Strauss, A.** (1987) *Qualitative Analysis for Social Scientists.* Cambridge: Cambridge University Press.

**Strauss, A. and Corbin, J.M.** (1988) *Shaping a New Health Care System: The Explosion of Chronic Illness as a Catalyst for Change.* London: Jossey-Bass.

**Strauss, A. and Corbin, J.M.** (1990) *Basics of Qualitative Research: Grounded Theory Procedures and Techniques.* Newbury Park: Sage.

Stroebe, W. and Stroebe, M.S. (1995) *Social Psychology and Health*. Buckingham: Open University Press.

Strong, P. (1990) Epidemic psychology: A model. *Sociology of Health and Illness*, **12**, 249–59.

Susser, M. (1985) Epidemiology in the United States after World War 2: The evolution of technique. *Epidemiological Review*, **7**, 147–77.

Svenson, O. (1981) Are we all less risky and more skilful than our fellow drivers? *Acta Psychologica*, **47**, 143–8.

Swain, J., Heyman, B. and Gillman, M. (1996) *Challenging Behaviour and Learning Difficulties*. Paper presented at the 3rd International Interdisciplinary Qualitative Health Research Conference, Bournemouth University.

Swain, J., Heyman, B. and Gillman, M. (1997) Public research, private concerns: Ethical issues in the use of open-ended interviews with people who have learning difficulties. *Disability and Society*, in press.

Szasz, T.S. (1961) *The Myth of Mental Illness: Foundations of a Theory of Personal Conduct*. New York: Dell.

Takei, N.G., Murray, G., O'Callaghan, E., Sham, P.C., Glover, G. and Murray, R.M. (1995) Prenatal exposure to influenza epidemics and risk of mental retardation. *European Archives of Psychiatry and Clinical Neuroscience*, **245**, 255–9.

Taylor, S.E. and Brown, J.D. (1988) Illusion and well-being: A social psychological perspective on mental health. *Psychological Bulletin*, **103**, 193–210.

Ternulf-Nyhlin, K. (1990) Diabetic patients facing long-term complications: Coping with uncertainty. *Journal of Advanced Nursing*, **15**, 1021–9.

The Diabetes Control and Complications Trial Reasearch Group (1993) The effect of intensive treatment of diabetes on the development and progression of long-term complications in insulin-dependent diabetes mellitus. *New England Journal of Medicine*, **329**, 977–86.

The President's Commission for the Study of Ethical Problems in Medicine and Biomedical and Behavioral Research (1983) *Deciding to Forego Life – Sustaining Treatment*. Washington, DC: US Printing Office.

The Royal Society (1992) *Risk: Analysis, Perception and Management. Report of a Royal Society Study Group*. London: The Royal Society.

Thoburn, J., Lewis, A. and Shemmings, D. (1995) *Paternalism or Partnership? Family Involvement in the Child Protection Process*. Studies in Child Protection. London: HMSO.

Thompson, N. (1995) *Theory and Practice in Health and Social Welfare*. Buckingham: Open University Press.

Thompson, P.B. (1986) The philosophical foundations of risk. *The Southern Journal of Philosophy*, **24**, 273–86.

Thorin, E., Yovanoff, P. and Irvin, L. (1996) Dilemmas faced by families during their young adults' transitions to adulthood: A brief report. *Mental Retardation*, **34**, 117–20.

Thorne, S.E. and Robinson, C.A. (1988) Reciprocal trust in health care relationships. *Journal of Advanced Nursing*, **13**, 782–9.

Thorne, S.E. and Robinson, C.A. (1989) Guarded alliance: Health care relationships in chronic illness. *Journal of Nursing Scholarship*, **21**, 153–7.

Thornicroft, G. (1993) Case management for the long-term mentally ill. In Bhugra, D. and Leff, J. (eds) *Principles of Social Psychiatry*. Oxford: Blackwell Scientific Publications.

Tingle, J.H. (1996) Clinical guidelines: Risk management and legal issues. *British Journal of Nursing*, **5**, 266–7.

Tones, K. and Tilford, S. (1994) *Health Education: Effectiveness, Efficiency and Equity*. London: Chapman & Hall.

**Toft, B.** (1996) Limits to the mathematical modelling of disasters. In Hood, C. and Jones, K.C. (eds) *Accident and Design.* London: UCL Press.

**Townsend, P.** (1962) *The Last Refuge: A Survey of Residential Institutions and Homes for the Aged in England and Wales.* London: Routledge & Kegan Paul.

**Townsend, P. and Davidson, N.** (1982) *Inequalities in Health: The Black Report.* Harmondworth: Penguin Books.

**Townsend, P., Phillimore, P. and Beattie, A.** (1988) *Health and Deprivation, Inequality and the North.* London: Routledge.

**Trostle, J.A.** (1988) Medical compliance as ideology. *Social Science and Medicine,* **12,** 1299–1308.

**Trussell, J.** (1988) Teenage pregnancy in the United States. *Family Planning Perspectives,* **20,** 262–72.

**Tuck, S.M., Yudkin, P.L. and Turnbull, A.C.,** (1988) Pregnancy outcome in elderly primigravidae with and without a history of infertility. *British Journal of Obstetrics and Gynaecology,* **95,** 230–7.

**Tudor Hart, J.** (1971) The inverse care law. *Lancet,* **i,** 405–12.

**Tversky, A. and Kahneman, D.** (1973) Availability: A heuristic for judging frequency and probability. *Cognitive Psychology,* **5,** 207–32.

**Tversky, A. and Kahneman, D.** (1974) Judgment under uncertainty: Heuristics and biases. *Science,* **185,** 1124–31.

**Tversky, A. and Kahneman, D.** (1981) The framing of decisions and the psychology of choice. *Science,* **211,** 453–8.

**Tversky, A. and Kahneman, D.** (1983) Extensional versus intuitive reasoning: The conjunction fallacy in probability judgment. *Psychological Review,* **90,** 293–315.

**UKCC** (1992a) *Code of Professional Conduct for the Nurse, Midwife and Health Visitor,* 3rd edn. London: United Kingdom Central Council.

**UKCC** (1992b) *Scope of Professional Practice.* London: United Kingdom Central Council.

**Unschuld, P.U.** (1986) The conceptual determination of individual and collective experiences of illness. In Currer, C. and Stacey, M. (eds) *Concepts of Health, Illness and Disease.* Oxford: Berg.

**Utian, W.H. and Kiwi, R.** (1988) Obstetrical risks of pregnancy and childbirth after age 35. *Maturitas Supplement,* **1,** 63–72.

**Veatch, R.M. and Fry, S.T.** (1987) *Case Studies in Nursing Ethics.* Philadelphia: J.B. Lippincott.

**Vesley, W.E. and Rasmuson, D.M.** (1984) Uncertainties in nuclear probabilistic risk analysis. *Risk Analysis,* **4,** 313–22.

**Victor, C.R.** (1994) *Old Age in Modern Society.* London: Chapman & Hall.

**Vieregge, P., Verleger, R., Schulzerava, H. and Kompf, D.** (1992) Late cognitive event-related potentials in adult Down's syndrome. *Biological Psychiatry,* **32,** 118–34.

**Vincent, C.** (1995) Pathways to litigation. *Managing Risk,* April 1.

**Vingard, E., Alfredsson, L., Goldie, I. and Hogstedt, C.** (1993) Sports and osteoarthrosis of the hip: An epidemiologic study. *American Journal of Sports Medicine,* **21,** 195–200.

**Viscusi, W.K.** (1992) *Fatal Tradeoffs: Public and Private Responsibilities for Risk.* New York: Oxford University Press.

**Wallsten, T.S., Fillenbaum, S. and Cox, J.A.** (1986) Base rate effects on the interpretation of probability and frequency expressions. *Journal of Memory and Language,* **25,** 571–87.

**Wallsten, T.S., Budescu, D.V., Zwick, R. and Kemp, S.M.** (1993) Preferences and reasons for communicating probabilistic information in verbal and numerical terms. *Bulletin of the Psychonomic Society,* **31,** 135–8.

**Wallsten, T.S., Budescu, D.V., Rapoport, A., Zwick, R. and Forsyth, B.** (1986) Measuring the vague meanings of probability terms. *Journal of Experimental Psychology: General*, **115**, 348–65.

**Walsh, M. and Ford, P.** (1992) *Nursing Rituals: Research and Rational Actions.* Oxford: Butterworth Heinemann.

**Walsh, J., Lythgoe, H. and Peckham, S.** (1996) *Contraceptive Choices: Supporting Effective Use of Methods.* London: Contraception Education Service/Family Planning Association.

**Ward, S., Viergutz, G., Tormey, D., DeMuth, J. and Paulen, A.** (1992) Patients' reactions to completion of adjuvant breast cancer therapy. *Nursing Research*, **41**, 362–6.

**Watney, S.** (1989) The subject of AIDS. In Aggleton, P., Hart, G. and Davies, P. (eds) *AIDS: Social Representations, Social Practices.* Basingstoke: Falmer Press.

**Webb, S. and Webb, B.** (1909) *The Minority Report of the Poor Law Commission, Vol. 1.* London: Longman Green.

**Webb, C., Addison, C., Holman, H., Saklaki, B. and Wagner, A.** (1990) Self-medication for elderly patients. *Nursing Times*, **186**, 46–9.

**Weber, E.U. and Hilton, D.J.** (1990) Contextual effects in the interpretation of probability words: Perceived base rate and severity of events. *Journal of Experimental Psychology: Human Perception and Performance*, **16**, 781–9.

**Weeks, J.** (1991) *Against Nature: Essays on History, Sexuality and Identity.* London: Rivers Oram Press.

**Weinstein, N.D.** (1980) Unrealistic optimism about future life events. *Journal of Personality and Social Psychology*, **39**, 806–20.

**Weinstein, N.D.** (1982) Unrealistic optimism about susceptibility to health problems. *Journal of Behavioral Medicine*, **5**, 441–60.

**Weinstein, N.D.** (1988) The precaution adaption process. *Health Psychology*, **7**, 355–86.

**Weinstein, N.D. and Klein, W.M.** (1995) Resistance of personal risk perceptions to debiasing interventions. *Health Psychology*, **14**, 132–40.

**Weir, M.W.** (1991) Towards an holistic understanding of health and illness. *Health Visitor*, **64**, 77–9.

**Weir, M.W. and Whittaker, C.** (1996) A new vision for healthcare. In Twinn, S., Roberts, B. and Andrews, S. (eds) *Community Health Care Nursing.* Oxford: Butterworth Heinemann.

**Weiss, N.E.** (1985) Can *not* smoking be hazardous to your health? *The New England Medical Journal*, **313**, 632–3.

**Wellings, K., Field, J., Johnson, A.M. and Wadsworth, J.** (1995) Provision of sex education and early sexual experience: The relation examined. *British Medical Journal*, **311**, 417–20.

**White, J.E.** (1989) *Introduction to Philosophy.* St Paul MN: West Publishing Company.

**Whitehead, M.** (1987) *The Health Divide: Inequalities in the 1980s.* London: Health Education Council.

**WHO** (1948) *World Health Organisation Constitution.* New York: World Health Organisation.

**WHO** (1973) *The International Pilot Study of Schizophrenia.* Geneva: WHO.

**WHO** (1980) *International Classification of Impairments, Disabilities and Handicaps: A Manual of Classification Relating to the Consequences of Disease.* WHO: Geneva.

**WHO** (1984) Health Promotion: A WHO discussion document on the concepts and principles. Reprinted in *Health Promotion*, **1**, 73–6.

**WHO** (1995) Collaborative study for cardiovascular disease and steroid hormone contraception. *Lancet*, **346**, 1575–82.

**Wilkinson, R.G.** (1996) *Unhealthy Societies: The Affliction of Inequality.* London: Routledge.

**Wilson, H.S.** (1989) Family caregiving for a relative with Alzheimer's dementia: Coping with negative choices. *Nursing Research,* **38,** 94–8.

**Wilson, J.** (1995a) Clinical risk modification. *British Journal of Nursing,* **4,** 667.

**Wilson, J.** (1995b) Caroline: A case of a pregnant teenager. *Professional Care of Mother and Child,* **5,** 139–40.

**Wilson, S.H., Brown, T.P. and Richards, R.G.** (1992) Teenage conceptions and contraception in the English regions. *Journals of Public Health Medicine,* **14,** 17–25.

**Winkler, G.M.R.** (1990) Necessity, chance and freedom. In von Furstenberg, G.M. (ed.) *Acting Under Uncertainty: Multidisciplinary Conceptions.* Boston: Kluwer Academic Piblications.

**Wishart, J.G.** (1993) The development of learning difficulties in children with Down's syndrome. *Journal of Intellectual Disability Research,* **37,** 89–403.

**Wolfensberger, W.** (1983) Social role valorization: A proposed new term for the principle of normalisation. *Mental Retardation,* **21,** 8–12.

**Woodcock, A.J., Stenner, K. and Ingham, R.** (1992) Young people talking about HIV and AIDS: Interpretations of personal risk of infection. *Health Education Research,* **7,** 229–47.

**Woodhouse, J.M., Pakeman, V.H., Saunders, K.J., Parker, M., Fraser, W.I., Lobo, S. and Sastry, P.** (1996) Visual acuity and accommodation in infants and young children with Down's syndrome. *Journal of Intellectual Disability Research,* **40,** 49–55.

**Woodroffe, C., Glickman, M., Barber, M. and Power, C.** (1991) *Children, Teenagers and Health: The Key Data.* Oxford: Oxford University Press.

**Woods, N.F., Yates, B.C. and Primomo, J.** (1989) Supporting families during chronic illness. *Journal of Nursing Scholarship,* **21,** 46–50.

**Wynne, B.** (1996) May the sheep safely graze? A reflexive view of the expert–lay knowledge divide. In Lash, S., Szerszynski, B. and Wynne, B. (eds) *Risk, Environment and Modernity: Towards a New Ecology.* London: Sage.

**Wynne-Harley, D.** (1991) *Living Dangerously: Risk-taking, Safety and Older People.* London: Centre for Policy on Ageing.

**Yearley, S.** (1992) Green ambivalence about science: Legal–rational authority and the scientific legitimation of a social movement. *British Journal of Sociology,* **43,** 511–32.

**Ylaherttuala, S., Luoma, J., Nikkari, T. and Kivimaki, T.** (1989) Down's syndrome and atherosclerosis. *Atherosclerosis,* **76,** 269–72.

**Zakay, D.** (1983) The relationship between the probability assessor and the outcome of an event as a determiner of subjective probability. *Acta Psychologica,* **53,** 271–80.

**Zimmer, A.C.** (1983) Verbal vs numerical processing of subjective probabilities. In Scholz, R.W. (ed.) *Decision-making under Uncertainty.* Amsterdam: Elsevier Science Publishers.

**Zohar, D.** (1991) *The Quantum Self.* London: HarperCollins.

**Zohar, D. and Marshall, I.** (1994) *The Quantum Society.* London: HarperCollins.

**Zureik, M., Courbon, D. and Ducimetiere, P.** (1996) Serum cholesterol concentration and death from suicide in men: Paris prospective study 1. *British Medical Journal,* **133,** 649–51.

# Author Index

# Subject Index